Emergency medical 3D printing

A case study during the COVID19 pandemic

Plateforme 3D COVID, Abbaye de Port-Royal, Hôpital Cochin, Paris, 21.I.2021. Encre de Chine sur papier, 50 x 65 cm. Collection particulière. © Christelle Téa

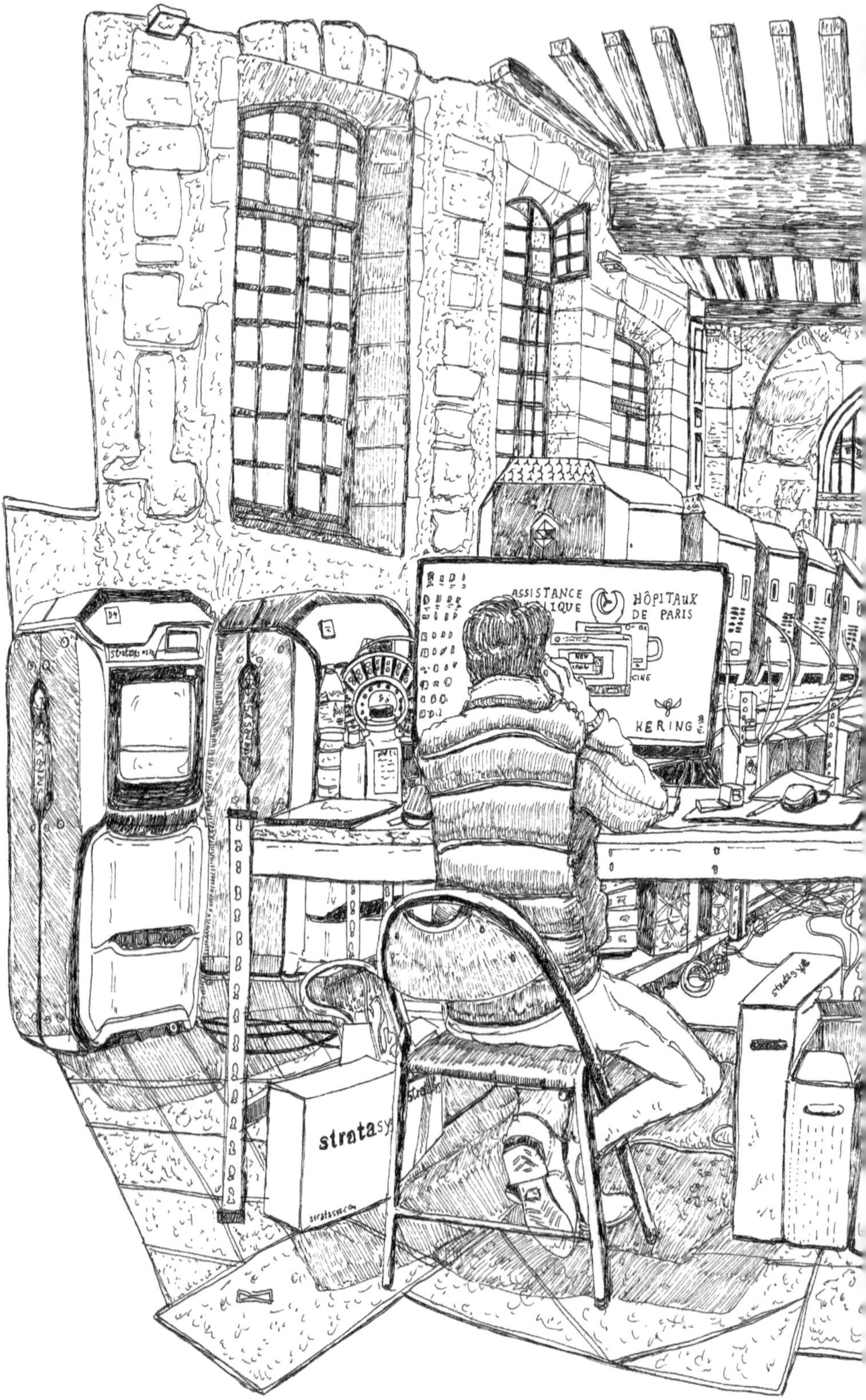

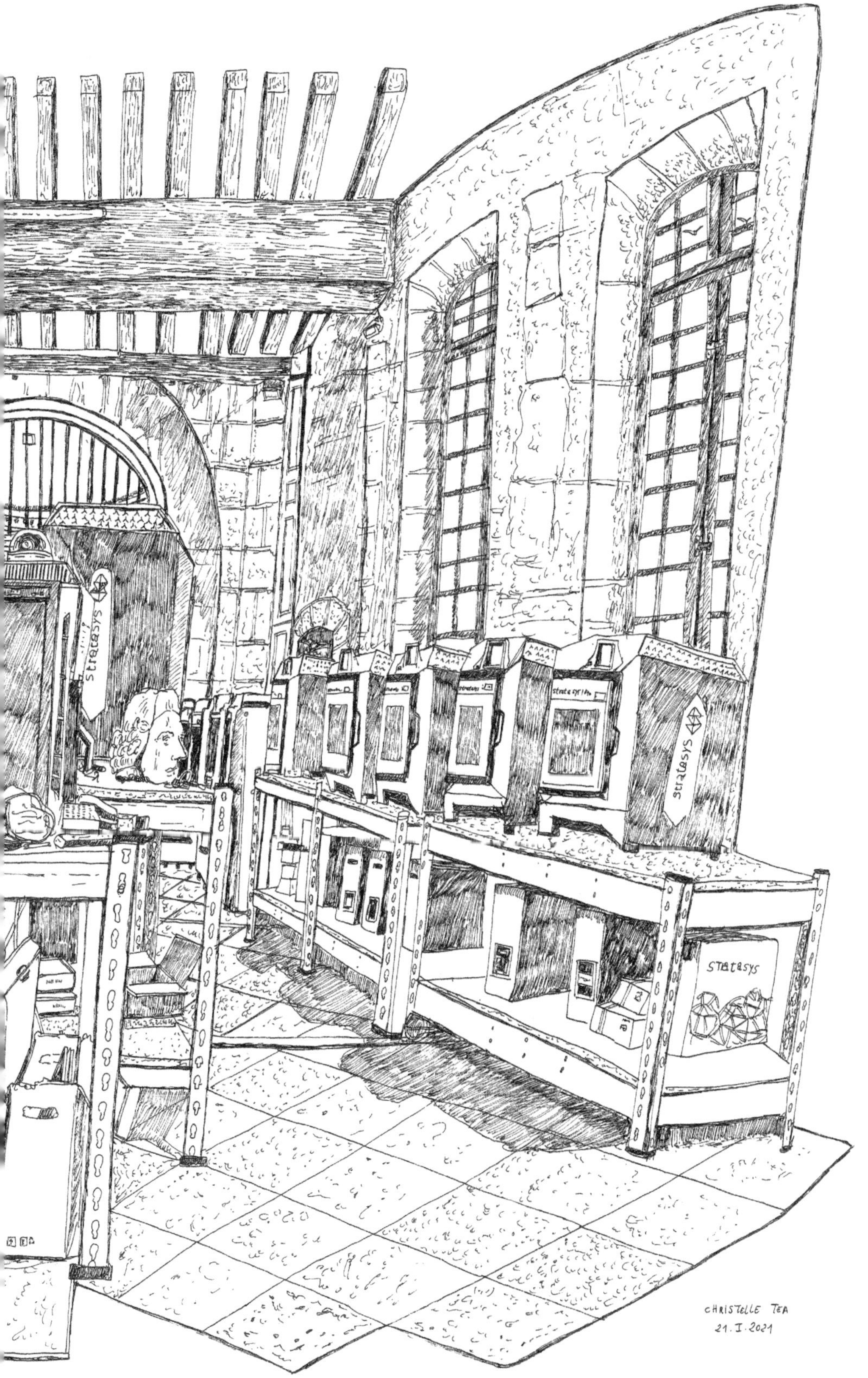
stratasys
stratasys
stratasys
CHRISTELLE TEA
21. I. 2021

Cover
3D COVID in the chapter rooms of Port-Royal Abbey

5-7, rue de l'École-Polytechnique ; 75005 Paris
http://www.editions-harmattan.fr
ISBN : 978-2-14-034775-7
EAN : 9782140347757

Roman Hossein Khonsari

Emergency medical 3D printing

A case study during the COVID19 pandemic

L'Harmattan

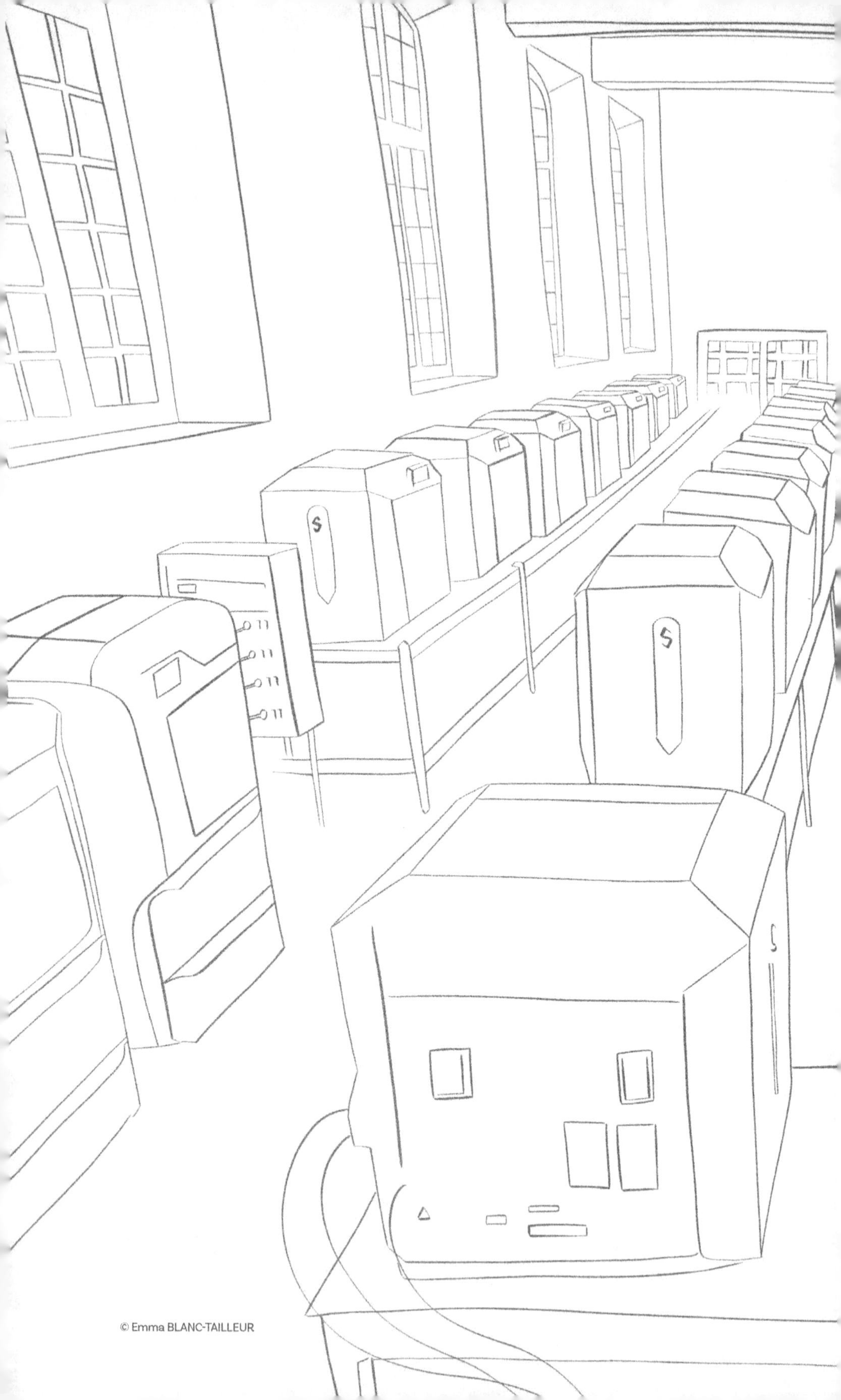

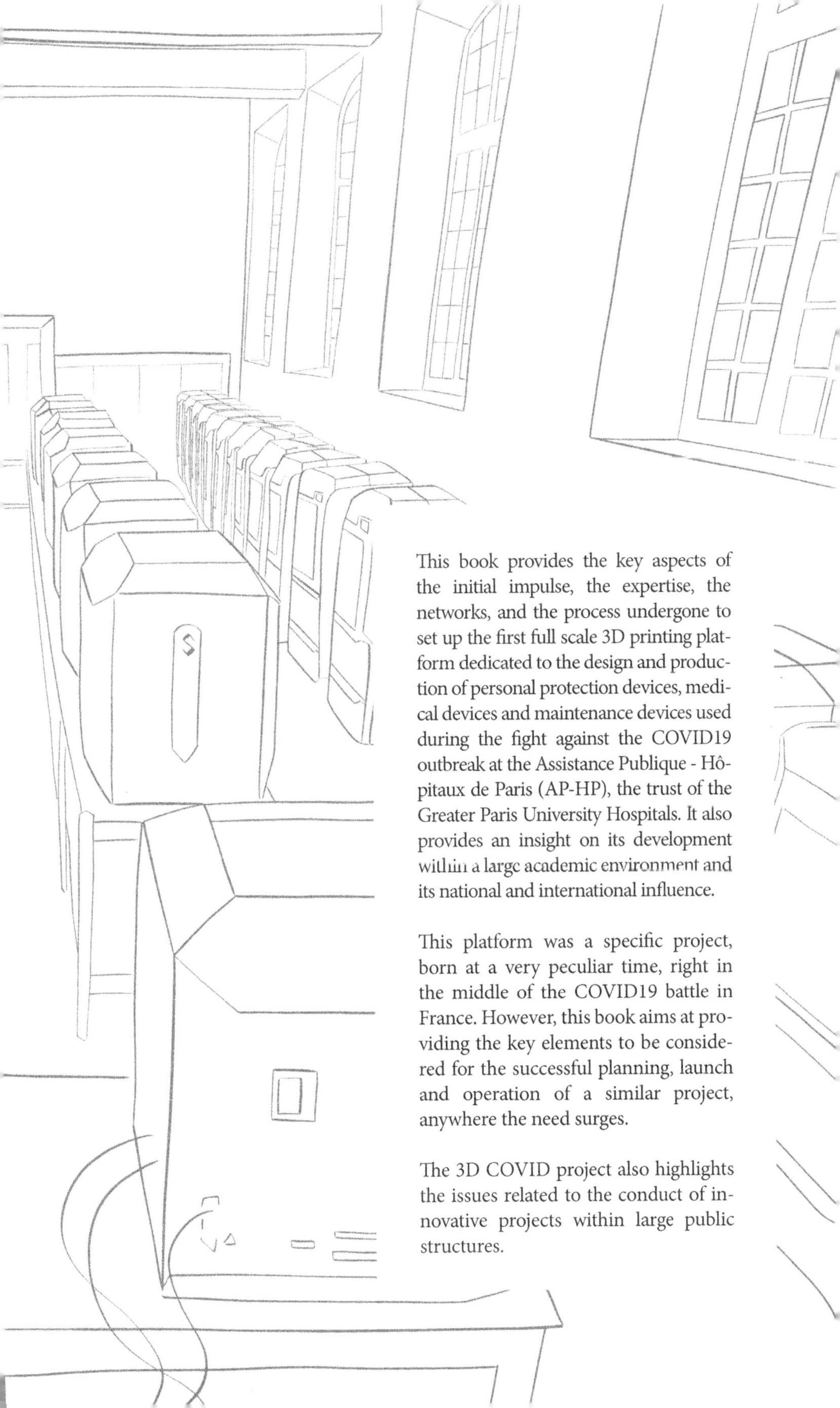

This book provides the key aspects of the initial impulse, the expertise, the networks, and the process undergone to set up the first full scale 3D printing platform dedicated to the design and production of personal protection devices, medical devices and maintenance devices used during the fight against the COVID19 outbreak at the Assistance Publique - Hôpitaux de Paris (AP-HP), the trust of the Greater Paris University Hospitals. It also provides an insight on its development within a large academic environment and its national and international influence.

This platform was a specific project, born at a very peculiar time, right in the middle of the COVID19 battle in France. However, this book aims at providing the key elements to be considered for the successful planning, launch and operation of a similar project, anywhere the need surges.

The 3D COVID project also highlights the issues related to the conduct of innovative projects within large public structures.

Table of contents

0. Project genesis

Here we describe the first steps of the project that led to the creation of a large-scale emergency 3D printing platform for all Greater Paris University Hospitals: how the initial ideas emerged, how key people met and how the institutional support was granted.

0.1 General context

Digital fabrication, including additive manufacturing, is a medical revolution, much more dramatic in its forthcoming consequences than most current health professionals envision. For the first time in history, practitioners have the potentiality to personally design and manufacture their own tools on their working site, following two technical steps that are becoming more and more familiar to a wide public: computer-assisted design and 3D printing. The recent advances in these fields have resulted in the release of user-friendly open-source design software and in the conception of cheap, reliable, printers – 3D printing is about to become a familiar companion in patient care and innovation for most health professionals. Three remaining limitations to the definitive adoption of 3D printing in medical practice are the object of current critical strategic decisions at political and local levels: (1) issues with regulation for the in-house production of medical devices, (2) questions of intellectual property related to the free diffusion of 3D designs, and (3) unclear business models when this new activity is introduced within hospitals. Short-sighted decisions in these three domains could limit the integration of digital fabrication into patient care and be detrimental to the quality of health services. In the case study we report in this book, 3D printing was used in a large hospital trust in the context of an international sanitary crisis, and the three aforementioned limitations were the trickiest issues to tackle. The next few years will be critical in preventing regulatory bodies to limit the deployment of in-house production while still ensuring patient safety – heavy lobbying is performed by the main industrial medical device manufacturers to complicate regulatory processes and limit access to design and production, while, in parallel, positive control processes are being designed to prevent the unfortunate production of dangerous devices – finding a balance in the regulation of the distributed production of medical devices is thus a major challenge. Other incoming challenges involve promoting a flexible conception of the sharing of production protocols and designs and encouraging reasonably risky strategies when considering the financial aspects of 3D printing platform implementation.

More generally, additive manufacturing will lead to a deep modification in our relationship with consumerism. By becoming both the creators and producers of a significant number of objects we use in our everyday life, we will challenge one of the bases of modern societies, the trade of manufactured goods. Nevertheless, the irruption of large-scale distributed production will be more than a gadget only if cheap raw materials are made available worldwide and if circularity can be introduced when dealing with the waste - a specifically relevant issue in healthcare as digital fabrication involves prototyping steps creating a large and unavoidable number of objects with a very limited period of interest. Furthermore, despite the increase of health professionals with a basic training in 3D design, the implementation of 3D printing in hospitals raises an educational challenge and the need to redefine the role of engineers within health institutions.

During the pandemic, outstanding financial and logistic support was obtained to settle an ambitious emergency sanitary 3D printing platform within the largest hospital trust in Europe, Assistance Publique – Hôpitaux de Paris. The 3D COVID project, which is exposed in all relevant details in this book, was motivated by the risk of shortages in critical medical supplies due to their extraordinary use in COVID units and to defective international supply chains. Based on our experience, additive manufacturing seems a convincing solution to tackle logistic issues in extreme situations such as sanitary crises, war zones, or in isolated territories. In this book, we analyze the outcomes of this specific project to outline our general conception of how 3D printing should be integrated into the everyday life of health practitioners, beyond its remarkable properties in dealing with disasters. We hope that in the near future, large hospital trusts will benefit from internal production platforms allowed to manufacture medical devices. Such platforms, which are the modern and expanded pendants of the prosthetics laboratories familiar to, among others, maxillofacial surgeons, dentists and orthopedic surgeons, will be sites of intense creativity with a central and new role played by biomedical engineers. This new generation of engineers, working together with health practitioners, will not only take part into the design and prototyping processes across different specialties and compile ideas arising from practical situations that could potentially benefit from unified solutions, but also train health professionals to distributed production, and contribute to define the involvement of designers and manufacturers in regulatory processes.

This book tells the story of a specific initiative started in 2020 in Assistance Publique – Hôpitaux de Paris, during the first wave of the pandemic. The goal of this report is to show that this peculiar situation was a laboratory where we defined the future principles for the integration of distributed medical device production within health institutions and attempted to anticipate the subsequent professional transformations that would result from this integration.

0.2 Specific situation

Before COVID19 became a fierce reality in France, in the medical sector there were already pioneers trying to leverage the promises of 3D printing technologies. These were early adopters for their personal and professional use, connected to the community of makers, with a working knowledge of the involved technology[1].

In-house production of 3D printed custom-made medical devices was a goal that many hospitals of the trust of Greater Paris University Hospitals (Assistance Publique – Hôpitaux de Paris, AP-HP) had the plan to reach in the short term at the beginning of 2020, generally under the lead of their maxillofacial and/or plastic surgery departments. A new European settlement with demanding pre-requisites was supposed to be applicable in May 2020 (delayed earliest September 2020 and then May 2021 due to the pandemic) and imposed a considerable amount of control processes in order to obtain the status of medical device manufacturer in a hospital environment[2]. In this context, many physicians within AP-HP were aware of both the potentialities and the barriers due to regulation issues related to medical 3D printing.

When AP-HP began to endure a rapid surge in the number of patients incoming to its dozens of hospitals in the Paris region, the supply of medical devices became quickly one of the bottlenecks, a challenge for the well-being of these patients and the ability of the institution to perform as expected in a context never seen before. Devices that could encounter shortage were the ones that were specifically used to manage COVID19 patients, but also devices for which the supply chains were defective due to the international sanitary situation.

Furthermore, personal protection devices were needed in extraordinary quantities and maintenance devices for the everyday life of hospitals were at risk of encountering shortage.

On the 15th of March 2020, a call for projects was made public by the Army (Direction Générale de l'Armement, DGA) two days before the first lock-down was imposed to the general French population[3]. The goal of the call was to identify initiatives that may alleviate the shortage of protection and medical devices during the COVID crisis.

In response, two initiatives that would secondarily converge to form the current project were submitted to this call.

1 For an insightful overview of the perspectives opened by additive manufacturing and digital fabrication in general: Greenfield A., Radical technologies: The design of everyday life. Verso, 2017.

2 Regulation (EU) 2017/745 of the European Parliament and of the Council of 5 April 2017 on medical devices: https://eur-lex.europa.eu/legal-content/ENG TXT/PDF/?uri=CELEX:32017R0745.

3 DGA call for COVID19-related projects: https://www.defense.gouv.fr/aid/appels-a-projets/appel-a-projets-lutte-covid-19.

1 An independent software developer and the AMC (Association des Amis des Malades de l'Hôpital Cochin[4]), helped by an independent accountant had the idea to settle the following structure:
→ an open source platform where independent makers would post medical device designs,
→ a social network call to the community of makers,
→ quality control on the supply chains.
Based on this, on the 23rd of March, a project named RACE2BREATH was submitted to DGA. The aim of this platform was to connect makers with healthcare workers in terms of demands and supplies.

2 A laboratory dedicated to the modelling of growth processes in the craniofacial region ('Craniofacial Growth and Form'[5], CGF) had recently purchased an advanced polyjet 3D printer (Stratasys J735), funded by the Fondation « Les Gueules Cassées »[6], and was in the process of applying to become a producer of in-house custom-made medical devices before the pandemic. This team was thus aware of the potentiality of 3D printing. With the CEO of BONE 3D[7], a Parisian start-up specialised in medical 3D printing with a experience in academic projects[8], the CGF laboratory team conceived three objects intending to limit viral contamination within hospitals (door openers, button pushers and pencil holders, Figures 1-2)[9]. The 16th of March, prototypes of these devices were printed in the CGF lab to be tested locally. Thanks to a private donation of 3000€ (Wisepops, Paris[10]), limited series of each of these devices could be produced and served as a proof of concept within Hôpital Necker - Enfants Malades, which led to applying to the DGA call with the project of extending the production of these devices by acquiring a larger scale internal production platform for AP-HP.

Simultaneously, JOGL (Just One Giant Lab) launched the Open Covid19 Initiative on its platform[11]. JOGL consisted in creating international open-source exchange groups focused on a specific scientific question, such as for instance the design of a simple syringe driver that could be produced in crisis situations. JOGL groups seemed particularly adapted to the quick design of specific devices in response to the pandemic. JOGL agreed to dedicate a specific space on his platform to the projects emerging from the soon-to-come AP-HP 3D printing initiative.

4 Association des Amis de l'Hôpital Cochin: http://amisdesmalades.com.
5 https://www.growthnform.com/
6 Fondation des 'Gueules Cassées', a prominent charity founded after World War I funding research projects dedicated to craniofacial science: https://www.gueules-cassees.asso.fr.
7 BONE 3D, a Parisian start-up specialized in medical 3D printing: bone3D.com.
8 Previous experience with BONE 3D in medical device conception: https://BONE 3D.com/en/actualite/bb-rhino-sous-contrat-de-licence-avec-lap-hp.
9 Paper on three types of protection devices: François PM, Bonnet X, Kosior J, Adam J, Khonsari RH. 3D-printed contact-free devices designed and dispatched against the COVID19 pandemic: the 3D COVID initiative. J Stom Oral Maxillofac Surg 2021;122:381-385.
10 https://wisepops.com/
11 Open Covid19 initiative on the JOGL interface: https://app.jogl.io/program/opencovid19.

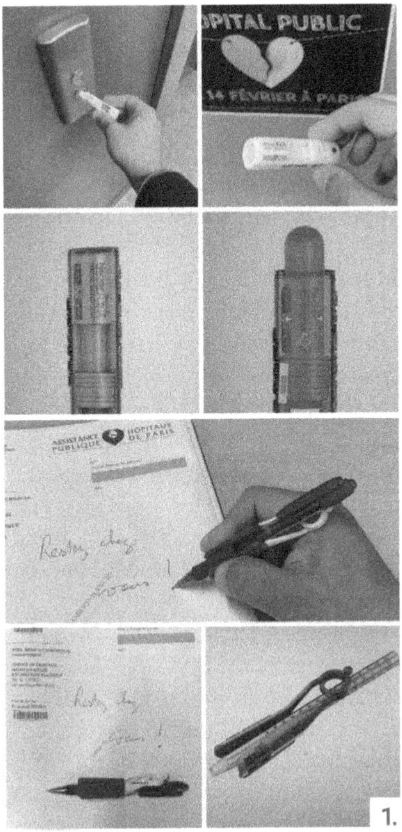

1.

Fig. 1. Two objects designed in March 2020 in collaboration with BONE 3D: button pusher and pencil holder and produced for Hôpital Necker - Enfants Malades thanks to private funding (Wisepops, Paris).

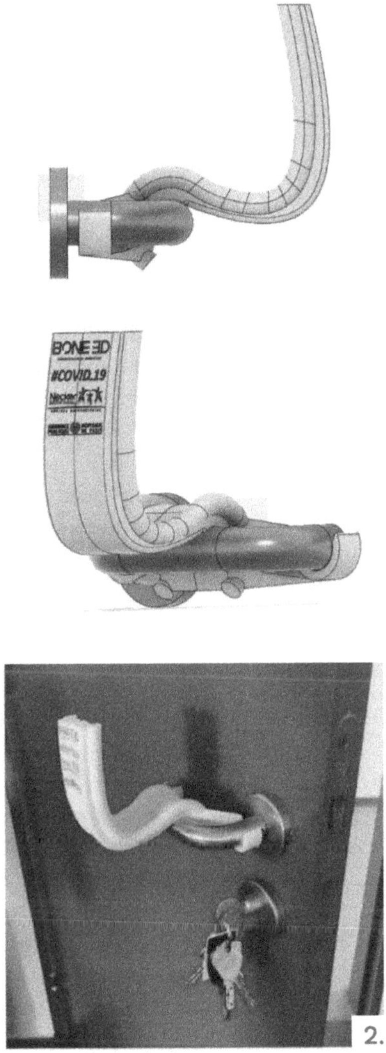

2.

Fig. 2. Initial design of the door openers, March 2020, tested in Hôpital Necker - Enfants Malades thanks to private funding (Wisepops, Paris).

The idea of fusing the three approaches (1. makers, 2. a group of university hospitals, academia, and industry, and 3. JOGL with open science) quickly emerged and laid the foundations of a profit and loss scheme for a larger project made ready to be presented to the AP-HP top management the 26th of March: the 3D COVID initiative was born.

A business plan[12] and a short abstract about the aims of the project – fast

12 See Supplementary Material (12.1)

R&D on COVID19-related questions followed by internal design and production – was transmitted to the head of the Medical Commission of AP-HP (Commission Médicale d'Établissement, CME) and to the dean of the Paris-Descartes Medical School renamed since Université de Paris and then Université Paris Cité, who transferred the proposal to the general director of AP-HP. The dean and the CME head stressed to the top management of AP-HP that the core of the idea consisted in using 3D printing technologies within AP-HP in order to improve autonomy and relocate medical devices production into French hospitals, with a supply line that would complement the classic procurement in the looming case of shortages.

Of note, the sections of the project involving makers and JOGL were not included into the proposal submitted to AP-HP: we had strong reasons to believe that AP-HP decision makers did not have the state-of-mind to interact with competent but non-academic individuals. The RACE2BREATH initiative of the Cochin team – soon to become Emergency.io – was thus in formally connected to the core 3D COVID project, as well as JOGL, but the frontline of the project that was presented to AP-HP officials was focused on the creation of an internal 3D printing facility.

By the meantime, with BONE 3D, we pressurized 3D printing suppliers in order to make sure printers and raw material would be available in case the project would be validated by AP-HP top management.

AP-HP top management validated the project on the 28th of March, which fueled parallel research for funding (see below).

Meanwhile, all proposals mentioned above were rejected by the DGA.

At this point, two key people were introduced into the project by AP-HP:
→ the former head of finances of this institution, and who would become the strategic lead of the initiative,
→ then current (at this time) head of finances of AP-HP, and who would be the main point of entry for the 3D COVID core team for dealing with practical and organizational issues during the project.

Fast forward: 1st April 2020. 60 high-end 3D printers from the Stratasys company are delivered to the Abbey of Port-Royal, a couple of footsteps away from the Hôpital Cochin main gate. The first prototype leaves the 3D farm the day after and the production starts.

Driven by the emergency of the sanitary situation and the impeding need of basic medical devices by French hospitals, the largest European platform of 3D printers has been envisioned, designed, funded, installed, and set to production in 10 days.

The following chapters describe each step of the project launch.

1. Team assembly

The 3D COVID project relied on a few key people gathered in the right environment during an unprecedented crisis. Here we describe the initial team and governance that gave rise to this initiative.

1.1 Expertise

3D COVID is first and foremost the reunion of a few people with decisive assets, being the 'core team' of the project.

Medical expertise
A physician familiar with 3D printing working within a university hospital, with an academic position in a large medical school, and previous experience in working with start-ups and regulatory bodies.

Engineering expertise
An engineering team that could handle the design, production, and maintenance of 3D printers, with strong medical experience and relationships with engineering schools.

Medical and healthcare professional staff involvement
A will to assess the designs with the highest standards by the very people who would eventually use them on the field, for the well-being of their patients.

Institutional support
Key leaders supporting the project in a huge institution, ready to give a formal green light to an innovative approach without tampering with endless paperwork.

Regulatory and pharmacological expertise
A specialist at ease with the regulation of medical devices, able to rationalize the production chains and manage the conditioning and the distribution of the output.

Project management
A financial expert able to present a budgeted project to AP-HP decision makers.

Computer science literacy
The ability to design a platform for connecting people along with their expertise and make it go live in a few days.

1.2 Networks

Aside from their expertise, the 'core team' previously defined added steam and torque to the project thanks to their access to various networks.

AP-HP network
An institution with 100,000 professionals, hundreds of thousands of medical acts every year in 39 hospitals, is easier to grasp and talk to with savvy connected insiders.

Academic network
Paris hosts several high-level medical and engineering schools – a precise knowledge of the potential connections to establish with these institutions, in terms of specific issues in design or device assessment, is key.

Charity
The ability to knock at doors ready to be opened for a decisive participation in the initial funding of the project.

Media and press
Both internal (AP-HP) and mass media coverage of the initiative is crucial for increasing the scope of the project and benefiting from the inputs of, among others, AP-HP health professionals and independent engineering.

Hundreds of passionate makers
The community of makers started way before the first COVID19 case hit the country to investigate the promises of 3D printing.

Independent volunteering engineers
Offering their services for free designs in the specific context of the sanitary crisis.

JOGL workgroups
As part of the Open Covid19 Initiative, several groups were ready to work on topics related to medical devices and COVID19.

1.3 Mindset

The core team and its connected networks had to go through a series of initial challenges before the first devices hit the end of the production line. Tackling these challenges was made possible for these people, despite their professional and personal constraints over a narrow time frame, with a specific mindset.

Highly reactive mindset
To speed up the processes and minimize the slowdown due to the instrumental validation steps, the whole team adopted a very reactive working mode, anticipating and preparing the forthcoming steps to be ready to proceed upon validation.

Focus on the patient and healthcare professionals
Every day since the beginning of the COVID-19 outbreak has been droned in the humming of a relentless body count. The whole point of such a project is to help professionals save lives therefore it is not enough to make it quick and dirty. In turn, a constant focus was set on a high standard of validation of the medical devices to be used above all for the well-being of patients, in close connection with the needs of the professionals of AP-HP.

Emergency mindset
Better safe than sorry, the 3D COVID core team believed from day one that solidarity, open information and sharing are the three pillars of a genuine strategy against the virus, when actual action turns into efficiency.

Specific focus on regulation
3D COVID was the first attempt to produce 3D printed medical devices in response to a sanitary crisis using a dedicated platform – regulation was the main reason why such an initiative had not been launched earlier and was central in the mindset of the core team.

Intellectual property and valorization

Even though all the designs produced by 3D COVID were available open source on the website of the initiative (see chapter 3.12), offers from the private sector and foreign countries that would eventually flow in after the launch of the project imposed connections with lawyers and valorisation specialists.

1.4 Organization

The mindset of the few individuals composing the core team is reflected upon the organization of the project that was built on the following items.

Organization of the onsite project core team

The team was organized around a duo formed by a medical coordinator – who took in charge the interactions with health professionals, AP-HP hierarchy and academia, and a prime contractor (BONE 3D) – who managed a group of engineers and took in charge maintenance and production. Onsite pharmacists would help to build quality control processes and take in charge both conditioning and distribution, following the instructions of both the medical coordinator and the prime contractor.

Links with the AP-HP and Université de Paris hierarchy

The main directions in terms of production priority were dictated by members of the executive committee of AP-HP, who had an eye on the supplies of the whole institution. The management of AP-HP supplies was supervised by a specific agency, the Agence Générale des Équipements et des Produits de Santé (AGEPS), who would have a central role in the initiative (see below).

Limited number of people involved in the decision-making process

As emergency preparedness and response experts know intimately, one of the key challenges in a crisis is to perform swiftly in a limited time. This calls for procedures that cannot be standard, low in process but high in information. To be as reactive as possible, it has been pivotal to reduce the number of interlocutors by having, for each step, an individual reference contact with the highest possible decision-making power. Another related key point is the presence of the decision makers on site – the critical person, on top of the duo medical doctor / engineer, being a pharmacist specialized in the regulation and production of medical devices.

Openness

Taking the time to inform about the project helps the team reinforce over time, by attracting people with similar values and will to participate. Scientific publications on the structure of the project and on the devices also contribute to legitimate and advertise the initiative.

2. Initial plan

The initial plan on which 3D COVID was based was defined early on and the institutions with which we would interact readily emerged. The dynamics of several of these interactions ended up being more complex than initially expected.

The core team had to go through the following steps:

1. Anticipate the type of supply (personal protection devices, medical devices, maintenance, academia) that will be requested during the crisis,

2. Identify the type of technology able to respond to such needs,

3. Quantify the necessary material (printers, consumables),

4. Quantify and identify the people that will be needed for design and production,

5. Write an abstract about the project and a business plan with predictions on production,

6. Onboard the institution(s) based on the abstract and various political supports,

7. Fund the project,

8. Find suppliers,

9. Define the type of contracts offered to the prime contractor and his team,

10. Find a location to install the platform,

11. Check local constraints in terms of power supply, network coverage, fire safety, access control, ground resistance, ventilation, furniture, storage space and water supply for post-treatment,

12. Coordinate the staff with the prime contractor and institutional actors,

13. Define processes for set up, production, supply chain management and distribution,

14. Provide a web platform for broadcasting the designs,

15. Set up registers for the follow-up of production and the record of various issues and problems,

16. Ensure the project unfolding.

In practical terms, BONE 3D deployed a team of engineers ensuring design, production, and maintenance. We relied on a scientific team of health professionals and engineers initially coordinated by a pediatrician from Robert Debré Hospital (available during the pandemic due to low workload in paediatric hospitals), and by pharmacists supervised by the pharmacy department of Hôpital Cochin. The main AP-HP structures interacting with the 3D COVID core team where:

→ Université de Paris for academic development

→ AGEPS for medical device validation

→ Licensing and technology transfer office (OTT&PI)[1]

→ AP-HP International[2], the AP-HP international subsidiary

These interactions and their outcomes will be detailed below.

1 Licensing and technology transfer office of AP-HP (Office du Transfert de Technologie et des Partenariats Industriels): http://ottpi.AP-HP.fr.

2 AP-HP International, a private fully state-owned subsidiary of AP-HP: https://www.aphp.fr/international/ap-hp-international-la-filiale-dap-hp-ap-hp-international-subsidiary-ap-hp

3. Processes and Interaction with the institutions

The aim of this section is to provide enough elements so that the 3D COVID experience can be reproduced in other environments and during other types of sanitary crises. In this key chapter, all the practical details and the main results of the initiative are reported, from the most trivial details of the setting (furniture for instance) to the trickiest aspects of regulatory and intellectual property issues.

3.1 Funding the project: the financial process

As mentioned earlier, none of the initial projects managed to obtain the DGA funding (see chapter 0).

Once the AP-HP was on boarded notably through the budgeted project validation by top management, the fundraising step started. At this time, the AP-HP head knew that large amounts of private money would be donated to AP-HP for crisis management, but the specific donator to 3D COVID had not been determined when the principle of the project was approved.

Multiple contacts were made with various partners, both from the public and private sphere. Among them, the dean of Université de Paris activated the communication consulting company Image7 through family connections[1]. Image7 manages the communication of several CAC40 companies and identified clients that could potentially be interested in supporting the project based on three elements:

→ Interest in financially supporting public projects linked to the current medical state of emergency,

→ Companies with headquartered in France to streamline the decision-making process,

→ Companies with a quick decision-making process – the decision could obviously not wait for a hypothetical board of Directors to validate the funding.

As a result of this process, the 3D COVID project was fully funded by the Kering Foundation for a total of 1.7 million euros. In particular, the Kering group was solicited together with other firms by Image7 through a half-page summary explaining the context, aim, needs and timing of the project. Astonishingly, the funds were released within 24 hours.

The Kering group did not ask for visibility or for a communication campaign on their participation to the project and let Image7 and the AP-HP communication office coordinated and managed the press-releases and media campaigns.

1 https://www.image7.fr

3.2 Finding the place: history and practical constraints

The discussions on the localization of the 3D COVID platform started on the 27th of March, when the financial issues were being solved. Two locations were considered: (1) Leriche building within Broussais Hospital, in the South of Paris, within a former AP-HP hospital now used for training and research purposes and (2) the chapter room of the Port-Royal Abbey, within Hôpital Cochin, more central and within a strikingly beautiful XVIIth century historical building (Figures 3-4).

The criteria for an eligible location forthe platform were defined as follows:

→ Central situation in Paris, close to the homes of the leaders of the project (the country was locked down),

→ Within a large university hospital with possible direct interactions with health professionals from different specialties,

→ On ground floor, without stairs,

→ Accessible to trucks for delivery,

→ Sufficient surface (> 150 m^2),

→ Sufficient power supply,

→ Nearby secondary room for post-treatment, with water supply,

→ Storage space for raw materials and production before distribution,

→ Good wireless network coverage,

→ Available 24h security service,

→ No specific fire-related risks,

→ Air conditioning or good ventilation.

Both locations seemed to fulfill these criteria, but Port-Royal was more central and was located close to Hôpital Necker - Enfants Malades, to the offices of BONE 3D[2] and to the personal homes of most of the members of the team – these were crucial details in a context of lockdown with limited rights to circulate within Paris.

Furthermore, Port-Royal was a beautiful place that would have a positive impact on 3D COVID members in terms of quality of life, but also in terms of communication for press and other media.

Extra support for settling in Port-Royal was provided by relatives of Jean-Denis Cochin (1726-1783), the founder of Hôpital Cohin, still active within AMC and thus with symbolic influence on the staff of this hospital. AMC (Association des Amis de Malades de l'Hôpital Cochin) is one of the oldest medical charities in France (founded 1922), involved in the everyday life of is hospital. AMC contacted the head of Hôpital Cochin, to support the project and obtained a formal agreement on the 30th of March.

2 Additional machines located in the CGF laboratory at Hôpital Necker - Enfants Malades and at BONE 3D headquarters were used, see below.

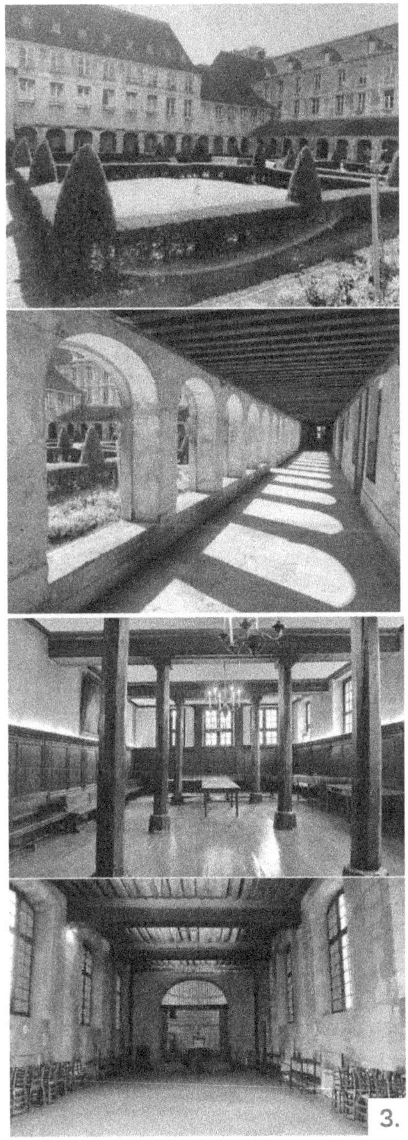

3.

Fig. 3. Port-Royal Abbey within Hôpital Cochin in central Paris. The chapter rooms were used as reception areas and were empty in March 2020.

Interestingly, the Port-Royal Abbey still hosts an active catholic church, with a mass celebrated daily at 5 pm, even during the confinement period (Figure 5). The Port-Royal Abbey had a long medical-related history. After the French revolution, the rooms in which we would settle the printers were turned into a prison. These spaces would then become a delivery room for the nearby Port-Royal hospital, which is still one of the most active maternity departments in Paris. A medical miracle has even been registered by the Catholic Church within these premises: the miracle of the Holy Thorn. Marguerite Périer (6 April 1646 – 14 April 1733) was a French nun and follower of Jansenism. She was the niece and goddaughter of Blaise Pascal. She was diagnosed with an eye condition, most probably a tear duct obstruction. On the 24th of March 1656 the child declared herself cured from placing her eye against a reliquary containing part of Christ's crown of thorns. The Port-Royal Abbey thus combined all the pre-requisites to shelter a pioneering medical initiative in a context of global sanitary crisis.

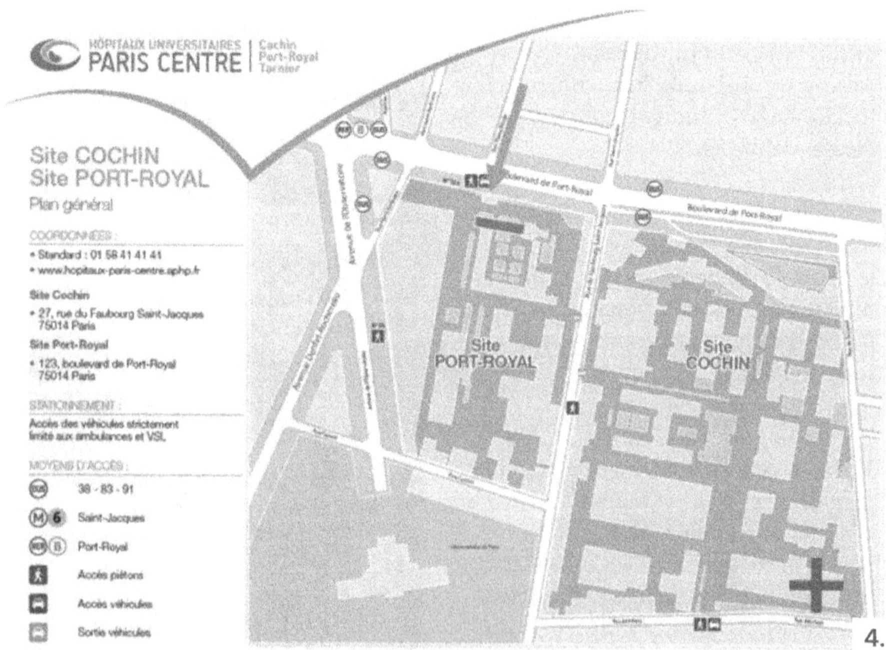

4.

Fig. 4. Chapter rooms of Port-Royal abbey within Hôpital in central Paris, located close to the main entrance (arrow) and to the main pharmacy with disinfection and sterilization facilities (cross)[3].

3 Adapted from: https://www.cochin-poa.com/informations-pratiques

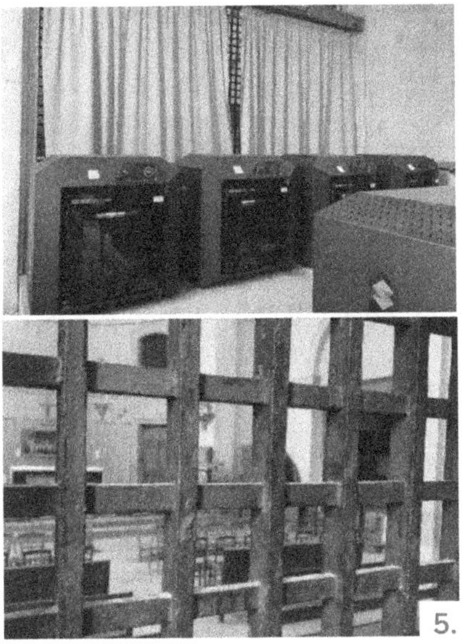

5.

Fig. 5. Behind the curtain in the main chapter room: an active catholic church. The grid originally separated the nuns from laymen attending religious ceremonies. The machines were positioned in the section initially reserved for nuns and now desacralized.

3.3 Choosing the machines: simple and reliable printers

The 3D printing technologies that were compatible with being settled quickly in a relatively non-controlled environment for large-scale production purposes were Fused Deposition Modeling (FDM), stereolithography (SLA) and polyjet. Polyjet was too expensive in terms of hardware and production costs. SLA was too complex to handle with demanding maintenance protocols. FDM seemed to be the ideal technology for fast and easy prototyping as well as the production of large quantities of devices.

Printer	Weight	Size (mm)	Int. temp.	Int. hum.	Sound	Max. ext. temp.	Max. ext. hum	Required power
F120	124	889x870x721	59° - 86°	< 30%	46 Db max. 35 Db when on standby	35°	20-90%	200-240 V 50 - 60 Hz
F170	227	1626x864x711						
F370								

1.

Table 1. Technical characteristics of Stratasys FDM printers from the F123 series. Int: internal; temp: temperature; hum: humidity; max: maximum; ext: external.

Based on the expertise of BONE 3D and availability during the crisis, three printers from the F123 series of Stratasys (Eden Prairie, MN, USA) were chosen: F120, F170 and F370 (Tables 1-2, Figure 6). The F123 FDM printers provide precise high-resolution printing thanks to extrusion heads mobilized by servo motors in closed insulated build chambers allowing temperature control and airflow design[4].

Printer	Wb size	Available material	Résolution	Racks
F120	254x254x254	ABSM30 ASA Support	ABS & ASA 0,12[1] - 0,17 - 0,25 - 0,33 mm	- 1 for plastic - 1 for support
F170		ABSM30 ASA PLA TPU94A Support	- same for ABS & ASA - PLA & TPU : 0,25 mm	
F370	355x254x355			- 2 for plastic - 2 for support

1 Not recommended by the manufacturer, many dysfunctions.

2.

Table 2. Printing characteristics of Stratasys FDM printers of the F123 series. Wb: workbench.

Stratasys was distributed in France by two companies: CADVision[5] and Seido Systèmes[6].

CADVision was the main and best-established distributor, with which both BONE 3D and the CGF laboratory at Hôpital Necker - Enfants Malades had already worked. The Stratasys machines available in Europe were stored in Stuttgart, Germany. According to the Stratasys commercial delegate, contacted by BONE 3D, the company had 90 machines from the F123 series available on the continent at the end of March 2020.

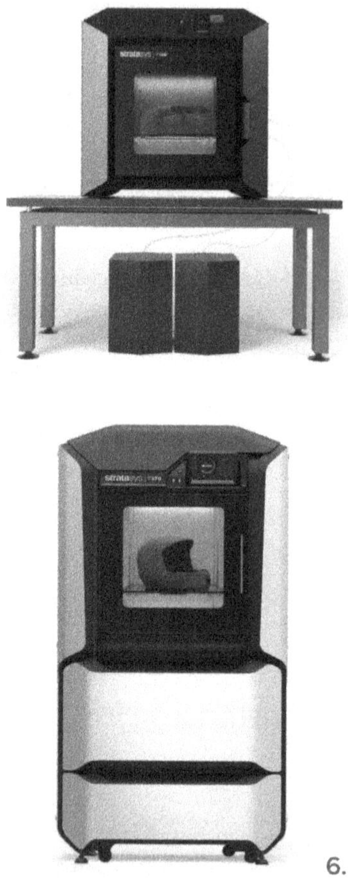

6.

Fig. 6. Stratasys F120 (top) and F170/F370 (bottom), two FDM printers from the F123 series[7].

4 Stratasys F123 FDM printers – technical characteristics: https://www.stratasys.com/content/Stratasys%20F120%20Experience/index.html.
Caution: this is a commercial video.
5 CADVision, the main Stratasys distributor in France: https://www.cadvision.fr.
6 Seido Systèmes, an alternative Stratasys distributor in France: https://www.seido-systemes.fr/.

7 Adapted from: https://www.stratasys.com/3d-printers/f123-series

Of note, approximatively at the same time, Dr Renato Favero designed with Isinnova, a company from Brescia, Italy, a 3D-printed connector allowing using Decathlon EasyBreath snorkeling masks[8] as ventilation devices[9]. This innovation benefited from a considerable press coverage that revealed the potential interest of additive manufacturing in the fight against COVID19. When the 3D COVID core team considered acquiring a series of F123 printers, the Italian Ministry of Health also consulted Stratasys on their hardware availabilities (Stratasys, personal communication). This potential threat to the availability of printers prompted the agreements with AP-HP and the settlements of the deals, even though it may have been a commercial argument used by Stratasys to speed up the purchase of the machines.

In usual situations, public contracts are mandatory between AP-HP and private companies, via a competitive call. Due to the sanitary crisis, the purchasing department of AP-HP commissioned the head of IT purchases to lead the acquisition of the printers. The IT purchase department trusted the expertise of BONE 3D and designed a specific deal based on sanitary crisis in order to avoid a call, with the support of the AP-HP legal department.

Machines			
Product	**Quantity**	**Unitary price (€)**	**Total price (€)**
J120	44	13,775 €	606,100 €
J170	14	20,333 €	284,662 €
J370	2	41,396 €	82,792 €
Post-treatment tank	3	6,950 €	20,850 €
Total Machines			**994,404 €**

3.

Table 3. Initial purchase of AP-HP from CADVision, March 30th, 2020.

8 Easybreath, a surface snorkeling mask extensively used as a protection and ventilation during the COVID19 crisis: https://www.decathlon.fr/p/masque-de-snorkeling-en-suface-easybreath-500-oyster/_/R-p-148873?mc=8485021&c=BLEU_TURQUOISE.

9 Isinnova, an Italian startup offering 3D-printing services: https://www.isinnova.it/easy-covid19-eng.

Consumables

Product	Quantity	Unitary price (€)	Total price (€)
Extrusion heads F120 / Support	15	895 €	13.425 €
Extrusion heads F170 / F370	5	895 €	4,475 €
Workbench F120	45	175 €	7,875 €
Workbench F170 / F370	15	175 €	2,625 €
ASA F170 / F370	45	595 €	26,775 €
ASA F170 / F370	50	199 €	9,950 €
Support F120	25	595 €	14,875 €
Support F170 / F370	25	199 €	4,975 €
Post-production solution	4	490 €	1,960 €
Total - consumables			86,935 €
Total			1 081,339 €

3.

3.4 Hiring the people: public contracts during a sanitary crisis

To define the terms of the BONE 3D contract involving design, production and maintenance, the IT purchase department had to settle a deal over the weekend of the 27th of March. The final terms of the contract were finalized during a late-night call (1.30 am on the 28th) with the head of IT purchases at AP-HP.

The contract between AP-HP and BONE 3D was based on a market termed « Providing conception and manufacture services for 3D printing »[10]. The initial duration of the contract was 4 months for a total amount of 536,391€ with a planned extension of 8 extra months. The 536,391€ included 213,191€ of re-billing to CADVision, one of the Stratasys distributors in France, which left a total sum of 323,200€ for the engineering services of BONE 3D for the initial 4-month period.

10 Marché 2020ACHC 203806 relatif à la fourniture de prestations de conception et fabrication de pièces sur imprimante 3D, opération d'impression 3D fournitures et prestations associées.

BONE 3D employed 4 full-time engineers dedicated to the project, under the direct supervision of the CEO of the company. Help with production and maintenance was provided by another specially commissioned BONE 3D technician. All were previous employees of BONE 3D (Table 4).
During the project, BONE 3D furthermore employed an engineering student (from the 17/04/2020), who was interning in the CGF lab before the crisis and steeled up the whole quality and regulatory system of the Necker 3D printing platform. This engineering student was employed a under limited term contract to support part of the quality and regulatory activity related to the platform. Later during the summer on 01/06/2020, another BONE 3D technician was added to the team under limited term contract to support production.

AP-HP furthermore had a contract with CADVision for advanced maintenance issues. Two senior technicians were commissioned to help with the installation of the machines, assisted by a junior technician. Commercial interactions with CADVision were led by their commercial delegate for the Paris region. The maintenance contract was signed for 3 years with AP-HP (Table 5).

	Monday	Tuesday	Wednesday	Thursday	Friday	Saturday	Sunday
6 am 2.30 pm	Technician 1	Engineer 1	Engineer 1	Technician 2	Technician 2	Technician 2	Technician 2
1.30 pm 10 pm	Engineer 2	Technician 1	Technician 1	Engineer 2	Technician 2	Technician 2	Technician 2
9 am 6 pm	Engineer 3	Engineer 3	Engineer 3	Engineer 4	Engineer 4	Engineer 4	Engineer 4
10 pm 6 am	Engineer 4 + Technician 1/2	Engineer 4 + Technician 1/2	Engineer 4 + Technician 1/2	Engineer 4 + Technician 1/2	Engineer 4 + Technician 1/2	Engineer 4 + Technician 1/2	Engineer 4 + Technician 1/2

4.

Machine type	Number of machines	Price / machine / year (€ HT)	Total price (€)
F120	2	5,983 €	35,898 €
F170	14	3,208 €	134,736 €
F370	44	3,208 €	423,456 €
Total (€ HT)			594,090 €

5.

Table 4. Initial schedule of BONE 3D employees dedicated to running 3D COVID.

Table 5. Maintenance contract between AP-HP and CADVISION for 3 years.

3.5 Practical installation of the machines: a factory within a hospital

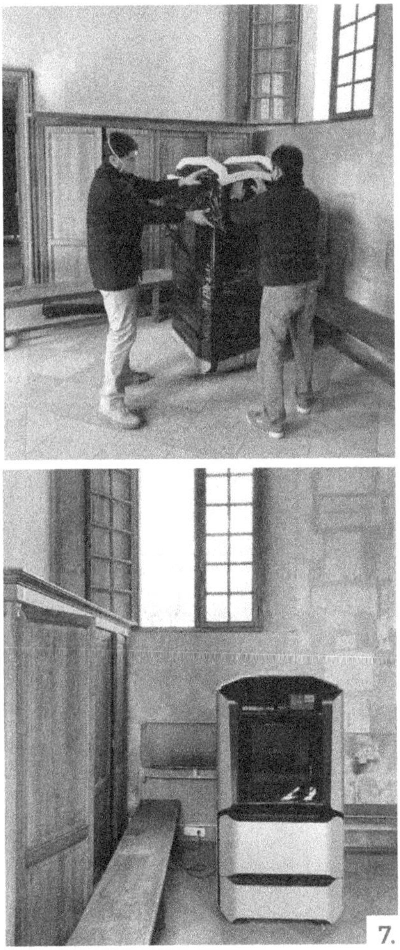

7.

Fig. 7. The first F370 printer, lend by CADVision on the 30th of March 2020, to test delivery possibilities to the chapter rooms of Port-Royal Abbey.

The delivery day for the machines was fixed on the 1st of April 2020. On Monday the 30th of March, CADVision agreed to lend a F370 machine to 3D COVID, in order to start testing delivery possibilities and installation issues (Figure 7).

The rest of the machines was delivered from 8AM to 2PM the 1st of April by 6 trucks arriving from Germany. Trucks could enter Port-Royal and park in front of a lateral entrance of the Abbey, in front of the main gate of the maternity. Care was taken to leave enough space for the circulation of a large ambulance lateral to the parked truck, in order to avoid interfering with patient care. This specific point should be considered whenever unusually large amounts of material are to be delivered within hospitals, especially to buildings that are not designed for this purpose.

Packages containing the machines were carried to the two chapter rooms by the team BONE 3D and a group of surgery trainees, with the help of the CADVision staff (Figure 8). The technical staff of the hospital supervised the delivery but did not actively take part into it. Two reel carriers were available, one provided by Hôpital Cochin and one by CADVision (Figure 9).

Printers were progressively dispatched between the two chapter rooms. All F170 and F370 printers were stored in the room that had a stone floor – the room with a wooden floor only had F120 printers. The heavier machines – F170 and F370 – were furthermore placed close to the walls of the room to minimize mechanical constraints on the floor.

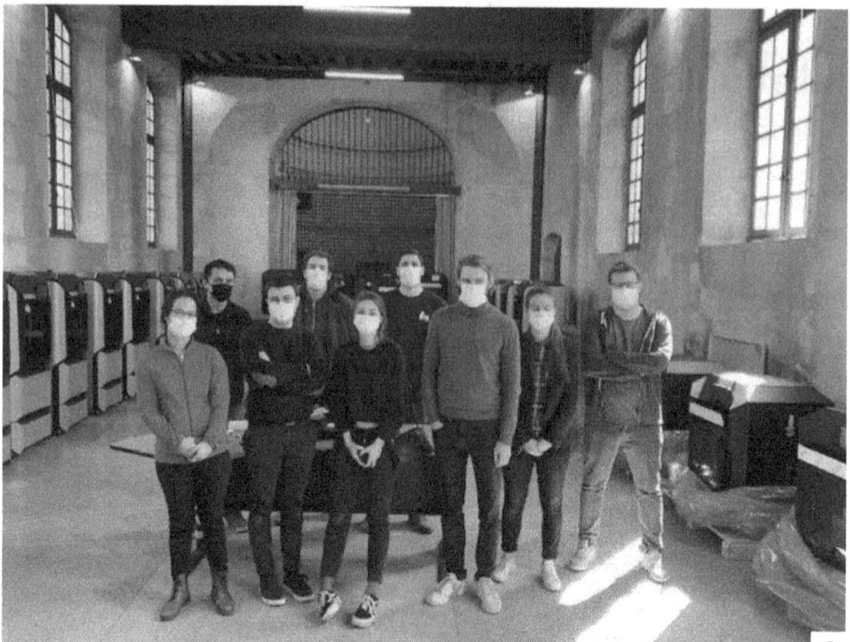

8.

Fig. 8. The team of engineers and surgery registrars that installed the 60 3D printers on the 1st of April 2020.

This installation led to the production of a massive quantity of waste that required a professional management. The local logistics of Hôpital Cochin declined managing this waste. Via the Robert Debré paediatrician assisting us for the project, who had direct contacts with staff members at the Paris city hall, we got in touch with the head of Waste Collection and Street Cleaning services of the XIVth district, where Port-Royal was located. Due to the lockdown and low workload, the Waste Collection service could send a waste truck to collect all the palettes and wrappings (Figure 10).

Fig. 9. (a) Trucks delivering printers and consumables. Line: necessary space for ambulances accessing the maternity department. Blue cross: main entrance of Port-Royal hospital. Blue arrow: path to the lateral entrance of the Abbey. (b) Transporting the printers using reel carriers.

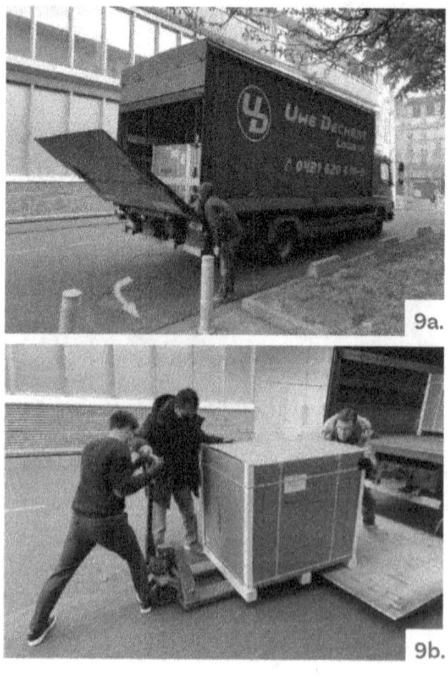

9a.

9b.

Fig. 9. (c,d) Entering the abbey with the reel carriers – the corridor could not be 1 cm narrower. (e) Opening the boxes in the chapter rooms. (f,g) Step-by-step installation of the printers.

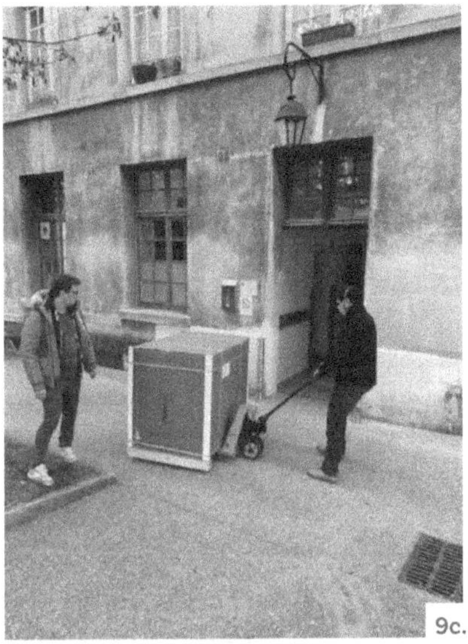

9c.

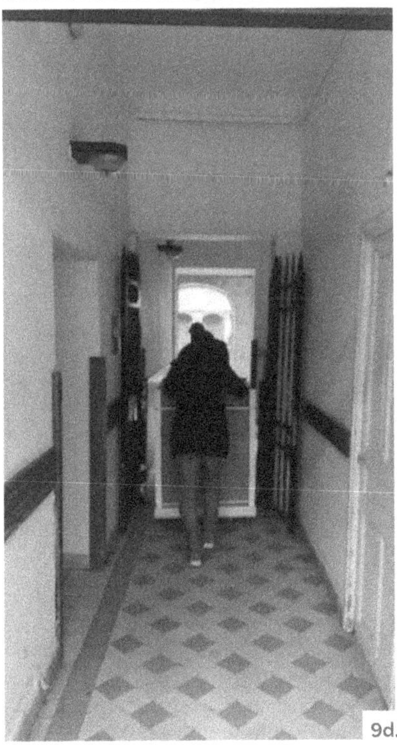

9d.

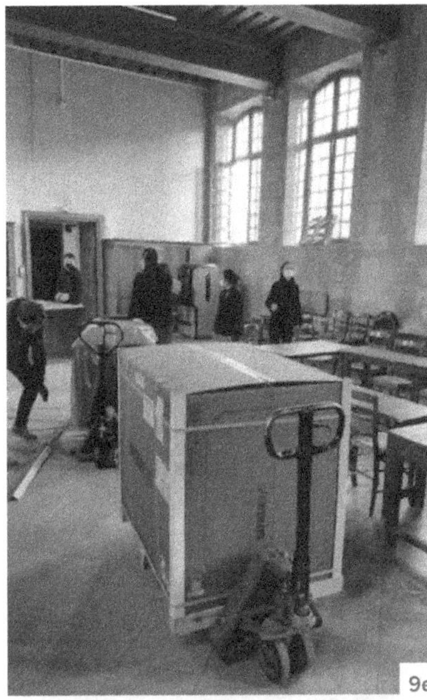

9e.

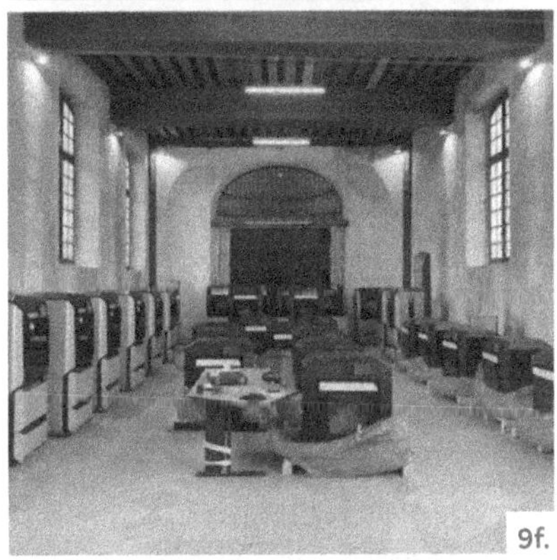

9f.

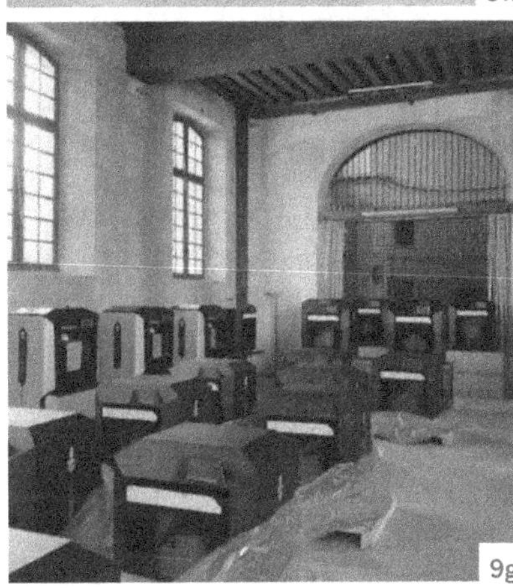

9g.

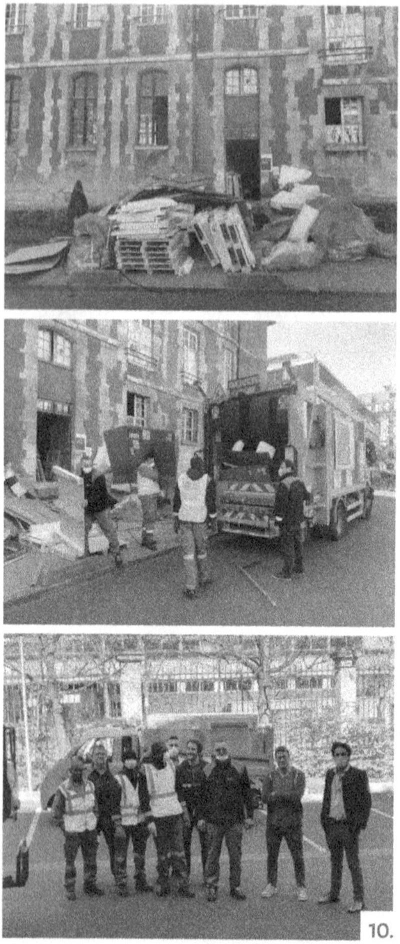

10.

Fig. 10. Waste Collection and Street Cleaning services of the XIVth district collecting the palettes and the wrappings from the 60 printers, on April 1st 2020.

F120 printers had to be positioned on tables. For this purpose, 34 2-level Mecalux[11] tables supporting 320 kg per level were purchased and delivered the 2nd and the 3rd of April 2020. The price per table was 136€, paid by BONE 3D and then secondarily billed to AP-HP.

11 Mecalux, Barcelona, Spain: https://www.mecalux.fr

Finally, a command computer was purchased by BONE 3D, in order to manage the 60 printers. This computer ran under Windows 10 Professional, had an Intel Core i9 4.60 Ghz with 64 GB of RAM and an Nvidia RTX 2080Ti graphics card.

On Friday mid-day, the full platform was settled (Figure 11). In parallel, issues with power supply and post-treatment were also managed.

Of note, Challancin[12], the company in charge of cleaning the premises in most AP-HP hospital including Port-Royal, refused to enter the two production rooms due to the presence of electrical cables on the ground and despite safety validation by the fire safety department (see section 3.8), so that the two rooms were cleaned daily by the medical and the engineering team.

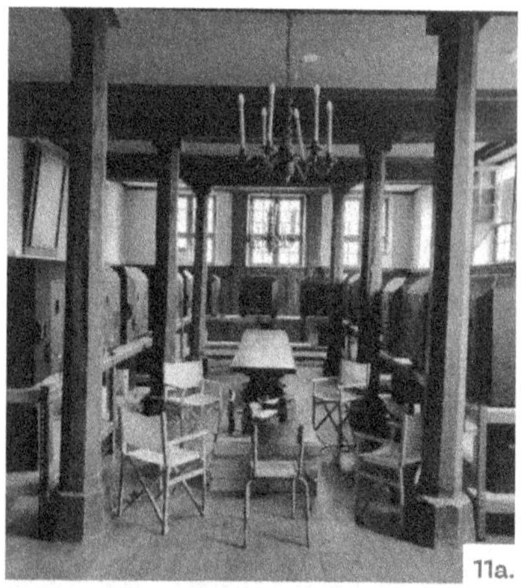

11a.

Fig. 11. (a) Final setting of 3D COVID in the chapter rooms of Port-Royal Abbey. A coffee table was designed using delivery palettes.

12 Groupe Challancin, Saint-Ouen, France : https://groupe.challancin.fr

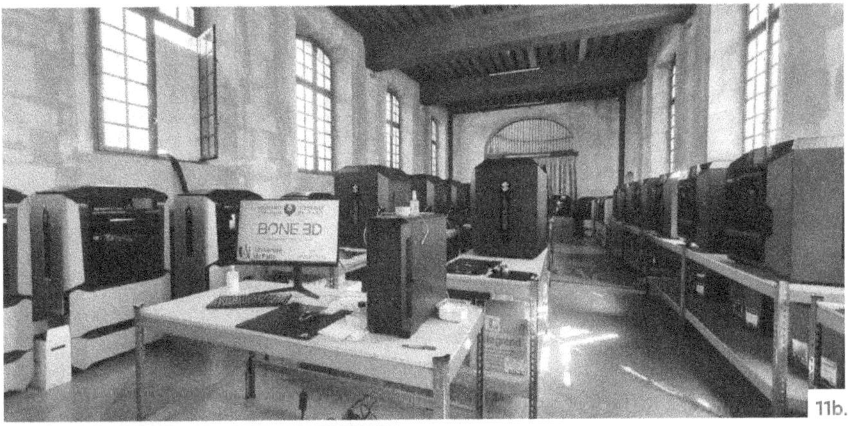

11b.

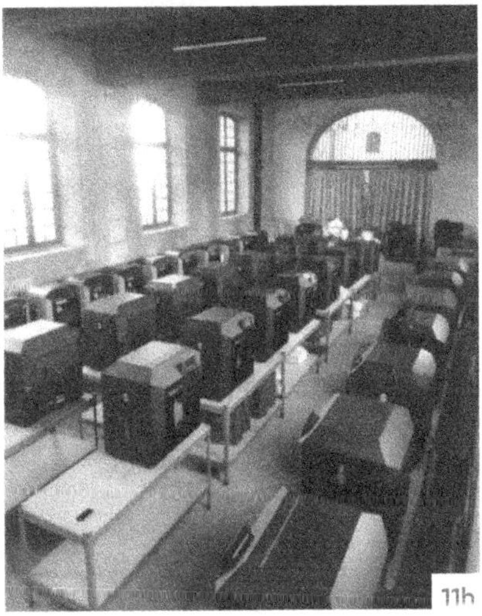

11b

Fig. 11. (b) The computer managing all printers was in the main room. The furniture (except tables for F123 printers) was temporarily lent by Hôpital Cochin.

3.6 Post-treatment: rehabilitation of an abandoned kitchen

The post-treatment room was settled in an abandoned kitchen a few meters away from the production center. An empty room next to this kitchen served as a storage facility for consumables. Three post-treatment tanks were settled (Cleanstation SCA-3600 support cleaning system, Stratasys, Eden Prairie, MN, USA). The water supplies were adapted to these tanks. Power requirement for each tank was 230 VAC +/- 10%, 50/60 Hz with amperage of 15A.

The 3D printed devices were subjected to post-treatment and secondarily rinsed using tap water (Figure 12). For medical devices, we planned to send the products to the central pharmacy of Hôpital Cochin for disinfection +/- sterilization and conditioning.

Water needs were estimated at 100 L per tank, changed every 2 weeks, which corresponded to 150 L per week. Post-treatment was performed at 70°C and post-treatment time depended on the amount of support.

Quantity of post-treatment product used was 13 Ecoworks bi-reactant cleaning agent tablets (Stratasys, Eden Prairie, MN, USA) per tank every two weeks, which corresponds to about 15 tablets per week.

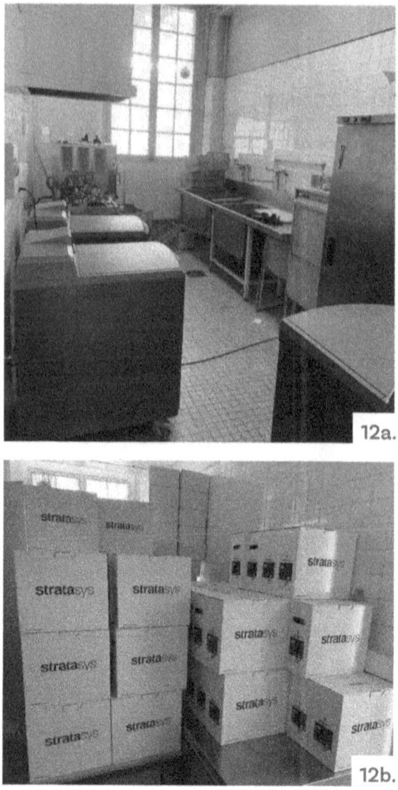

12a.

12b.

Fig. 12. Three post-treatment tanks settled in an abandoned kitchen with a sink for rinsing the devices (a), and an adjacent storage room for consumables (b).

Many volunteers helped for post-treatment, during different phases of the 3D COVID project, including engineering students, scouts, and medical students.

3.7 Power supply: feeding hungry machines

The power supply required solving two specific issues:

→ Bringing enough power to the chapter rooms,

→ Building enough electrical cabinets to distribute this power to all the machines in the two rooms.

The main power supply was redirected from the nearby maternity building using high-tension cables (Figure 13). These cables were connected to a main electrical cabinet, which dispatched power to two secondary cabinets (Figure 14)[13].

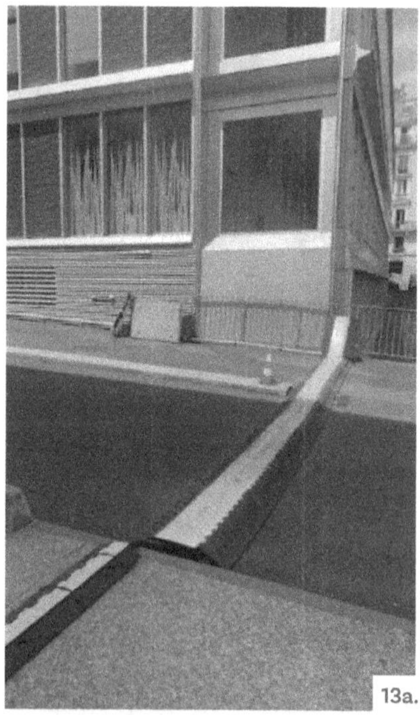

13a.

Fig. 13. (a). High-tension cables redirected from the nearby maternity building and entering the chapter room through a window to be connected to the main electrical cabinet.

13 Wiring and manufacture of electrical cabinets was performed in a record time by TBES – Travaux, Bâtiments, Électricité, Sécurité: https://www.tbes.fr.

Fig. 13. (b) The main electrical cabinet. (c, d)The two secondary cabinets were connected to the main cabinet by the wiring described on Figure 14.

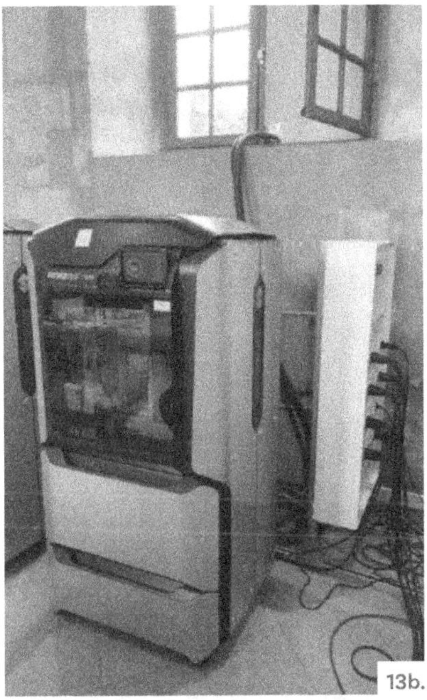

13b.

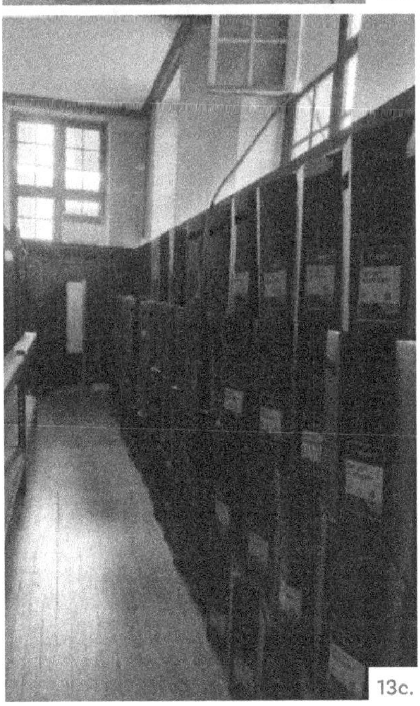

13c.

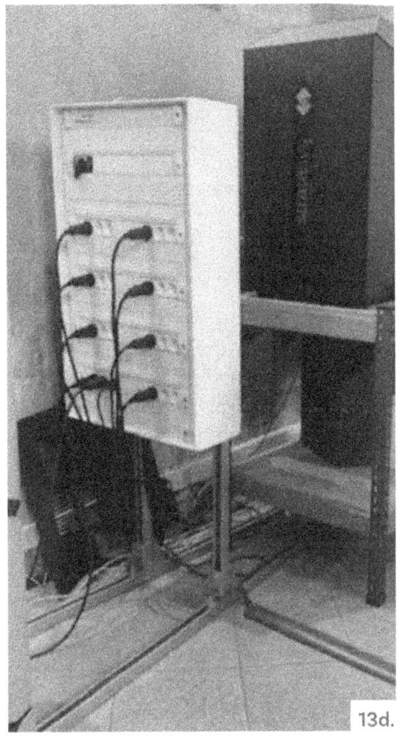

13d.

Fig. 14. Wiring of the three electrical cabinets.

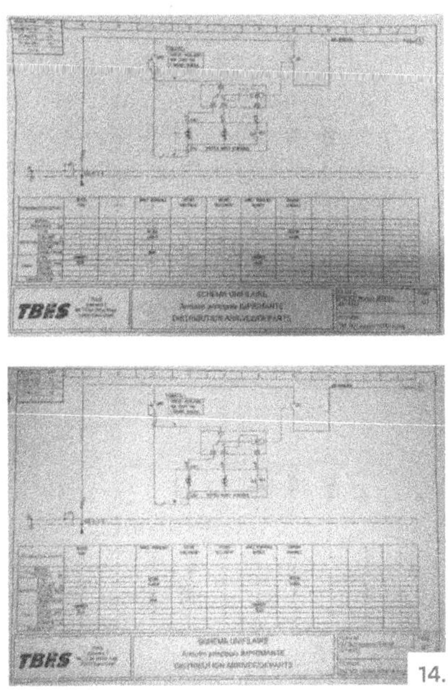

14.

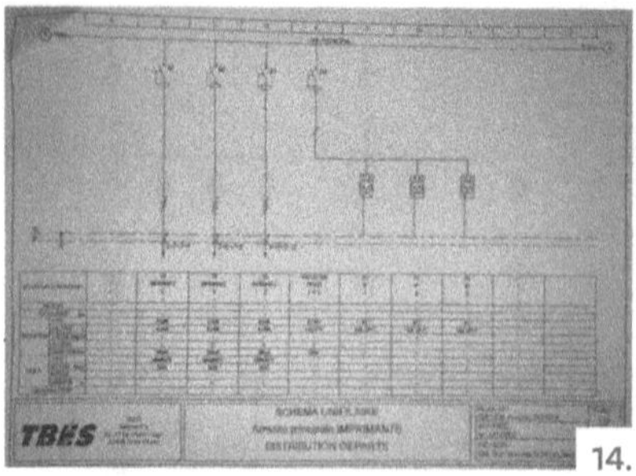

14.

Each machine of the F123 series required 200-240V of power with a theoretical amperage of 7A. In France, the amperage is defined at 10A minimum - here the amperage was set at 16A.

3.8 Security issues: protecting expensive machines in a public place

The main entrance of the Port-Royal Abbey was facing the main security post of the hospital, with a 24/7 duty. A list of the main participants to 3D COVID was established and provided to the head of Security and Safety at Hôpital Cochin, who then provided a copy of the list to his team. Security agents would deliver the keys of the Abbey to team members anytime of the day and night based on this list.

Due to the large number of people willing to see the facilities, the team decided to systematically close the doors when working on the machines.
A security breach occurred on the 27th of May 2020, when an unknown individual who was not listed managed to convince security to get the keys and attempted to login the main computer controlling the machines at 8.05 pm. After this unfortunate event – the abused agent eventually lost his job – two cameras were positioned in each of the chapter rooms with constant supervision by central security (Figure 15).

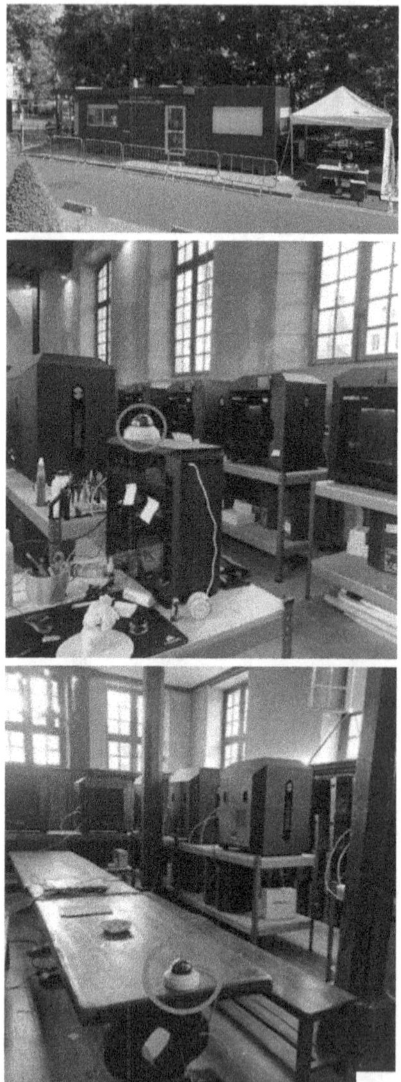

15.

Fig. 15. Security headquarters in front of the entrance of the abbey open 24/7. Two cameras (circles) positioned after a security breach on the 27th of May.

Regarding fire safety, only one fire extinguisher was available for the two rooms when the initiative started. On the 2nd of April, 5 extinguishers were added: class A and B extinguishers for electrical fires (CO_2) and fire with a combustion agent (here, wood) (water with additive) (Figure 16). Furthermore, all team members benefited from 1h of fire safety training on the 8th of April 2020.

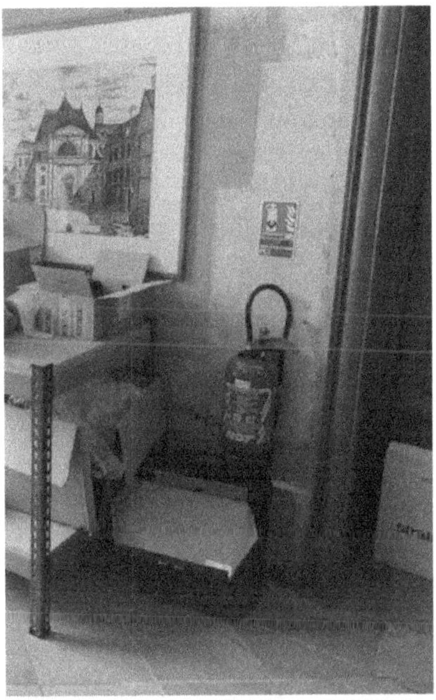

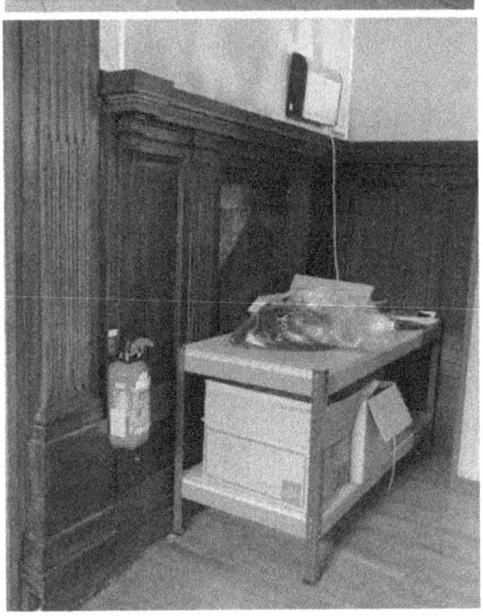

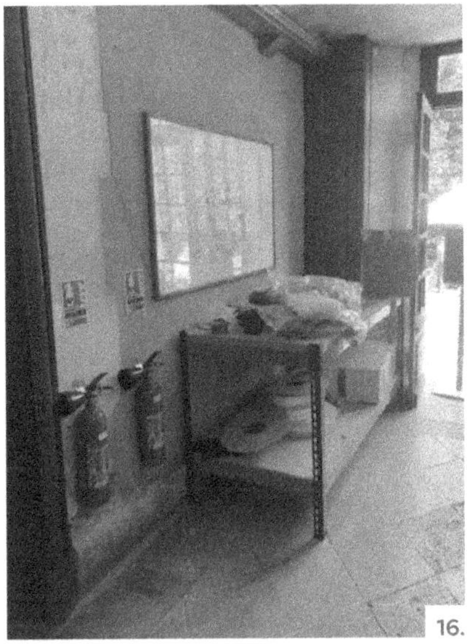

16.

Fig. 16. Different types of fire extinguishers added after the settlement of the printers in order to comply with fire safety regulations.

3.9 Rationalizing the production chain: professional batch follow-up

One of the basic requirements of medical device regulation is batch follow-up that allows efficient quality control on the production. Establishing this type of follow-up is the competence of pharmacists. The lead of the sterilization platform at Hôpital Cochin immediately showed a spontaneous interest for our initiative and commissioned one senior registrar and one resident to follow-up the project. This team of pharmacists and BONE 3D engineers worked together to lay the bases of the quality control of the production of 3D COVID:

→ Each printer was identified, and production lines were defined,
→ Each lot of consumables was identified by its serial number,

→ Production batches were defined and identified (Figures 17-18).

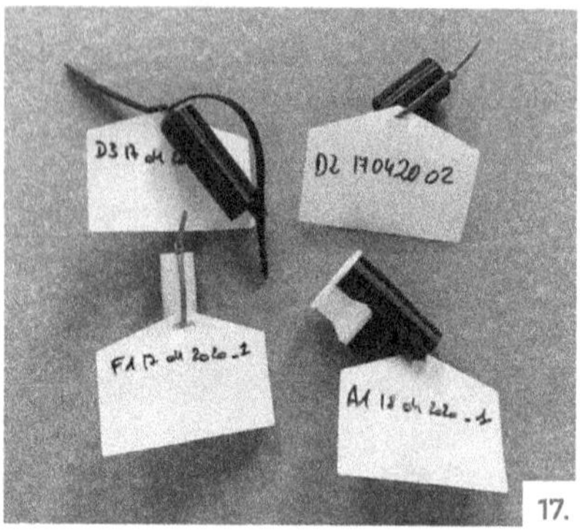

17.

Fig. 17. Identification of batches for follow-up and quality control.

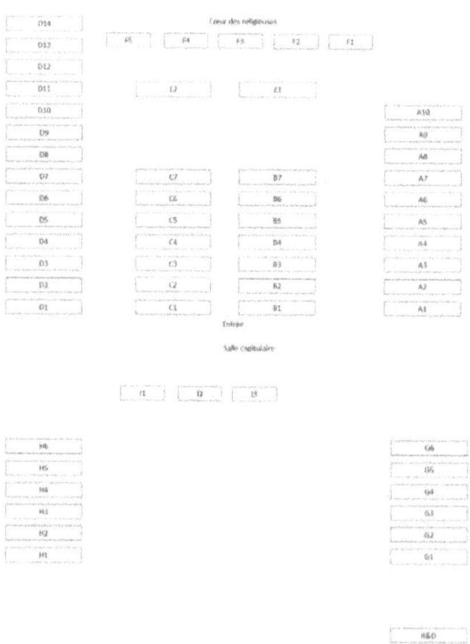

18.

Fig. 18. Distribution of production lines in the two production rooms.

3.10 Hygiene issues: preparing the dispatching of medical devices

Disinfection and sterilization processes were defined in collaboration with the head of the sterilization platform. 86.68 Getinge (Getinge, Sweden) washer-disinfectors with a specific cycle compliant with the EN ISO 15883-1 norm were used[14]. The cycle was set as follows:

→ Rinsing with softened water at 20°C with TH < 7°F for 1 min,

→ Wash with softened water at 55°C during 5 min with detergent NEODISHER MEDICLEAN FORTE at 0.4% (Dr Weigert, Hamburg, Germany),

→ Rinsing with softened water at 20°C with TH < 7°F for 2 min,

→ Thermic disinfection with reverse-osmosis-purified water à l'eau osmosée (resistivity < 15 µS/cm²/20°C) for 10 minutes at 70°C with a drying surfactant NEODISHER MEDIKLAR SPECIAL at 0.03% (Dr Weigert, Hamburg, Germany),

→ Drying 30 min at 70°C.

The follow-up of the hygiene processes was performed using the T-Doc software (Getinge, Getinge, Sweden).

14 Washer-disinfectors, Part 1: General requirements, definitions and trials (ISO/DIS 15883-1: 2006).

The effects of this cleaning protocol were assessed by analysing the 3D shape of selected devices before and after disinfection. For this, three devices produced by 3D COVID (Figure 19) were micro-CT-scanned before and after disinfection, with a resolution of 0.1 mm, at the Institut de Biomécanique Humaine Georges Charpak, École Nationale Supérieure des Arts et Métiers, Paris, France. Surfaces were superimposed using global registration under 3-Matic (Materialise, Leuwen, Belgium) and point-surface distances were computed between surfaces before and after disinfection, and the with the original CAD model (Table 6).

More precisely, the devices analysed were printed 3 times each during a single printing cycle, on the same F120 machine, with a layer thickness of 0.25 mm.

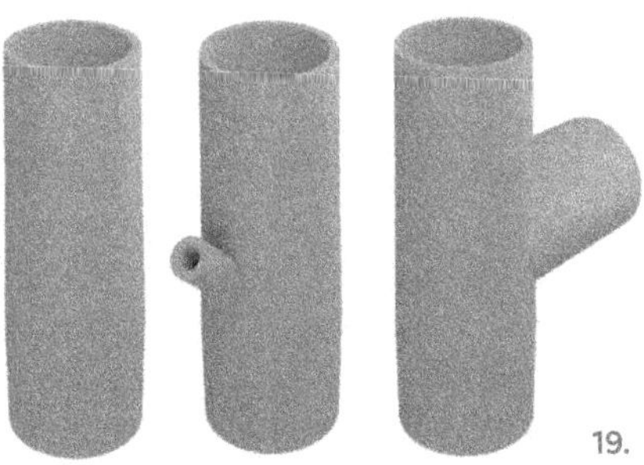

19.

Fig. 19. From left to right, F22M22 long, M22 F22 T and F22M22M22 (see section 7.2).

	F22 M22 long			M22 F22 T			F22 M22 M22		
	№1	№2	№3	№1	№2	№3	№1	№2	№3
Before disinfection	0,048 ± 0,046	-0,008 ± 0,045	0,006 ± 0,045	-0,052 ± 0,104	0,048 ± 0,108	-0,020 ± 0,068	0,022 ± 0,040	0,027 ± 0,038	0,020 ± 0,092
After disinfection	0,024 ± 0,032	-0,006 ± 0,040	0,030 ± 0,040	-0,012 ± 0,070	0,026 ± 0,036	-0,010 ± 0,095	0,018 ± 0,042	0,010 ± 0,089	0,001 ± 0,090

6.

Table 6. Distances between device and CAD model before and after disinfection (average values ± standard deviation).

Before disinfection, the maximum distance between the actual object and the CAD 3D object was 0.052 ± 0.104 mm. After disinfection, this maximum value was 0.030 ± 0,040 mm, which showed little global effect of disinfection on the 3D shape of ABS-printed devices.

Differences between models and devices mostly concentrated on corners and regions perpendicular to the main axis of the object: for F22M22M22, a maximal distance of 0.32 mm was found within the lateral T-shaped extrusion (Figure 20).

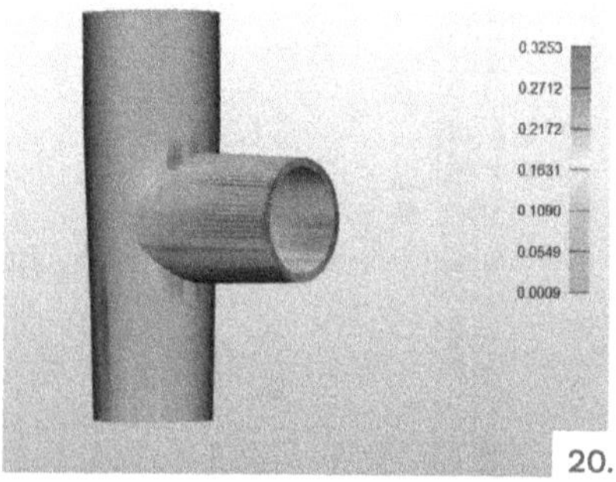

20.

Fig. 20. Distribution of the distance between F22M22M22 after disinfection and the original CAD model, in mm.

3.11 Identifying the designs: numerous sources for innovating ideas

By locating a prototyping and production center within a hospital in a context of sanitary emergency, we created a place where many individuals with innovating ideas would converge to interact with our engineering team, from all the different professional backgrounds working in public hospitals and public institutions.

Furthermore, during the first phases of the crisis, numerous independent designers posted open-access files of various quality online, offering prototypes for protection and medical devices. Independent designers and industrials companies (such as Dassault Systems for instance) spontaneously offered us their pro bono assistance shortly after our initiative got advertised.

These offers were generally very generous, but sometimes more patronizing, with incentives by several large private companies to use their internal platform for storing our designs, arguing that we would not be able to handle our production without professional supervision, but failing to describe all the implications of the use of their interface in terms of intellectual property.

One example of design arising from an independent engineer was the Boussignac valve, on which an independent engineer volunteered to worked by interacting directly with its inventor Georges Boussignac[15]. Boussignac eventually passed away before the completion of the project, but the engineer had the opportunity to print various prototypes of his valve on the machines of the platform.
Other designs were directly proposed by

15 Georges Boussignac passed away in May 2020 at the age of 76. This great inventor was homeless when he arrived in France from Croatia and rose to the level of one of the best experts worldwide in ventilation. We are proud to have worked directly with him in adapting his concepts to 3D printing.

AP-HP staff, either by physicians, such as neo-natalogists at Port-Royal hospital, who required a specific design for a joint allowing to connect filters to pediatric ventilators, or by a paramedic (head nurse of a large intensive care unit) who had the idea of a head rest for patients requiring prolonged prone position in intensive care. In all cases, the designs were assessed, redesigned/corrected by BONE 3D engineers before prototyping.

We also benefited from JOGL[16] groups that put together independent designers and academics willing to help, to promote open science and innovation on specific design questions related to the pandemic. Within the OpenCovid19 initiative[17], several relevant workspaces were opened, towards which we could direct many volunteers that contacted our group with interesting designs and ideas that we could not process in the immediate crisis context. Examples of such projects were an open-source low-cost syringe pump adapted to hospital uses (24 members in the JOGL workgroup)[18], Easy Breath connectors (13 members in the JOGL workgroup)[19], and the open-source face-mask challenge (54 members in the JOGL workgroup)[20]. All groups had French and international members. These JOGL groups did not lead to the development of medical or protection devices that reached production stage during the first pandemic wave. Nevertheless, these groups had highly beneficial effects in terms of brainstorming on hot topics in a context of sanitary emergency.

The dynamics of the low-cost syringe pump group were interesting as a case study of the use of open science during a sanitary crisis. The JOGL group on the syringe pump put together several prominent engineers including a professor from EPITA (École pour l'Informatique et les Techniques Avancées)[21], a top-level Parisian engineering school. A pump prototype was progressively designed based on regular interactions within the JOGL workgroup, using several pieces initially designed for the Makair ventilator, an open-source ventilator project launched independently in response to the pandemic[22]. This innovative approach using available pieces from another initiative was nearly reaching its goal when another independent project emerged, led by Electrolab, a non-academic group of makers supported by several academic institutions, such as the Fondation de l'Académie de Chirurgie.[23,24] The Electrolab group did not accept to collaborate with the JOGL group, even though including Makair pieces into an emergency design was a very promising approach. On the 25th of April 2020, Electrolab tweeted false information about the presumed fact that EPITA had contacted the regulatory authorities in charge of medical devices (Agence nationale de sécurité du médicament et des produits de santé, ANSM) about their own pump project and had pretended that they were working with Electrolab to promote their own interests. This insulting tweet clearly stated that EPITA teachers were giving wrong examples of professional practices to their students regarding the ethics of open science. Despite formal protests from EPITA and

16 Jogl.io
17 https://app.jogl.io/program/opencovid19
18 https://app.jogl.io/project/185
19 https://app.jogl.io/project/184
20 https://app.jogl.io/project/150
21 https://www.epita.fr
22 https://makair.life
23https://forum.electrolab.fr/viewtopic.php?f=16&t=1870#p11197
24 https://fondationacademiechirurgie.fr

proof that the tweet was wrong, Electrolab refused to erase this message. Because of this situation, the two projects did not fuse and none of them reached the status of medical device during the active phase of the pandemic. This case study is an illustration of both the great perspectives of collaborative science and, unfortunately, the persistence of wrong behaviors related to the characteristics of open-source projects. In the specific case of interactions between maker organizations and academic institutions, mutual lack of consideration – suspicion towards institutional science on the maker side and patronizing attitude of academia towards highly competent but self-made technicians – led to a sub-optimal use of promising open-science tools that could have resulted in much faster innovation.

3.12 Interactions with users: Covid3D.org

Interactions with users were mostly relying on two pathways: (1) direct contacts and (2) contacts via a dedicated website – covid3D.org.

Direct contacts occurred initially mostly with teams from Port-Royal and Hôpital Cochin, where 3D COVID was implanted. Hospitals in which the core 3D COVID team had colleagues (Pitié-Salpêtrière, Lariboisière, Robert-Debré, Necker – Enfants Malades) also immediately collaborated, as well as local public institutions (for instance primary schools in the 5th district, facing the 3D COVID premises). Other contacts were established via BONE 3D and their previous partners in various AP-HP hospitals (Beaujon hospital in Clichy for instance).

Nevertheless, an orchestrated internal communication campaign at the level of medical doctors and administration would most probably have had considerably increased the initial scope of activity of 3D COVID. It is noteworthy that even with a subset of AP-HP hospitals, a convincing proof of concept of the importance of an internal 3D printing platform was established within a few weeks. After a few months of successful interactions within AP-HP, mostly based on word of mouth, but also due to the diversification of our production, our partners within AP-HP considerably increased; at the end of 2020, the team interacted with most of the 39 AP-HP hospitals.

The Covid3D.org website was designed by an independent volunteering developer during the first two weeks following the installation of the platform. The AMC charity offered to host the website for free. The terms of service were written by a lawyer specialized in intellectual property who worked pro bono.

The site offered two options (Figure 21): an entry point for health professionals in need for devices and another entry point for engineers and makers willing to help 3D COVID. Engineers and makers were directed towards JOGL and Emergency.io (Figure 22 and section 3.13). All the sponsors and the partners of 3D COVID were also listed on the main page of the website (Figure 23).

All devices produced by 3D COVID had their own page on which the printing characteristics were detailed and where a copy of the STL file could be freely downloaded. For further information or inquiries of missing devices, users could write to 3D.covid@aphp.fr, an email address to which the core team of the project had access.

A scientific committee was furthermore defined, mostly by the core members of the project and its composition was listed on the website. This committee nevertheless had no specific role in the management of the initiative. Despite its non-official role, several personal issues were raised by people not included into this committee. Issues were raised again after committee members were reduced in number without previous notice in May 2020 to fit the list with people actively collaborating with the platform. This was obviously a management mistake that led to numerous misunderstandings. Based on this experience, more care was taken when selecting the members of the strategic committee of the 'Phase 2' of the initiative that would consist in the post-COVID platform.

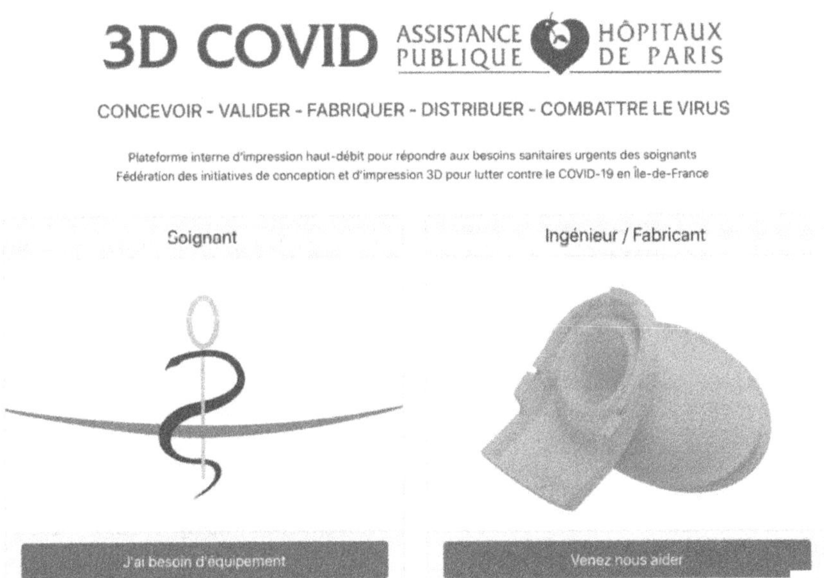

21.

Fig. 21. Front page of the website, directing users towards (1) the list of available devices and (2) projects on which engineers and makers could help via JOGL and Emergency.io

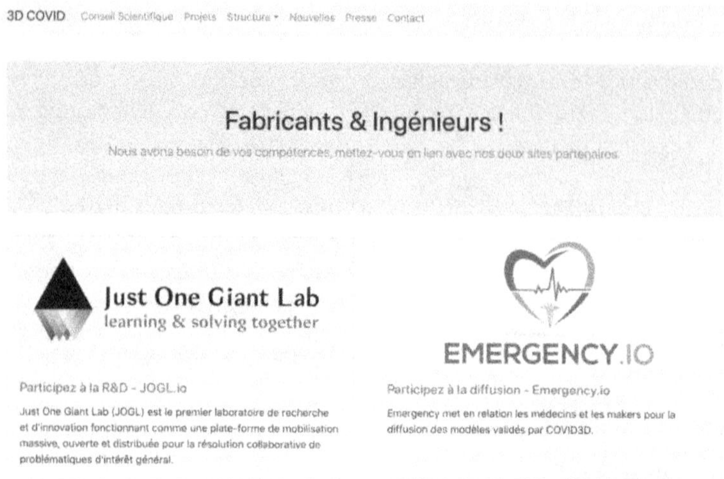
3D COVID Conseil Scientifique Projets Structure Nouvelles Presse Contact
Fabricants & Ingénieurs !
Nous avons besoin de vos compétences, mettez-vous en lien avec nos deux sites partenaires
Just One Giant Lab
learning & solving together
Participez à la R&D - JOGL.io
Just One Giant Lab (JOGL) est le premier laboratoire de recherche et d'innovation fonctionnant comme une plate-forme de mobilisation massive, ouverte et distribuée pour la résolution collaborative de problématiques d'intérêt général.
EMERGENCY.IO
Participez à la diffusion - Emergency.io
Emergency met en relation les médecins et les makers pour la diffusion des modèles validés par COVID3D.

22.

Fig. 22. Two partner websites that engineers and makers could use to help the 3D COVID initiative: JOGL and Emergency.io.

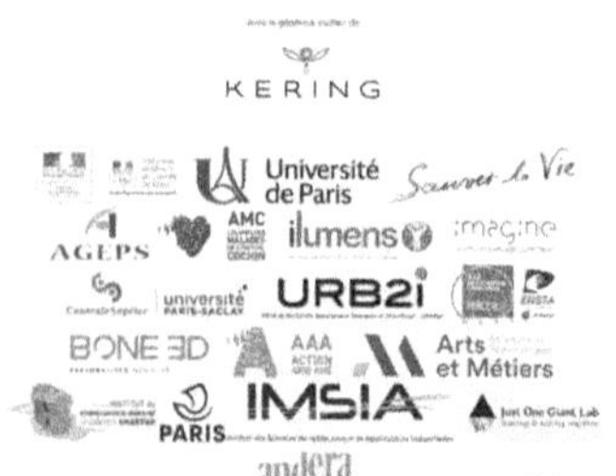
KERING
Université de Paris
Sauver la Vie
AGEPS
ilumens
URB2i
BONE 3D
Arts et Métiers
IMSIA
PARIS
andera

23.

Fig. 23. Logos of the main partners of the 3D COVID initiative as listed on the front page of the website covid3D.org.

3.13 Interations with makers: emergency.io

When the pandemic wave hit France, many makers volunteered to print protection devices and medical devices that would be secondarily distributed to health professionals and hospitals. These initiatives were difficult to monitor in terms of quality control, especially to produce medical devices.

Groups such as 3D4Care[25] invested lots of time and energy in regulating the manufacture processes of makers, with good results for protection devices.

As 3D COVID was receiving daily offers of individuals wishing to be involved in printing various types of devices, Emergency.io was dedicated to establishing links between makers and health professionals. The 3D COVID core team then systematically directed all makers or maker associations wishing to help 3D COVID to both 3D4Care and Emergency.io.

The idea behind the interactions between 3D COVID and Emergency.io was that the 3D COVID team would set the standards: we would determine which device could or could not be printed by makers, and with which technical characteristics. Emer-

25 3D4Care.org

gency.io would furthermore connect makers with health professionals, including private practices, in order to adapt production to actual needs.

The Emergency.io team was not able to provide precise metrics on how many makers / health professionals used their platforms, but the numbers were low. This failure was due to internal organization issues within the Emergency.io team that led to delays in website design and management. The 3D4Care initiative was much more successful in this field and provided many head shields to the greater Paris region by managing the production of a large number of makers.

While producing medical devices based on maker networks proved impossible due to regulatory issues, the results obtained by 3D4Care tend to show that makers can still strongly contribute to production in crises situation. Several maker groups fused during the pandemic with a strong incentive to provide common responses in case of potential future crises[26]. Coordination with these initiatives will be a key element when building the 'phase 2' of the 3D COVID initiative for the post-COVID years. One key issue will be whether a central initiative such as 3D COVID should provide financial help to makers in order to assist them in their production.

More generally, interactions with amateurs is a crucial question in 3D printing. There are a few fields in science and technology - such as astronomy for instance - where amateurs play a critical and beneficial role in the progress of research and in augmenting the scale of industrial projects. Makers have available time for design and for working on technical aspects of 3D printing by manipulating the printers. They furthermore hold a significant pool of machines, and are often organized into active associations. Their support can thus be crucial in crisis situations such as epidemics when large quantities of devices have to be produced and distributed over large territories. In this context, one role of platforms such as 3D COVID could consist in the definition of standards and in the formal or informal validation of designs and printing characteristics[27].

3.14 Validating the designs: the regulatory process

At the beginning of the crisis, the in-house (that is, inside hospitals) production of custom-made medical devices was about to be regulated by a new European settlement[28]. In short, this new settlement imposed a strict supervision of the production lines based on quality control and risk management. This implied the mandatory use of CE-marked devices for design and production (including

26 Strong groups have gathered the leader of the Réseau Français des FabLabs (fablab.fr), with whom 3D COVID has established positive professional interactions.

27 For an insightful analysis of the role of amateurs in the progress of science (based on the example of astronomy): Dyson F., Imagined worlds, Harvard University Press, 1997.

28 Regulation (EU) 2017/745 of the European Parliament and of the Council of 5 April 2017 on medical devices: https://eur-lex.europa.eu/legal-content/ENG/TXT/PDF/?uri=CELEX:32017R0745

design softwares) but did not impose the individual CE-marking of each custom-made device. On the other hand, the mass production of standard medical devices was subjected to different and much more demanding rules, including an individual CE marking of each device and measures of increasing complexity based on the class of the device.

The production of non-custom-made medical devices in moderate quantities (several hundreds to several thousands) using 3D printing, in response to a sanitary crisis, had thus to follow the same rules as the mass production of any medical device. The requirements for settling a mass production line of medical devices, using 3D printing or not, were not compatible with a crisis context. The 3D COVID initiative was thus facing an intrinsic regulatory issue that required close collaboration with competent French regulatory bodies.

Within AP-HP, the agency responsible for selecting medical devices and checking their conformity was AGEPS (Figure 24), which employed a team of pharmacists specialized in this type of assessment. Within the first days after the settlement of 3D COVID, we established close contacts with AGEPS, notably with the head of sales within this agency (see below).

At a national level, the structure able to authorize the release of a new medical device was the Agence Nationale de Sécurité du Médicament et des Produits de Santé (ANSM), with a specific department dedicated to medical devices (Figures 25-26). ANSM only could provide authorizations for placement on the market (Autorisation de Mise sur le Marché, AMM), the unavoidable step before any practical use of a medical device outside the scope of a clinical study.

3D COVID was thus confronted to a

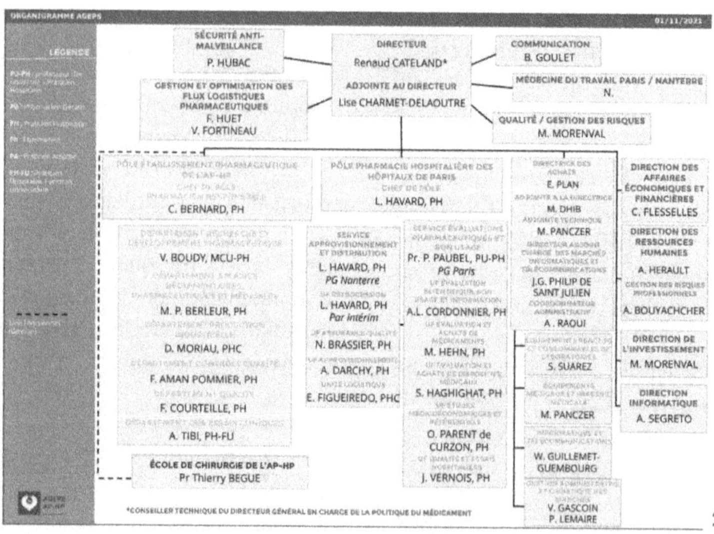

24.

Fig. 24. AGEPS hierarchy[1].

1 Adapted from : http://ageps.aphp.fr/wp-content/blogs.dir/64/files/2021/10/Organigramme-au-01-11-2021.pdf

difficult question: would it be possible, in collaboration with AGEPS and ANSM, to obtain exceptional AMMs for specific 3D printed devices related to the COVID19 crisis? To make long stories short, we failed, and we will see why in the following.

Of note, for PPEs, similar issues were encountered. The French PPE regulations were monitored by the Ministry of Labor (Ministère du Travail), and not the Ministry of Health (Ministère des Solidarités et de la Santé), as it was the case for medical devices. Similarly, strict norms applied to PPE production. When we investigated the topic before starting head shield production at 3D COVID, there was a significant level of uncertainty on the qualification of certain PPEs: the protection googles used in operating rooms were for instance references by AGEPS as medical devices while similar devices were also referenced as PPE in the catalogue of several manufacturers and subjected to the Ministry of Labor regulations. Furthermore, at the beginning of the crisis, several large-scale initiatives arised to promote the production of PPEs (mostly head shields) by networks of makers – some of these initiatives were academic and clearly non-profit[29], like 3D4Care that we previously mentioned, while others were grieved by personal conflicts of interest and mostly designed for self-promotion[30]. In all cases, PPE regulations were mostly ignored until the end of April 2020, even though networks such as 3D4Care spontaneously established professional quality control and disinfection procedures. 3D COVID, as well as the numerous networks of makers, were thus in need of specific instructions on the applications of specific COVID19-adapted production norms for PPE, and even more, for medical devices.

29 3D4Care, an academic initiative for promoting the production of face shields by networks of makers in the Paris region, with strict quality control and disinfection protocols: http://www.3d4care.org/

30 COVID3D, a personal network managed by an independent blogger, mostly focused on self-promotion https://www.covid3d.fr/

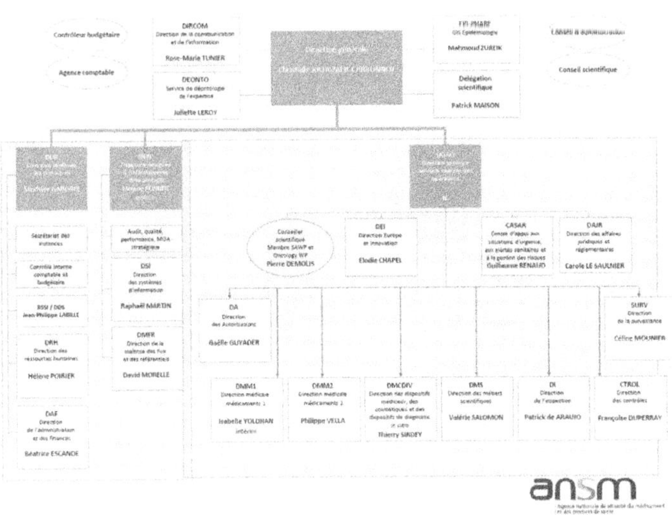

25.

Fig. 25. ANSM hierarchy[1].

1 Adapted from : https://archiveansm.integra.fr/L-ANSM/Organisation/L-organisation-interne/(offset)/0

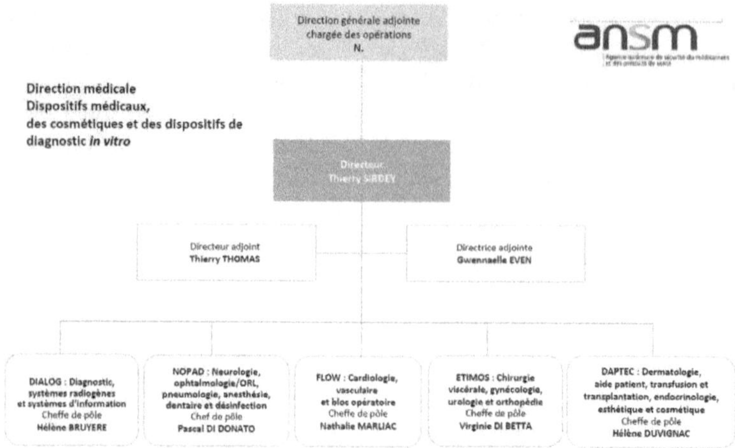

26.

Fig. 26. Hierarchy of the ANSM division dedicated to medical devices[31].

An EU commission recommendation (2020/403) released the 13th of March 2020 established the specific conditions for producing both medical devices and PPEs during the pandemic,[32] by considering both regulations 2016/425 and 2017/745. This recommendation stated the following: 'Where market surveillance authorities find that PPE or medical devices ensure an adequate level of health and safety in accordance with the essential requirements laid down in Regulation (EU) 2016/425[33] or the requirements of Directive 93/42/EEC or Regulation (EU) 2017/745, even though the conformity assessment procedures, including the affixing of CE marking have not been fully finalised according to the harmonised rules, they may authorise the making available of these products on the Union market for a limited period of time and while the necessary procedures are being carried out'. The market surveillance authorities mentioned in this recommendation were, in our case, ANSM at the national level and AGEPS at AP-HP level. Following the 2020/403 recommendation, several official documents were released in France to transpose locally these validation conditions for PPEs (23th, 30th April 2020)[34,35], and for medical devices (10th of April 2020)[36].

The regulatory bases were thus established as early as April 2020 to expect a resolution of the specific issues related to the production of medical devices by 3D COVID.

31 Adapted from : https://archiveansm.integra.fr/L-ANSM/Organisation/L-organisation-interne/(offset)/0
32 Commission recommendation (EU) 2020/403 of 13 March 2020 on conformity assessment and market surveillance procedures within the context of the COVID-19 threat: https://eur-lex.europa.eu/legal-content/eng/TXT/PDF/?uri=CELEX:32020H0403&from=EN
33 Regulation (EU) 2016/425 of the European Parliament and of the Council of 9 March 2016 on personal protective equipment: https://eur-lex.europa.eu/legal-content/EN/TXT/?uri=CELEX:32016R0425

34 See Supplementary Material 11.2
35 See Supplementary Material 11.3
36 https://ansm.sante.fr/var/ansm_site/storage/original/application/5815bdac1a0df00eb1d08ba1a0e459fa.pdf and Supplementary Material 11.4

Interactions between 3D COVID and AGEPS started at the end of March 2020, based on regular exchanges with the head of sales. Both the core members of 3D COVID and AGEPS were unaware at this time of the regulatory efforts at the EU level. The initial unformal agreement with AGEPS was that 3D COVID would supervise the clinical assessment of the various devices produced by the platform with clinicians from AP-HP, and have the final versions of the prototypes approved (or not) by pharmacists at AGEPS – the process was initially planned to take place within 48 hours. 3D COVID also had the duty to centralize all the demands arising from AP-HP health professionals, as, at this point of the crisis, AGEPS was overflown by the screening for alternative markets for the various devices that were progressively missing. The issue of final ANSM assessment had not been discussed at this time.

The massive media coverage of the 3D COVID initiative, with clear and premature mentions of the involvement of the platform in medical device production led AGEPS to organize a formal control of our premises by two pharmacists the 10th of April 2020, in order to accelerate the settlement of a coordination protocol. It came out from this visit that AGEPS had no precise knowledge of 3D printing technologies but was willing to build a proper regulated workflow that would eventually lead to authorizations for placement on the market from ANSM.

In parallel, in collaboration with the Central Pharmacy of Hôpital Cochin and more specifically its sterilization platform, production lines, disinfection and sterilization protocols had been settled (see 3.9 and 3.10). These spontaneous initiatives from our side helped in showing AGEPS pharmacists that 3D COVID was proactive in complying with proper production processes. The on-site AGEPS visit was mostly uneventful and our team waited for further instruction from regulatory bodies while continuing design and production at a fast pace. It was agreed that AGEPS would quickly send to the team a set of formal assessment forms for the various medical devices that were being developed at this time (connectors, ventilation masks), in order to standardize their clinical validation. Assessment documents for ventilation masks were send to the team the 16th of April.

Meanwhile, a set of connectors for ventilators produced by 3D COVID was being tested in vitro at Pitié-Salpêtrière Hospital, the largest of AP-HP hospitals, under the supervision of AGEPS. Our team did not have accessed formal AGEPS assessment forms for this category of device. Initial tests at Pitié-Salpêtrière showed that connectors printed using FDM single layer settings had significant leaks. These disappointing results led to the modification of the printing parameters (thicker layers, use of coating – a specific post-treatment method) and to the production of other sets of connectors using polyjet printers expected to leak less. The 3D COVID core team believed that this was a good example of the importance of the accelerated exchanges between engineers and clinicians, leading to the fast improvement of the initial designs. But this opinion was not shared by AGEPS.

The initial disappointing tests performed on our connectors were in fact perceived very negatively by AGEPS: the 17th of April 2020, one of the pharmacists of this institution sent an alarming email to prominent members of AP-HP – without warning 3D COVID core members – to denounce the lack of professionalism of the 3D COVID initiative (based only on the failure of the initial testing of the connectors), and insisted on poor relevance of 3D printing, which was not, according to AGEPS, adapted to the production of medical devices in general. AGEPS members also accused BONE 3D of dealing with several AP-HP hospitals and offering them private contracts, thus betraying the initial commitments of the 3D COVID initiative to provide all their productions for free to public institutions. This email was in contradiction with the efforts of many members from AGEPS to work on validation procedures with 3D COVID but was nevertheless a demonstration of the global lack of understanding of several AGEPS decision makers regarding the core of the 3D COVID initiative. It was also a brilliant example of administrative violence.

After this unfortunate event, AGEPS top management commissioned two pharmacists from OMEDIT IDF (Observatoire des Médicaments, des Dispositifs médicaux et de l'Innovation Thérapeutique d'Île-de-France[37]) to work on the regulatory interactions between 3D COVID and AGEPS. OMEDIT was a private regional organization, fully state-owned, that offered counseling services on drugs and medical devices, mostly to regional health agencies (Agences Régionales de Santé, ARS).

The 18th of April 2020, the two core members of 3D COVID offered an accelerated training on the principles of 3D printing to the two OMEDIT pharmacists, who had expertise on the regulations of drug production but no specific knowledge of additive manufacturing or medical devices production. The next day, the two OMEDIT members were officially in charge of 3D printing at AGEPS with the creation of a 3D printing working group within this institution that had the duty to monitor the collaboration with 3D COVID.

More precisely, the two main missions of the two OMDEIT pharmacists, as formalized by AGEPS top management the 24th of April 2020, were to (1) write a procedure for the use of 3D printing during the COVID19 crisis (due April 24th) and (2) build the framework for submitting 3D printed medical devices to ANSM in order to obtain authorizations for placement on the market (due May 4th)[38]. During all this time, we could not progress in assessing the medical devices we were designing daily as the team was waiting for instructions from AGEPS on the procedure to apply for such assessment.

The immediate result of the work of OMEDIT at AGEPS was the release of a protocol, on the 24th of April, detailing the steps that could eventually lead to the production of medical devices, strongly inspired by the recent recom-

37 A state-owned agency commissioned by AGEPS to work on the interactions with 3D COVID regarding reglementary questions: OMEDIT http://www.omedit-idf.fr

38 Supplementary material 12.4

mendations of ANSM on 3D printing during the COVID19 crisis (see above)[39]. In brief, the protocol established unilaterally by AGEPS involved the seven following steps.

→ Analysis of needs in specific medical devices
1. Directly by AGEPS
2. By health professionals from one of the AP-HP hospitals, assisted by their local central pharmacist
The conditions for a need to be eligible were (1) total shortage, (2) absence of any potential alternative market and (3) vital necessity of the device in the context of the sanitary crisis.

→ Prototype request by AGEPS to 3D COVID, including a list of the mandatory characteristics for device that had to be reproduced (for instance: transparency, weight, thickness)

→ Feasibility study by 3D COVID in terms of, among others, chemical properties, biocompatibility, or physical properties, without the right to produce prototypes before authorization by AGEPS.

→ Statement of AGEPS on the opportunity to produce a prototype based on the feasibility report from 3D COVID.

→ Production of a prototype by 3D COVID that was directly transmitted to AGEPS without possibility to interact with AP-HP medical professionals.

→ Evaluation of the prototype by AGEPS based on various tests in relevant AP-HP units, and collection of relevant reports, without interaction with the 3D COVID team.

→ Decision on the opportunity to launch production taken directly by the head of AGEPS.

This procedure was a long-awaited formalization of the interactions between 3D COVID and AGEPS based on the ANSM recommendations mentioned above. Nevertheless, it was grieved by serious flaws that were immediately reported to the head of AGEPS by the 3D COVID core team. The two most critical issues were:

→ The impossibility for 3D COVID to freely work on research and development of new devices without an initial formal visa of AGEPS – that is the impossibility to anticipate potential shortage by starting to investigate tricky issues in additive manufacturing in collaboration with various universities, engineering schools and AP-HP health professionals,

→ The end of the fast and productive direct interactions between AP-HP health professionals and 3D COVID engineers during the prototyping phase – this constituted the core of the initiative and was placed under the total control of pharmacists by the AGEPS protocol.
In brief, the protocol proposed by AGEPS showed a total misunderstanding on what we considered as the core principles of fast prototyping.

After these recommendations, all medical device projects were paused, and the team expected clear instruc-

39 Supplementary material 11.6

tions from AGEPS on which medical devices should still be developed with which level of priority. From this point, only contradictory information was released by this institution:

→ the 24th of April, the team was asked to work on a set of connectors for ventilators and on ventilation masks,

→ the 28th of April, the work on connectors was strongly discouraged by a pharmacist from AGEPS,

→ the 4th of May, a prototype of ventilation mask, developed as requested by AGEPS, that is without any interaction of 3D COVID with AP-HP clinical teams, was assessed by a large intensive care unit at Hôpital Européen Georges Pompidou (AP-HP) but could not be properly tested as the assessing team was not aware of the specificities of FDM 3D printed objects in terms of transparency and did not have the appropriate connectors – as a result, as no interaction between 3D COVID and the assessing team was permitted by AGEPS, the testing of the ventilation mask was a fiasco,

→ the 5th of May, the connectors were requested again by AGEPS but no mention of numbers and types were provided,
→ the 20th of May, the connectors were not requested anymore but ventilation masks were ordered again to the 3D COVID team without precise feedback provided on the previously failed tests on the 4th of May.

Of note, the episode with the ventilation mask and the issue of its transparency was repeatedly used by AGEPS administration in the following months as an illustration of two supposedly severe dysfunctions within our team: (1) our little awareness of the specific characteristics of medical devices[40] and (2) the deliberate lack of interactions between our team and AP-HP health professionals.

These complications led the 3D COVID team to stop working on medical device design and production. The team requested numerous times to AGEPS to reconsider the protocol and discuss it with the core members, but these requests were not considered. Furthermore, AGEPS progressively stopped interacting with the medical coordinator and limited its work exchanges with BONE 3D members, using the argument that the medical coordinator did not have an official administrative appointment at the head of the 3D platform. As a result, COVID 3D fully focused on protection material and various maintenance objects.

Nevertheless, under the incentive of AP-HP management, 3D COVID continued interacting with AGEPS in order to obtain a placement authorization for at least one device, as a proof of concept. The chosen device was a suture holder for cardio-thoracic surgery. The contents of the files prepared for ANSM submission by 3D COVID consisted in 3 core documents and 18 supplementary files:

1. A formal request for an exceptional authorization for placement on the

40 Regarding this transparency issue, Belgium approved an 3D printed non-transparent ventilation mask during the first wave: https://www.materialise.com/en/blog/3d-printed-peep-mask-alleviate-ventilator-shortage

market, with the following sections
→ conception of the device
→ software for design, printing and follow-up
→ manufacturing - printers, 3D model of the device, techniques used, disinfection and sterilization
→ maintenance of the process
→ specificities of the device
→ precise description
→ disinfection and sterilization
→ evaluation of the device properties
→ plan for continuous improvement

2. A clinical evaluation form

3. A physical evaluation form

4. And a total of 18 supplementary documents
→ map of the localization of the printers on site
→ register of all machines and consumables used since the launch of the initiative
→ follow-up of the activity of the platform since the launch of the initiative
→ mechanical properties and security documents for ABS (one set for each color)
→mechanical properties and security documents for silicon one set for each type)
→ CE marking documents of the silicon
→ Security documents on chemicals used for post-treatment of ABS
→ 3D geometric assessment of shape conservation after disinfection and sterilization
→ Device-specific risk analysis
→ Device-specific technical document
→ Device-specific assembly notes and instruction.

Here again the interactions were complex: after a phase of collaboration between OMEDIT pharmacist and engineers at 3D COVID, leading to the production of the files listed above, the files were retained by AGEPS members, who continued working on the project independently without interactions with 3D COVID members. AGEPS then submitted the files to ANSM without willing to share their final version. Despite numerous emails by the 3D COVID core team to the AGEPS head, no answers were provided on the work achieved on the files, or on the responses of ANSM. The formal arguments provided by AGEPS for justifying this attitude were that this phase of the project was too technical for medical doctors and should be fully managed by pharmacists and regulatory specialists. In this context, it was decided that our team was not entitled to be informed of the potential feedback of ANSM on the submission of our project.

The 12th of June, a virtual meeting organized by AGEPS and bringing together most people involved in the 3D COVID initiative led to the conclusion that a limited list of medical devices had to be submitted to ANSM for assessment within short delays, in order to prove that our initiative was solid and well-managed.
For this, AP-HP management asked AGEPS to transfer the answer of ANSM on the submission of the suture holder application to the 3D COVID team, in order to start working on potential issues raised by ANSM and tackle them. The queries of ANSM were finally sent to 3D COVID the 8th of July, a few minutes before another meeting organized by AGEPS and du-

ring which it was unanimously stated that the current management of the 3D COVID team was not competent enough to embrace the production of medical devices. Our team could only acknowledge these conclusions and insisted on the fact that internal regulatory competence, with a pharmacist dedicated to production on site, was crucial in order to finally solve our regulatory issues.

More precisely, the content of the answer of ANSM released by AGEPS on the 8th of July (and which had been sent to AGEPS by ANSM a month prior) was that the current setting of the 3D COVID platform was per se not compatible with the production of any type of medical device, due to the production and post-treatment conditions (and notably the use of a kitchen for post-treatment). This statement had been pronounced by ANSM without having performed any on-site visits, and only based on the indirect reports of AGEPS. Clearly, better communication between parties (3D COVID, AGEPS and ANSM) would have left considerable space for improvement of our production chain and would have avoided this failure in the production of medical devices.

In brief, our attempts to produce medical devices in a crisis context failed, with shared responsibilities from all parties involved. It took 3 full months to obtain clear feedback from the administration that our platform would never be allowed to produce any kind of medical device (Figure 27).

The practical conclusion of this section is that an internal regulatory specialist, located on site, is a key person when intending to produce medical devices in a crisis context. Of note, in 2022, a report assessing leakage in the ventilation fitting produced by 3D COVID demonstrated that FDM technology with coating, as well as polyjet technology, both allow obtaining satisfactory devices regarding leaks[41].

41 Khonsari RH, Oranger M, François PM, Mendoza-Ruiz A, Leroux K, Boussaid G, Prieur D, Hodge JP, Belle A, Midler V, Morelot-Panzini C, Patout M, Gonzalez-Bermejo J. Quality versus emergency: How good were ventilation fittings produced by additive manufacturing to address shortages during the COVID19 pandemic? PLoS One 2022;17:e0263808.

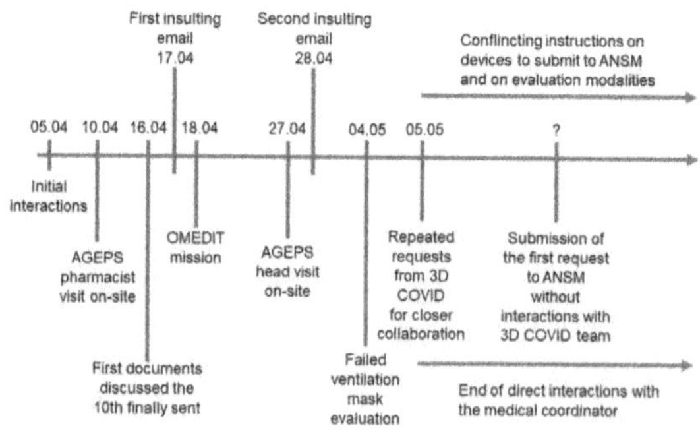

27.

27. Timeline of the interactions of 3D COVID with AGEPS showing the difficulties to establish a reglementary framework for 3D printing in a large state institution.

3.15 Running the 3D Farm: raw materials and production numbers

Everyday production was managed by the BONE 3D team, who interacted with CADVISION for placing orders of missing raw materials and technical issues with the printers. All orders were processed by the head of IT sales and finally validated by the 3D COVID core team (Table 7).

This contract ran until the 31st of December 2020 and no anticipation measures could be obtained from AP-HP so that all new projects were stopped at this date. BONE 3D agreed to pursue ongoing developments, but AP-HP did not clarify the financial plan for 2021 until long-term decisions were taken on how to proceed with the 'Phase 2' of the project (see below).

Table 7. Successive amounts billed by BONE 3D to AP-HP. For consumables, orders were placed by BONE 3D to CADVision and then billed at the same exact price to AP-HP. Tax rate was 20%. Prices in euros.

Service	Price / months before tax	April (30.04.20)	May (26.05.2020)	June (29.06.20)	July (27.07.20)	August / September / October 27.10.20	November (27.1100)	Total
Coordination of the platform	5000	+	+	+	+	+ (x3)	+	40000
Design	15000	+	+	+	+	+ (x3)	+	120000
Management of printing	15000	+	+	+	+	+ (x3)	+	120000
Post-processing	33000	+	+	+	+	+ (x3)	+	264000
Dispatching	6000	+	+	+	+	+ (x3)	+	48000
Maintenance	6000	+	+	+	+	-	+	48000
Training	800	+	-	-	-	-	-	800
Hardware	-	3311 (computer) 4632 (furniture)	-	-	-	-	-	7943
Subtotal before tax	-	89543	80000	80000	80000	24000	80000	649543
Subtotal after tax	-	107451.6	96000	96000	96000	288000	96000	779451.6
Raw materials before tax	-	43435	46938	51180.70	5970	-	-	147523.77
Raw materials after tax	-	52122	56325.60	61416.92	7164	-	-	177028.52
Total after tax	-	159573.5	152325.60	157416.92	103164	288000	96000	956480.02

7.

Machine reference	Machine type	Hours	Minutes
A1	F120	530	06
A2	F120	404	02
A3	F120	526	23
A4	F120	451	20
A5	F120	421	01
A6	F120	414	18
A7	F120	159	15
A8	F120	311	53
A9	F120	303	45
A10	F120	270	29
B1	F120	433	49
B2	F120	426	36
B3	F120	400	21
B4	F120	443	48
B5	F120	400	20
B6	F120	380	55
B7	F120	297	05
C1	F120	378	33
C2	F120	373	38
C3	F120	NA	NA
C4	F120	394	50
C5	F120	388	37
C6	F120	319	01
C7	F120	346	08
D1	F370	NA	NA
D2	F370	291	17
D3	F370	210	31
D4	F170	316	55
D5	F170	249	53
D6	F170	249	39
D7	F170	263	07
D8	F170	210	17
D9	F170	247	16
D10	F170	220	48
D11	F170	188	08
D12	F170	214	53
D13	F170	173	43
D14	F120	190	30
E1	F120	282	52
E2	F120	235	56
F1	F170	240	46
F2	F120	145	35
F3	F120	184	32
F4	F120	190	20
F5	F120	237	54
G1	F120	421	12
G2	F120	396	48
G3	F120	412	09
G4	F120	391	58
G5	F120	383	05
G6	F120	397	15
H1	F120	333	20
H2	F120	386	31
H3	F120	432	49
H4	F120	422	06
H5	F120	401	42
H6	F120	427	34
I1	F120	393	10
I2	F120	379	18
I3	F120	423	06

8.

Table 8. Hourly activity per machine on the 6th of June 2020.

The total amount spent on the platform for manpower and raw materials after 8 full months of work was 956480.02 euros with tax, which corresponds to a monthly rate of 119560 euros for all 39 AP-HP hospitals, and thus fees a bit over 3000 euros per month per hospital. This contract with BONE 3D ran until the 31st of December 2020.

The total working time of each machine was registered at the beginning of June and showed variable values, with higher values for the F120 machines, the ones that were mostly used for production (Table 8). A similar discrepancy between the uses of the different F123 models was also seen when plotting the number of devices produced per machine (Figures 28-30).

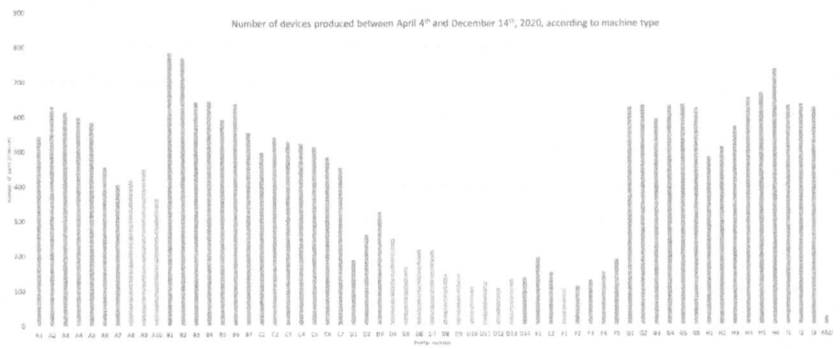

28.

Fig. 28. Number of devices produced per machine until December 14th, 2020. The most active machines were F120, intended for mass production.

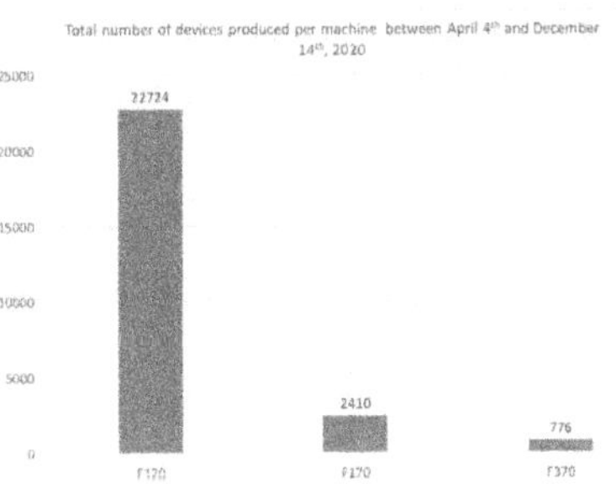

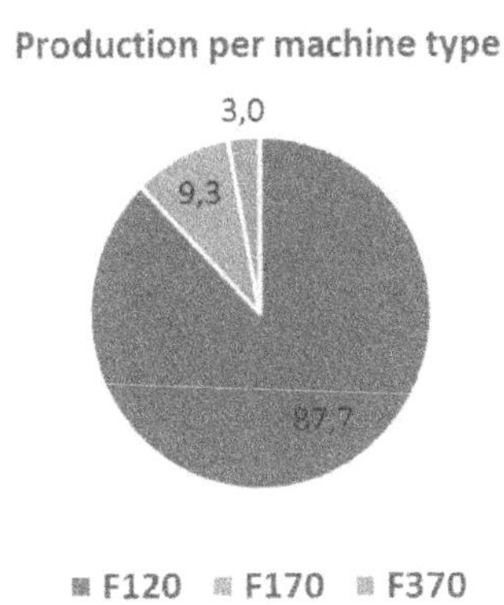

29.

Fig. 29. Production according to machine type until December 14th 2020.

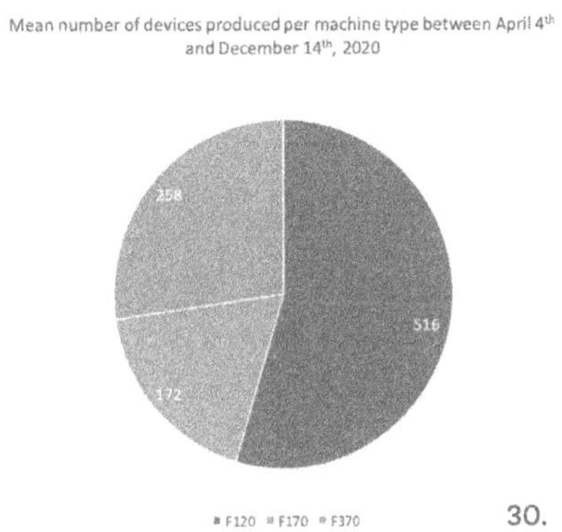

30.

Fig. 30. Average number of devices produced per machine until December 14th: F120 were used for larger scale production but F170 and F370 also produced significant amounts of devices.

Interestingly, mostly from April to June, the total number of devices produced per month decreased due to the end of the epidemic peak, but the type of devices produced changed, with a switch from protection devices to maintenance devices until the end of 2020. A moderate rise in protection devices was nevertheless associated with the second pandemic peak (Figures 31 & 32).

In brief, the production was initially focused on protection devices, for which important stocks were made during the early summer (thus leading to low production numbers in September and October). A clear diversification of the production, mostly after the summer, witnessed the integration of the platform within the AP-HP medical and academic ecosystem. Also, within Hôpital Cochin, which acted as a proof-of-concept academic hospital, data show that very diverse units interacted with 3D COVID, including medical departments, paramedics, administration, and technical staff.

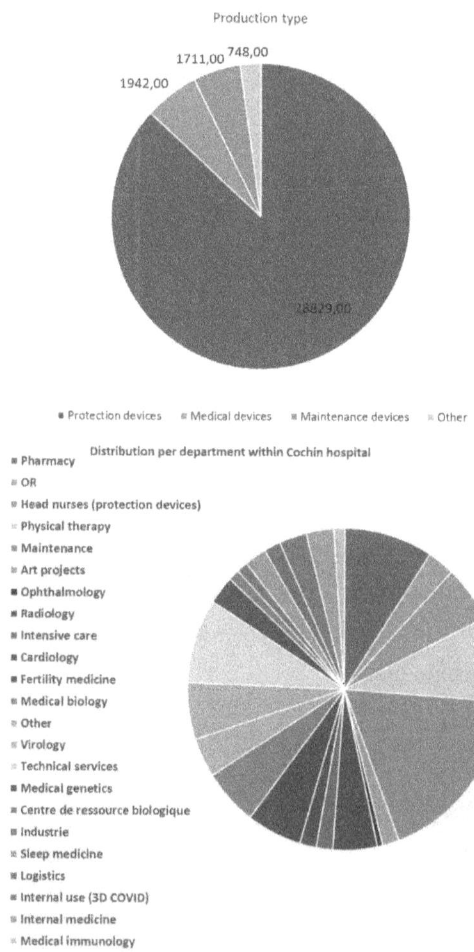

31.

Fig. 31. (upper chart) Production type until December 14th: strong preponderance of protection devices. (lower chart) Distribution of devices per department within Hôpital Cochin: most units of this large academic hospital worked with our team.

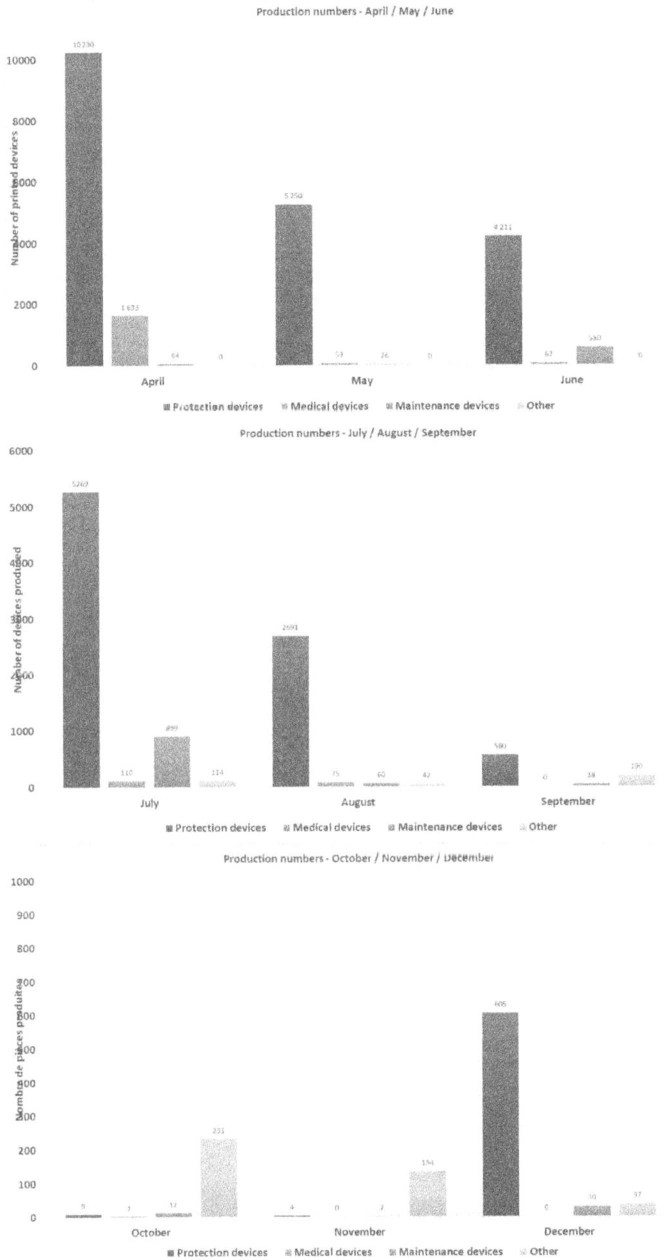

32.

Fig. 32. Progressive decrease of protection device production after the first pandemic peak and rise of maintenance devices & other designs (academic for instance). The production of medical devices was quickly stopped, except for a very limited amount of prototypes, due to ongoing regulatory issues.

3.16 Major technical problems: issues and solutions

Given the number of machines, the printing platform faced numerous technical issues. The technical issues were solved based on internal actions by the BONE 3D technical team and by CADVISION experts when required, for instance when the motherboard of the machines had failures. We recorded the occurrence of technical issues over time and noticed a global decrease, most probably related to the decrease in production (Figure 33).

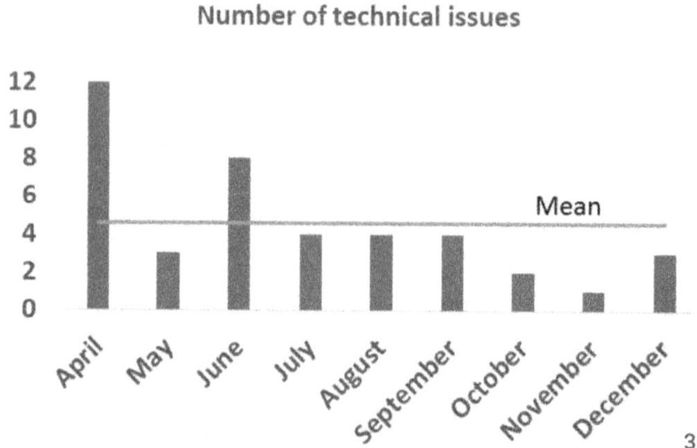

33.

Fig. 33. Number of technical issues over time. Most common issues were printing head problems, motor overcurrent and heater issues. The mean number per month from April to mid-December is low (approx. 4/month).

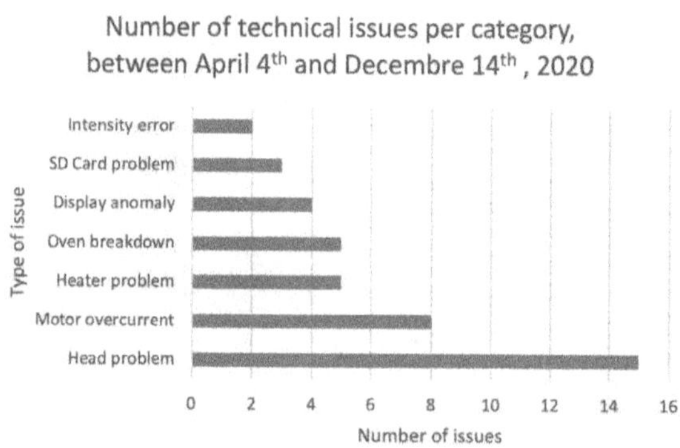

34.

Fig. 34. Distribution of technical issues per type. Most issues affected F120 printers, which were also the most active ones. All figures tended to show, expectedly, that the occurrence of technical issues was directly related to the intensity of use of the machines.

Number of problems per printer type, between July 16th and December 14th, 2020

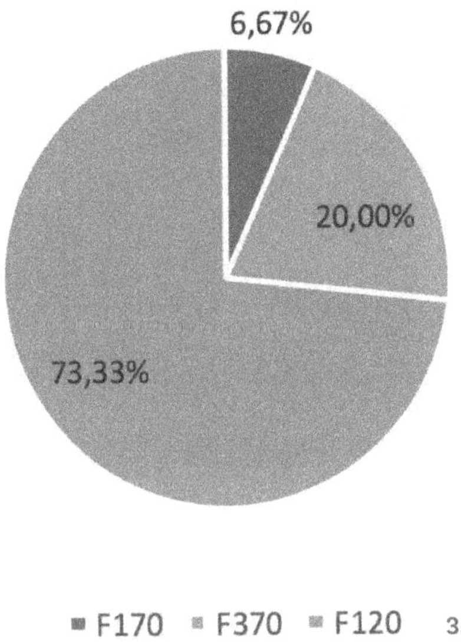

35.

Fig. 35. Distribution of technical issues per machine type: F120, the most active machines, were also the ones mostly subjected to technical issues.

In conclusion, our experience showed that FDM machines from the F123 Stratasys series had frequent technical issues but that these issues could be dealt with internally in most cases (Figure 33-35).

3.17 Recycling and sustainabilty

Due to active prototyping, 3D COVID produced a significant amount of unused devices. Furthermore, several (>5) unexpected power supply cuts also led to production losses.

As printed ABS remains pure plastics, we discussed the possibility to use these unused or partially printed devices to manufacture fresh raw materials. Stratasys did not easily allow this we got in touch with initiatives that could harvest the unusable ABS from 3D COVID and dispatch it to various centers who had the facilities to process it. Via Precious Plastics[42], we got in touch with Ateliers Samji[43] in Paris but we could not finalize the collection of the plastic waste. Internal recycling facilities will be major elements in the final setting of the platform (« Phase 2 », see below), as the production of unused devices is inherent to the research and development missions of our platform.

3.18 Everyday life at the emergency platform: basic needs

Every day, AP-HP provided 10 portions of food lunch to the COVID 3D team (Figure 36), including during weekends. At the beginning of the initiative, food was also delivered in the evening but after 10 days we indicated to the logistic services of AP-HP that lunch was sufficient.

Furthermore, for 5 weeks, two charity initiatives offered good quality products to 3D COVID members:

→ an operational director at Franprix, groupe Casino, who organized the delivery of fresh food to the team (Figure 37),
→ Lenôtre, a elite grocer owned by

42 https://preciousplastic.com/
43 https://www.facebook.com/AtelierSamji/

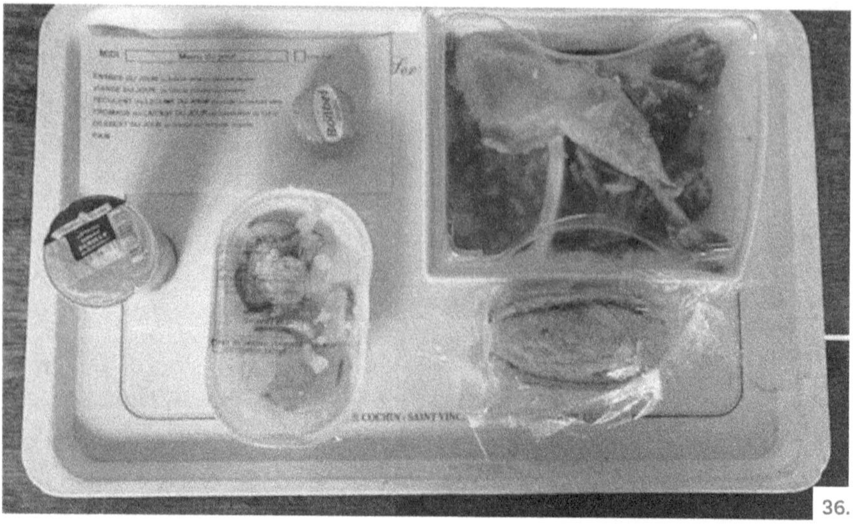

36.

Fig. 36. Food provided daily by AP-HP.

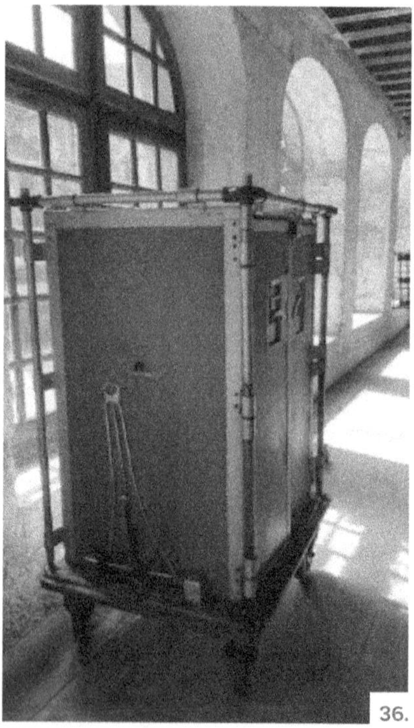

36.

Sodexo, the company providing the basic AP-HP food (Figure 36) delivered five portions of high-quality lunch.

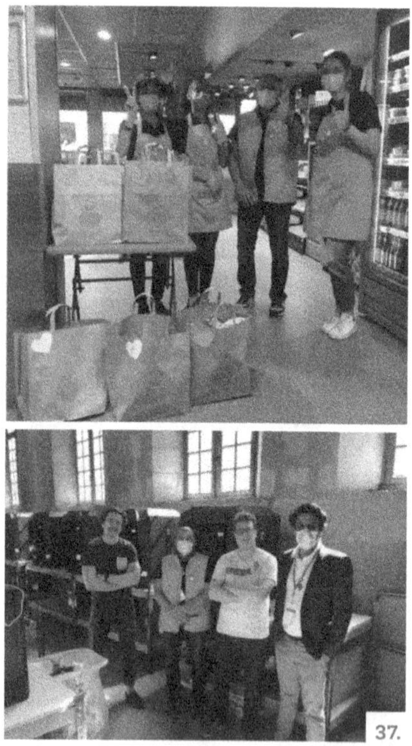

37.

Fig. 37. The Franprix team delivering food on Fridays to 3D COVID for 5 consecutive weeks.

Other charitable initiatives also benefited to the 3D COVID team:
La Roche Posay delivered numerous samples of moisturizers on the 7th of April 2020, which were used by the team in a context of constant application of hydro-alcoholic gel (Figure 38).

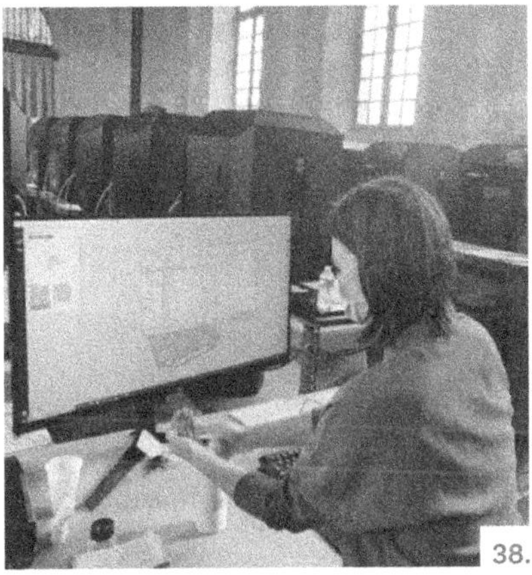

38.

Fig. 38. 3D COVID member moisturizing hands with cream offered by La Roche Posay.

3.19 Distribution: AP-HP networks and internal solutions

In the initial discussions with the administration, logistics was supposed to be a duty of AP-HP. After several attempts of organizing the dispatch of the production with the sales department, the 3D COVID team decided to use its internal workforce to perform the deliveries. A dedicated car - Renault Kangoo (Figure 39) was provided by the logistics services of Hôpital Cochin and was extensively used to cover the territory of the Greater Paris region. Specific authorizations were provided by the 3D COVID core team to allow the staff to circulate during the confinement period (Figure 40).

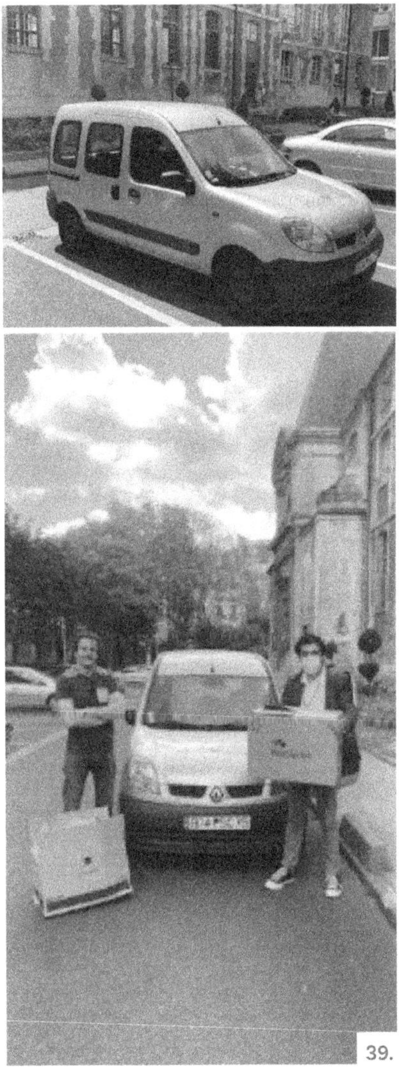

39.

Fig. 39. A Kangoo provided to 3D COVID by Hôpital Cochin and used for delivery. Delivering door handles to the elementary schools of the 5th district in Paris.

Besides direct deliveries using the Kangoo car, two courier services were used by 3D COVID team:

→ Coursier.fr[44] provided one free courier delivery a day to the 3D COVID team over a period of 6 weeks, thanks to the support of its co-founder and chief operating officer,

→ Stuart[45] was used when needed without specific financial arrangement, the fees of the deliveries being paid personally by members of the team or by BONE 3D.

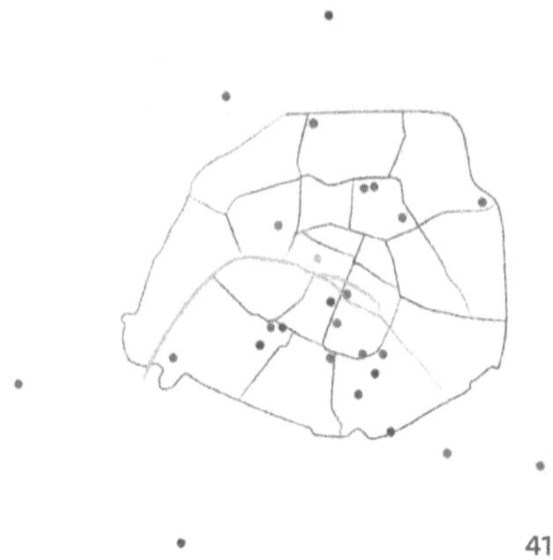

41.

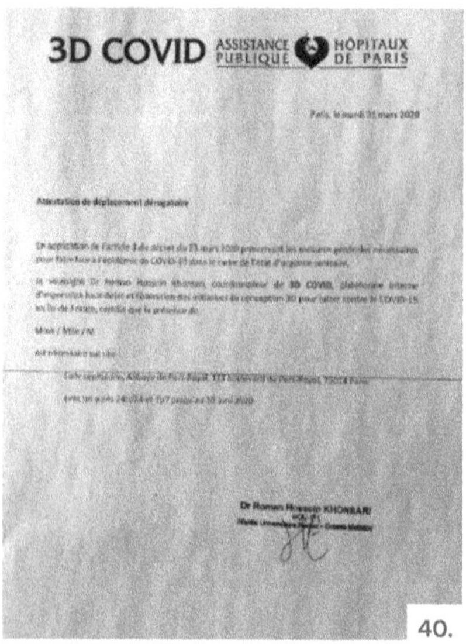
3D COVID ASSISTANCE PUBLIQUE HÔPITAUX DE PARIS

40.

Fig. 40. Circulation authorisation delivered to 3D COVID staff during confinement.

Fig. 41. Area covered by 3D COVID projects: most AP-HP hospitals, public institutions, and cultural institutions. Blue dots: hospitals; dark grey dots: public institutions (schools, city halls); and: academic centers; black dot: headquarters of BONE 3D; light grey dot: Louvre museum.

3.20 Intellectual property and valorization

It is noteworthy that AP-HP is an institution which does not solely takes care of hundreds of thousands of patients every year. It is also a major French center for education, research and professional training in the field of medicine, which in turn has created over decades major innovations and clinical and industrial patents. Academic health professionals working at AP-HP are all co-employed by this institution and by one of the medical universities of the Greater Paris region. The 3D COVID project takes therefore part in this history of innovations, as a project launched by AP-HP and Université de Paris, the largest European medical university by number of students.

Everything that is produced in the context of this project belongs to AP-HP. Intellectual property comes naturally either from contractual bounds

44 https://www.coursier.fr/corporate
45 https://stuart.com/fr

(for instance, BONE 3D is a AP-HP subcontractor) or from the basic fact that 3D COVID is a project supported by the AP-HP top management, and the AP-HP/DEFIP (Finance, Investment and Patrimony).
AP-HP seems to see value on the specific validation process and the definition of the role of AGEPS rather than on the designs themselves.

As a result, open-source designs incoming from the community of makers (and potentially redesigned by BONE 3D), once validated by the team, are bound to be broadcasted and used where there is a need.

In this context, the founder and medical coordinator of the project, being an employee of AP-HP, has no property on the designs or on the skills acquired during this experience. All the potential benefits of this initiative will go solely to public institutions. For instance, the international extension of the platform, based – for its medical component – on the experience of the core 3D COVID team, will most probably create substantial financial benefits that will go to the subcontractors (BONE 3D, CADVISION for instance), and to AP-HP, without involvement of the health professionals that carry the practical skills marketed by AP-HP (see chapter 4). 3D COVID is the first emergency large-scale 3D printing medical platform ever settled within a hospital. Based on this innovative aspect of the project, AP-HP is has been seeking for the last 2 years to define how the institution should benefit from the numerous projects in which BONE 3D has been involved worldwide since the initiative was launched.

4. International expansion: reproducing the Paris model

3D COVID had an international audience thanks to an efficient communication plan and wide media coverage. Here we outline the export perspectives of the expertise of the team.

BONE 3D and AP-HP International worked together, under the supervision of OTTPI, to build a partnership in order to help settling 3D printing factories in hospitals all over the globe. This partnership is an interesting potential source of valorization. For instance, the French annual market for hospital 3D printing platforms was estimated at 20 M€ in 2020. This market worldwide was estimated at 1,3Md€, also in 2020.

Initially, the most structured international expansion project is 3D Print for Africa, a private initiative launched by Elisabeth Moreno[1], including prominent intellectual personalities from various West-African French-speaking countries. This project was structured along consecutive phases (Figure 41):

7.1.Settling a 3D farm in Paris in order to produce protection devices for African countries, until mid-2021,

7.2. Dispatch the printers of the Paris farm between 5 large African cities, Kinshasa (Democratic Republic of the Congo) being the first chosen site,

7.3. Create a network of academic medical 3D printing centers in close association with local medical and engineering schools,

7.4.Build long-term relationships with the Paris AP-HP / Université de Paris platform for training African 3D printing specialists

The engineering partner of this project was BONE 3D and the French medical expertise is provided by AP-HP International. Nevertheless, clear deals with AP-HP International could never be settled and the project was independently persued by BONE 3D.

Similar projects have been deployed in parallel, independently, by BONE 3D, for instance in La Réunion, without the direct involvement of AP-HP despite repeated attempts by BONE 3D to include AP-HP into these secondary initiatives. The bases of the intellectual property of AP-HP in the process have not been defined yet, even though platforms are being installed in several sites by our industrial partner, based on the experience gained during the COVID19 crisis in Paris within AP-HP premises.

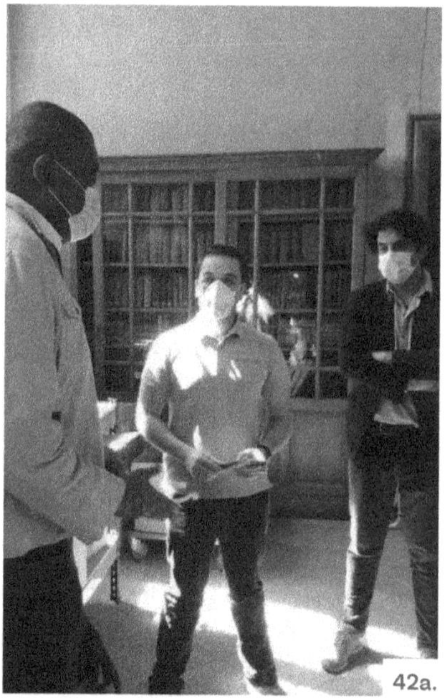

42a.

Fig. 42. (a) Visit of the chief information officer of the France Telecom Orange Group in DRC and special advisor to the president, at the AP-HP 3D platform, to discuss the 3D Print for Africa project with the 3D COVID core team.

1 Elisabeth Moreno serves as Minister Delegate for Gender Equality, Diversity and Equal Opportunities at the Prime Minister's Office in the government of Prime Minister Jean Castex since 2020. She was vice-president and managing director for Hewlett-Packard in South Africa from 2019 until 2020 and president of Lenovo France from 2017 until 2019.

Notably, a project of installing a platform in Yerevan, Armenia, is currently being developed with a team of physical therapists, in order to manufactures prostheses for the 2nd Artsakh war victims. This conflict raged between Armenia and Azerbaijan from September to November 2020. On the Armenian side, the project is coordinated by a physical therapist and a 3D designer. In all these international projects, the constant issue remains the qualification of the role of AP-HP and the nature of the valorization project. Two years of exchanges after the initial launch of the project have not led to clear solutions.

The 'Phase 2' of the project will most probably be ultimately associated with an expertise offer. The current French regulations do not allow a subsidiairy of AP-HP to work in France, so that the expertise offer will be targeted for an international audience, with prospects in Armenia and Ukraine to support war victims, mostly in the field of physical therapy.

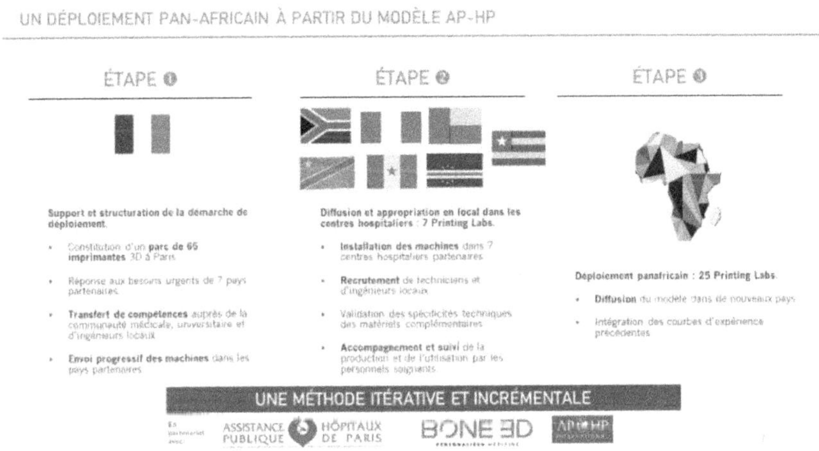

Fig. 42. (b) Organisation of the 3D Print for Africa initiative.

5. Strong points / weak points in brief: experience gained

3D COVID was a globally successful experience but several of its initial goals were not reached. Here, the strong and the weak points of this initiative are listed in order to provide basis for improved further experiences.

What is in our sense the core of our experience?

1. 3D COVID was the first emergency medical 3D printing platform ever developed within a hospital. We provide a unique proof of concept of a process that will be reproduced and improved in numerous locations.

2. The interaction between healthcare providers and engineers was the core of this initiative, via direct contacts and/or a dedicated website, with the aim of designing, prototyping, assessing and producing various devices in a record time in a context of sanitary crisis.

3. The process was relying on three key components: medical expertise, engineering skills and regulatory knowledge. Work within the platform was performed in collaboration with the intellectual property and technology transfer teams of our institution. This setup provided both the flexibility required in such emergency situations, and the guarantees of safety when working on medical material.

4. 3D COVID had a very positive public image in a context of severe crisis and provided a modern and pro-active image of AP-HP and Université de Paris.

What are the weaker aspects of our experience? And what are simple solutions to these issues?

1. Quality control and risk management were part of the initial concerns of the project but these aspects still require improvement as the platform was discarded at once as a medical device producer by ANSM.

2. Interactions between 3D COVID and regulatory bodies (AGEPS) were not fluid and let to considerable delays both in design and production. A pharmacist within the platform was a key missing aspect of our initiative. This pharmacist position should be supported by the regulatory bodies, with clear on-site delegation of power.

3. Interactions between 3D COVID and different departments and hospitals within the huge network of AP-HP were not optimal. Most of the devices were initially designed for hospitals with which 3D COVID members had personal links, or for Hôpital Cochin, which was located next to Port-Royal. Here, the missing link was an administrative person who would regularly reach clinical departments and screen for demands and would also supervise dispatching. Our network finally extended all over AP-HP hospitals, but better logistics would have favoured this process.

4. Another cause for the lack of diffusion of our initiative within the full range of AP-HP hospitals was the lack of internal communication. Despite impressive national and international media coverage, most AP-HP health professionals were not aware of 3D COVID outside Hôpital Cochin and the main South bank university hospitals. The situation improved after the summer thanks to word of mouth. Internal communication campaigns, supported by the administrative person in charge mentioned above, would have increased the scope of our initiative.

6. Next steps: 'Phase 2' platform and partnerships

Based on the 3D COVID experience, guiding principles for building an emergency sanitary 3D printing platform are defined, including technical, legal, administrative and financial aspects. The future of 3D printing at AP-HP, the largest hospital trust in Europe, is also drafted.

Besides support during the pandemic, a clear outcome of 3D COVID is the fact that AP-HP now owns a large set of professional 3D printers and has a unique experience in emergency 3D printing. The second phase of this project is currently being formalised. In September 2020, the AP-HP head designated one of the AP-HP Deputy Director Generals (who is also professor in intensive care medicine) as the main coordinator of the project for its future developments.

The two designated executive directors were a member of the 3D COVID core team and the newly appointed vice-director of AGEPS, with a health administrator background. Interestingly, the organisms that had actively slowed down the 3D platform project got appointed at this head after the crisis. Nevertheless, AGEPS is central in the placement of orders of medical devices within AP-HP and it was logical, although somehow unfortunate, that this structure would have a central role in the further phases of the initiative.

Besides these 3 people being at the head of the 3D platform project, an executive committee was created by AP-HP head management. A first meeting of the committee was held the 21st of September 2020.

The members of this committee were:
→ the head of AGEPS
→ the head of purchases of the Paris-Saclay hospital trust and promotor of a local 3D printing project at Hôpital du Kremlin-Bicêtre in the South of Paris, mostly focused on maintenance
→ the head of gynecology at Hôpital Beaujon and co-director of the Paris Nord iLumens[1] platform, an academic simulation platform hosting several 3D-printing projects
→ a pediatric intensive care physician at Hôpital Raymond Poincaré, familiar with 3D printing
→ a pediatric ENT surgeon working on several 3D printing projects with the 3D COVID core team
→ the head of IT sales at AP-HP
→ a pharmacologist, specialized in business models related to 3D printing
→ a hepatobiliary surgeon, head of an innovation center within Hôpital Paul Brousse (BOPA[2])
→ the head of the technology transfer and innovation office of AP-HP

1 http://ilumens.fr/
2 Chaire d'innovation Bloc Opératoire Augmenté (BOPA): www.chaire-bopa.fr

(OTT&PI)
→ the project leader at the central AP-HP data warehouse[3].

The following people were invited as external guests to the 21st of September meeting:
→ the CEO of Bone 3D and main contractor of 3D COVID,
→ the co-founder of Humaniteam and working as an advisor for the customer experience of the Kremlin-Bicêtre 3D platform (see above)
Two core members of the executive committee could not attend the first meeting:
→ the head of the AP-HP CME,
→ a pharmacologist from AGEPS.

The conclusions of this first strategic meeting were that the financial issues of Phase 2 needed further investigation and that a final location had to be determined (see 11.7). The medical director of 3D COVID took the engagement to submit a 5-year plan describing the principles of 3D printing at AP-HP and discuss this plan with AGEPS before circulating it to the strategic committee. This 5-year plan was sent within a week to the vice-director of AGEPS (see 11.8) but no answer had was obtained until mid-December, when it was decided that another meeting was necessary in January.

The principles of this 5-year plan were based on 5 initial facts:
1. AP-HP is the largest hospital trust in Europe,
2. AP-HP is a cluster of academic hospitals involved in patient care, teaching and research,
3. There is no current strategy regarding 3D printing at AP-HP level,
4. 3D printing is currently a routine technique for patient care, education and research,
5. The experience gained during the crisis provides the bases for a unique initiative at the trust level.

Furthermore, this 5-year plan considered that 3D printing in hospitals had 5 core missions both in design and production:
→ custom-made medical devices,
→ devices for healthcare professionals (not registered as medical devices)
→ small series of standard medical devices,
→ maintenance devices,
→ teaching and research material.

Considering these 5 initials facts and knowing these 5 missions, 6 guiding principles were defined.

Principle №1 – Central design and production unit

Bringing together engineers and healthcare professionals within a single location, with groups working on devices as diverse as maintenance objects and complex surgical instruments, will lead to fruitful collaborations and unexpected innovations. AP-HP is a huge trust with few creative interactions, suffering from a severe lack of attractivity due to heavy administrative constraints and non-competitive salaries. A central platform allowing innovation and contact with the latest technological innovations in the field of manufacturing will be a booster for innovation, but also open perspectives for financial valorization at

3 Entrepôt de Données de Santé de l'AP-HP: eds.aphp.fr

the institutional and individual levels. Furthermore, the complexity of regulations for the production of medical devices (RE 2017/745) is strongly in favor of a centralized production platform. Local initiatives will be encouraged but will benefit from the legal background and design task force of the central platform, with the initial choice of 5 satellite platforms within the network of AP-HP hospitals, with specific fields of excellence.

Principle №2 – Healthcare professional + Engineer duo

The core of the innovation process is a duo formed by a healthcare professional and an engineer. From the first steps of this process, three other major partners are required:
→ regulation specialist (for instance a pharmacist),
→ intellectual property specialist (OTT&PI),
→ logistics specialists (for instance a head nurse).

Principle №3 – Partnership with private companies

The current sharpest expertise in 3D printing is private. Partnerships with companies specialized in medical 3D design and 3D printing, preferably locally based, will provide access to the best engineers, and to competent people involved in the maintenance and management of the printers. These partnerships will lead to develop shared intellectual property and to the delegation of production if innovations developed within the platform become large-scale industrial products. The private partner will also have to duty to train internal AP-HP engineers in order to envision an internal transfer of competence within a range of 3-5 years.

An alternative to these private partnerships is hiring dedicated engineers (preferably two positions for a start), with then the need to adapt posts to offer competitive salaries. In any case, the platform will benefit from projects conjointly led with private partners.

Principe №4 – Fulfillment of the 5 basic missions of a healthcare platform

See above: centralization and interactions with competent industrial partners will allow fulfilling the 5 basic missions defined previously, including the trickiest one in terms of regulation – the production of standard medical devices in small series.

Principe №5 – Academic and social role

The role of the AP-HP 3D platform will include:
→ national and international training for 3D design and 3D printing for healthcare professionals and engineers, in collaboration with Université de Paris and École nationale supérieure des Arts et Métiers,
→ design and production of teaching material for healthcare professional and students (see chapter 8).

This mission will lead to the progressive transition of a technical platform towards a proper academic department, hosting medical students, post-graduate medical trainees and researchers.

Furthermore, the connection of the platform with its international secondary derivatices (such as 3D Print for Africa, see chapter 4) will lead to its evolution towards an international training center hosting guests from various 3D printing initiatives, starting from Kinshasa and Yerevan, and most probably Ukraine.

Finally, the co-localization of 3D printers, healthcare professionals and medical data will be of great interest for artists, that will be encouraged to develop projects involving AP-HP staff and patients (see chapter 9).

Principle №6 – Valorization

The AP-HP 3D platform is an innovation and valorization booster for the institution for at least three straightforward reasons:
→ the principle of an emergency platform is by itself an innovation and may lead to licenses for the various international developments, in collaboration with BONE 3D,
→ teaching offers will be developed for medical doctors, dentists, pharmacists, physical therapists and other categories of healthcare professionals with two focuses
→ teaching 3D printing by itself (design, production, regulation)
→ use of 3D printed products in teaching sessions (anatomical models, surgical simulators)
→ the devices developed on the platform will eventually lead to valorization, with the support of OTTPI.

In the memo sent to AGEPS, the 3D COVID core team furthermore argued in favor of the fact that printers should be kept in a single location. This location should be characterized by the following facts:
→ a central attractive place within Paris, inside a university hospital,
→ on ground floor, with a strong enough flooring to allow the potential installation of heaving production machines (such as titanium printers)
→ with the required characteristics in terms of ventilation and access to allow a free diversification of production methods (SLA, SLS, metal), on top of the adequate flooring
→ anticipation of the possibility to comply with the requirements to produre medical devices.

The 3D COVID core team evaluated the cost of adapting a standard office space to these standards at 200k€.
For extending the range of the production, two options can be considered:
→ Option 1 – selling the current machines (60 FDM machines) owned by AP-HP to a private company and loaning machines in order to benefit from flexibility in the choice of the technologies (SLA, SLS, SLM) and share the production with the private partner,
→ Option 2 – invest in machines in order to expand the current FDM platform: SLA : 15k€ ; SLS : 150k€ ; SLM : 350k€.

For managing the platform, the private partner will have to provide:
→ 4 full-time jobs for design, production and distribution (Principes №2-6),
→ 2 part-time jobs for more complex design and maintenance questions,
→ Management of raw materials

Construction work	200
Diversification of the production equipment	0/500
Management contract (/year)	1200
Regulatory work for complying to medical device production	200
Paperwork for 3 custom-made medical devices	450
Paperwork for 3 standard medical devices	90
Art and social projects	50
Total	2190/2690

The cost of this task has been estimated by the 3D COVID core team at a monthly fee of 100k€, which represents about 3,000€ per month per AP-HP hospital.

These considerations led to the following proposal submitted to the vice-director of AGEPS by the 3D COVID core team in September 2020.

AP-HP top management did not follow-up on this proposal and stopped paying the BONE 3D staff on the 31st of December 2020, even though clearly identified private sponsors were ready to fund the 'Phase 2' of the project. A new proposal was sent to AP-HP and AGEPS top management by the 3D COVID core team on the 12th of January 2021 but no answer could be obtained to this second proposal, which was similar to what had been proposed in September 2020. Finally, and surprisingly, when all the initial team of the project was convinced that AP-HP would stop supporting the idea of a long-term 3D-printing initiative, the situation totally changed in spring 2021, when an administrative head to 'Phase 2' was appointed by AP-HP top management to lead the project on its institutional aspects – a staff member for AP-HP head – while the initiator of the project were formally appointed scientific and medical director of this 'Phase 2'. With the support of the Fondation de l'AP-HP[4], funding for a project leader was secured and recruitment started in September 2021, with a job effectively starting November 2021.
The new organization of 'Phase 2' was the following.

1. Coordination committee – planned meetings every 3 months
→ an AP-HP Deputy Director general
→ 'Phase 2' medical and scientific director
→ 'Phase 2' administrative head
→ 'Phase 2' project leader
→ representatives from the following bodies: AGEPS, DST[5], DRCI (OTT&PI), start-ups, Fondation de l'AP-HP, AP-HP purchases department
→ representative for two innovative approaches: 3D-printing of drugs and bio-printing
→ AP-HP users' representatives
→ 3D representative for each AP-HP sub-unit[6].

4 https://fondationrechercheaphp.fr/

5 Direction de la Stratégie et de la Transformation

6 AP-HP is formed of 4 academic sub-units.
1. AP-HP. Centre - Université de Paris including Hôpital Corentin Celton, Hôpital Européen Georges Pompidou, Hôpital Vaugirard Gabriel Pallez, Hôpital Necker - Enfants Malades, Hôtel Dieu, Hôpital La Collégiale, Hôpital Broca and Hôpital Cochin.
2. AP-HP. Sorbonne Université including Hôpital Tenon, Hôpital Saint-Antoine, Hôpital Rothschild, Hôpital Armand Trousseau, Hôpital Pitié-Salpêtrière, Hôpital La Roche-Guyon and Hôpital Charles Foix.
3. AP-HP. Nord - Université de Paris including Hôpital Louis Mourier, Hôpital Beaujon, Hôpital Bichat Claude Bernard, Hôpital Bretonneau, Hôpital Lariboisière, Hôpital Fernand Widal, Hôpital Saint Louis and Hôpital Robert Debré.
4. AP-HP. Université Paris Saclay including Hôpital Sainte Périne, Hôpital Ambroise Paré, Hôpital Raymond Poincaré, Hôpital Antoine Béclère, Hôpital Bicêtre, Hôpital Paul Brousse and Hôpital Maritime de Berck.

2. Full committee – planned to meet twice a year
→ all the members of the coordination committee
→ representatives of the three Parisian medical schools – Université de Paris, Sorbonne Université, Université Paris Saclay
→ representative of iLumens (see above)
→ representatives of professional schools (nursing schools, midwife school, Ecole de Chirurgie[7])
→ AP-HP International (see above).

In brief, after a very dynamic initial initiative dedicated to the fight against the pandemic with contrasted outcomes (massive production but inability to produce medical devices), and after a phase of uncertainty regarding the future of 3D printing at AP-HP, the largest hospital trust in Europe has decided to launch an ambitious plan aiming at federating 3D printing within all its 39 health centers and produce medical devices according to the new European regulations. The people involved in this 'Phase 2' project combine several of the initiators of the first project, backed by solid institutional representatives in order to anchor the long-term project into more classical boundaries but keep its energy and will for innovation. The first step of 'Phase 2' will be either to hire a private contractor who will manage the printers and oversee the regulatory work, based on the rules of the French public market (call for competitive procedure), or to hire a local dedicated team of engineers and legal specialists, after adapting salaries in order to be competitive on this very dynamic job market. The aim of 'Phase 2' is to produce the first AP-HP in-house 3D-printed medical devices at the end of 2023[8].

Two meetings of the 'Phase 2' committee have been organized between November 2021 and May 2022, with an agreement on the choice of the final location of the new platform and its duties. The final location will be the Leriche (since renamed Ady Steg) building, lower ground floor, in the former AP-HP Broussais hospital, with a total surface of approximatively 200 m^2. A preliminary phase with pilot projects took place during the summer 2022, with 3 goals.

1. Build a solid process for producing fast-track anatomical models in traumatology, in partnership with one of the most active trauma centers of AP-HP - the objective being to produce the model (in FDM) and deliver it to the clinicians in 12-18 hours.

2. Build a similar fast-track process with a cardiac surgery unit for the production of patient-specific heart models for the repair of congenital malformations (using polyjet printers).

3. Build the reglementary network for the validation of these models, which are class 1 medical devices under 2017/745, with a preliminary step involving ISO 13485 certification[9].

7 The 'Ecole de chirurgie' is a unique structure within AP-HP, founded in 1832, providing all AP-HP full-time surgical staff with free fresh human bodies for training and teaching purposes: http://ageps.aphp.fr/ecoledechirurgie/

8 https://sfscmfco.fr/recommandations-de-bonnes-pratiques/

9 www.iso.org/standard/59752.html

For numerous practical reasons related to the complexity of the maintenance contracts of the 3D printers, these three initial goals could not be achieved during summer 2022 but the 'Phase 2' platform was still inaugurated as planned early January 2023. The final organizational choice was to employ two engineers, with competitive salaries, and to externalize the reglementary expert. The two engineers had design and manufacture backgrounds, one of them being a former employee of BONE 3D who had personnaly worked on the 3D COVID project (BONE 3D went bankrupt in February 2023). The aim of producing the first in-house medical device (most probably class 1) in 2023 was maintained. From January 2nd 2023, all AP-HP health professionals were offered to submit design projects via a dedicated internal online platform[10]. Projects were assessed by a team of experts representing the different academic subunits of AP-HP and the administrations involved in innovation, during a short online weekly meeting. After approval of the project, the project leader was directed towards the engineering team for initial exchanges and prototyping. At the end of February 2023, after only a few weeks of activity, one new project was deposited every 48h, from very various backgrounds (surgery, education, maintenance, and others), confirming the positive dynamics observed during the 3D COVID project. The outcomes of the platform will be monitored in collaboration with Hospinomics, a research chair co-created by AP-HP and the Paris School of Economics[11], in order to shape the long-term business plan.

10 plateformeprojets.aphp.fr

The 2023 challenges of the 'Phase 2' platform are massive:

→ define an long-term economical model as current charity funding will allow the platform to function for 24 months only from January 2023,

→ comply with EU regulation for the production of medical devices, starting with class 1 devices - class IIb and even class III production are considered within 24 months,

→ launch an AP-HP online platform to share designs, notably all designs resulting from the fight against the pandemic, while respecting intellectual property,

→ federate a group of 3D platform managers from the main French academic hospitals in order to share designs nationwide and operate lobbying at French (ANSM) and EU levels to adapt the regulatory framework to efficient patient care,

→ be recognized as a training center for 3D design and 3D printing by launching educational programs and welcoming interns[12],

11 www.hospinnomics.eu

12 For instance: Diplôme d'Université 'Planification chirurgicale et médecine personnalisée : du traitement de l'image à la gestion des risques', Université Paris Cité.

→ work on marketing our expertise in settling 3D platforms at the national and international levels, most probably by creating an AP-HP subsidiairy, with a first project in Ukraine[13].

→ interact with local innovation initiatives, such as BOPEX[14], which consists in commercial offers for companies willing to develop medical devices including medical expertise, clinical trials and reglementation-compliant production.

In brief, the 'Phase 2' platform was conceived as a new type of clinical department, available to all the health professionals of AP-HP in order to offer engineering expertise for design and manufacture. All the designs we will produce are not intended to be 3D printed, as physical interfaces will tend to be progressively marginalized with the development of virtual reality, augmented reality and haptics, associated with the increase in the price of raw materials and the imperative to build circular production systems.

In this context, the new AP-HP platform no only offers to design all types of printable and non-printable 3D objects, but also intends to offer a new type of clinical service, that is quantification solutions; for instance volume measurements in oncology or result assessments in surgery - when based on 3D imaging. In fact, 3D engineers trained in computer are specifically skilled for such approaches, and the need for quantification will be major in most specialties, especially when medical imaging is available.

In brief, at the beginning of 2023, the new AP-HP 3D platform is in the process of becoming one of the first Health Engineering and Quantitative Medicine unit located within a hospital trust, with services available for all health professionals.

---

13 superhumans.com

14 BOPEX derives from BOPA (chaire-bopa.fr) and was funding as a 'Tiers-lieu d'expérimentation en Santé' by the national investment plan France 2030.

7. Inventory of all designs produced by 3D COVID

Many designs were produced during the 3D COVID initiative, mostly using FDM printers, but also occasionally involving polyjet technology. In the following, all designs have been listed with production quantities and technical characteristics.

7.1 Personal protection equipment and comfort equipment

7.1.1 Large elastic holder

Personal protection PP1

Elastic holder designs have been released online from the first days of the pandemic. The current design has been performed by BONE 3D based on available open-source data and technological optimisation. The 3D rendering represents an improvement of the initial design, which had a risk of fracture (see below the broken elastic holder of Hirsch, head of AP-HP). The final model, more flexible was secondarily developed, the 18th of April 2020 and then systematically produced.

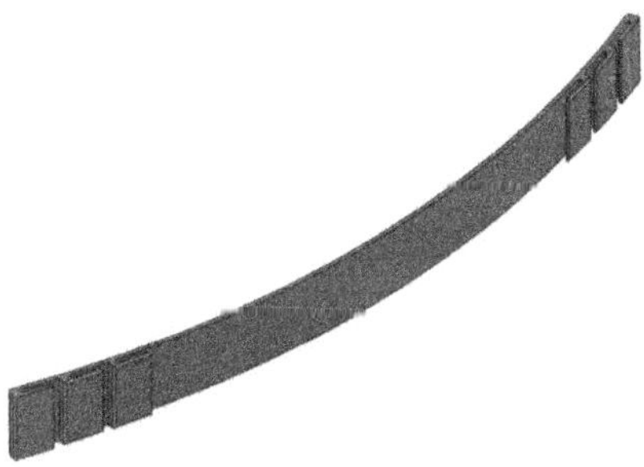

Date of first request	April 2020
Origin of the request	Nurses from Hôpital Cochin and Hôpital Necker - Enfants Malades
People involved in design	BONE 3D engineers
Quantity produced	5661
Destination	Necker/Bichat/Cochin/Pitié Hospitals

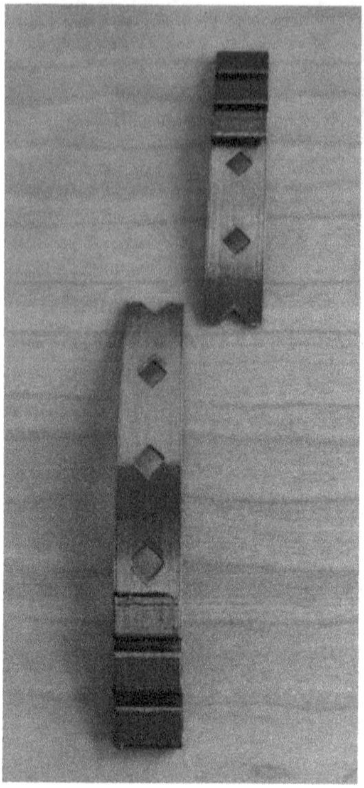

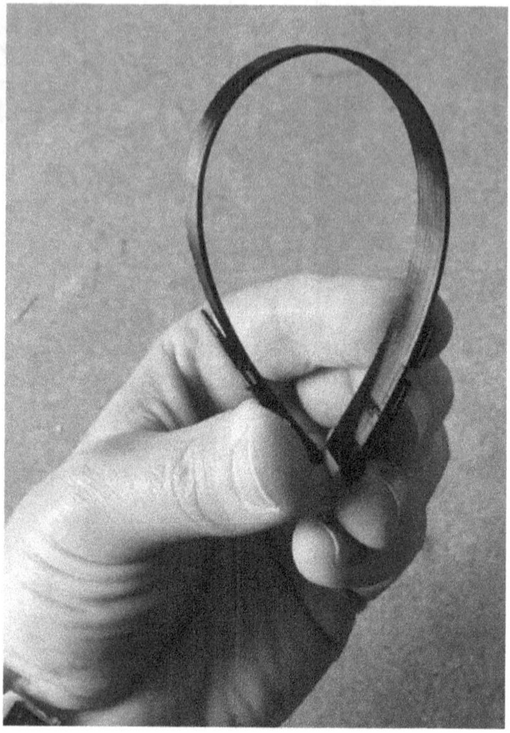

	One large holder	40 large holders
Layer thickness (mm)	0,33	0.33
Filling density	32%	32%
Wall thickness	1.52	1.52
Print duration	17 min	7 h 41 min
ABS quantity (cm3)	6.81	193.90
Support quantity (cm3)	2.07	47.31
Raw material costs (€)	1.70€	43.80€

7.1.2 Small elastic holder

Personal protection PP2

This smaller size was developed secondarily to fit FFP2 masks.

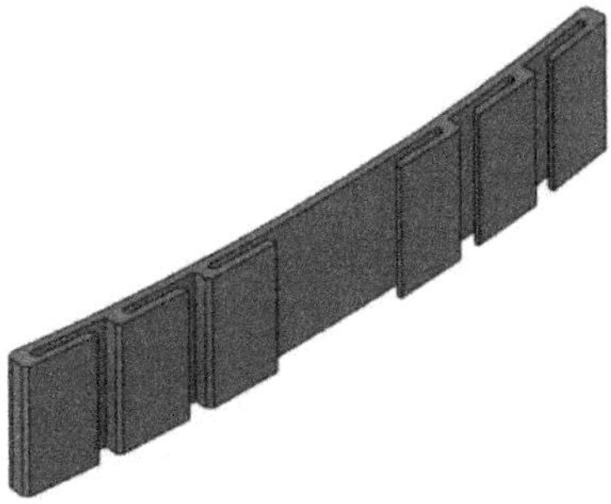

Date of first request	April 2020
Origin of the request	Nurses from Hôpital Necker - Enfants Malades
People involved in design	BONE 3D engineers
Quantity produced	5661
Destination	Necker/Bichat/Cochin/Pitié Hospitals

	One small holder	80 small holders
Layer thickness (mm)	0,33	0.33
Filling density	43%	43%
Wall thickness	1.52	1.52
Print duration	12 min	8 h 02 min
ABS quantity (cm3)	5.31	187.12
Support quantity (cm3)	1.22	39.06
Raw material costs (€)	1.19€	41.07€

7.1.3 Protection for slit lamps

Personal protection PP3

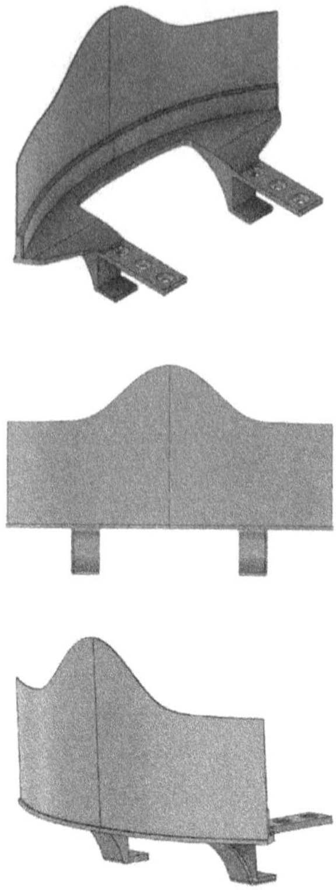

Slit lamp protections were initially required by the ophthalmology department of Percy hospital (a military hospital that does not belong to AP-HP), via a maxillofacial surgeon working part-time at Pitié-Salpêtrière Hospital. The model was developed in collaboration ophthalmologists at Percy. This specific model has been designed to fit on Height Streit BQ 900 slit lamps. The initial plan was to design a support fixed to the chin rest on which a transparent plastic layer would be fixed, but a one-piece full design was preferred.

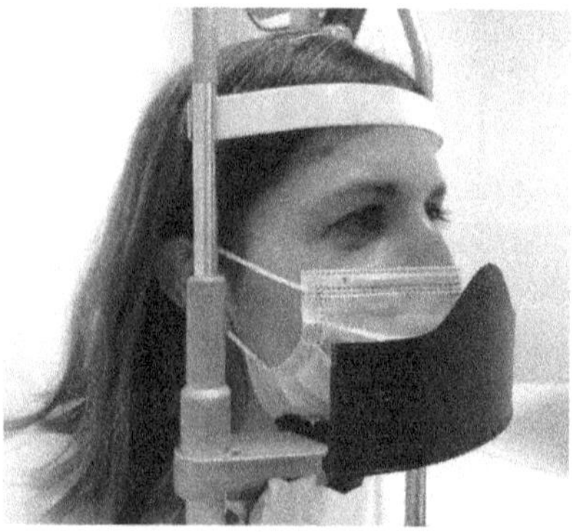

Scientific publication

Delbarre M, François PM, Adam J, Caruhel JB, Froussart-Maille F, Khonsari RH. 3D-printed shields for slit lamps produced during the COVID19 pandemic: the 3D COVID initiative. Ann 3D Printed Med 2021 1:100004.

Date of first request	April 2020
Origin of the request	Military surgeons (Percy Hospital)
People involved in design	BONE 3D engineers
Quantity produced	20
Destination	Necker/Cochin/Pitié Hospitals

	One shield	3 shield
Layer thickness (mm)	0,33	0.33
Filling density	32%	32%
Wall thickness	1.98	1.98
Print duration	2 h 32 min	6 h 18 min
ABS quantity (cm3)	50.66	124.90
Support quantity (cm3)	35.31	101.90
Raw material costs (€)	15.61€	41.04€

7.1.4 Button pusher

Personal protection PP4

Button pushers were designed before the 3D COVID project for internal distribution within Hôpital Necker - Enfants Malades. An initial production of button holders was funded by Wisepops (Paris) and was the initial impulse to the current project, that would then be supported by AP-HP on a larger scale (see section 0). These objects can only be printed using polyjet technology. Attempts using FMD printers were unsuccessful (no possible sliding of the inner part of the device). The device was printed as a single piece and required long manual post-treatment.

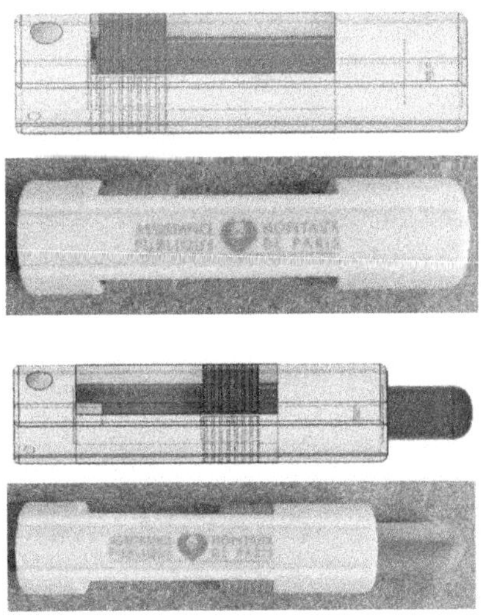

Date of first request	March 2020
Origin of the request	Hôpital Necker - Enfants Malades
People involved in design	BONE 3D engineers
Quantity produced	1300
Destination	Hôpitaux Necker - Enfants Malades/Cochin/ Pitié + all Greater Paris registrars

		One pusher[1]	60 pusher[2]
Layer thickness (mm)	Printing with Polyjet	NA	NA
Filling density		NA	NA
Wall thickness		NA	NA
Print duration		35 min	6 h 01 min
Resin quantity (g)	Veroblack	17	927
	Verocyan Vivid	7	341
	Veropure White	6	289
	Total (+ purge)	36	1632
Support quantity (g)		23	1289
Raw material costs (€)		11.34€	531€

Scientific publication

François PM, Bonnet X, Kosior J, Adam J, Khonsari RH. Scientific publication 3D-printed contact-free devices designed and dispatched against the COVID19 pandemic: the 3D COVID initiative. J Stom Oral Maxillofac Surg 2021;122:381-385.

1 On a Stratasys J735 polyjet printer.
2 High-speed settings on the J735 printer.

7.1.5 Multipurpose Ariane hook

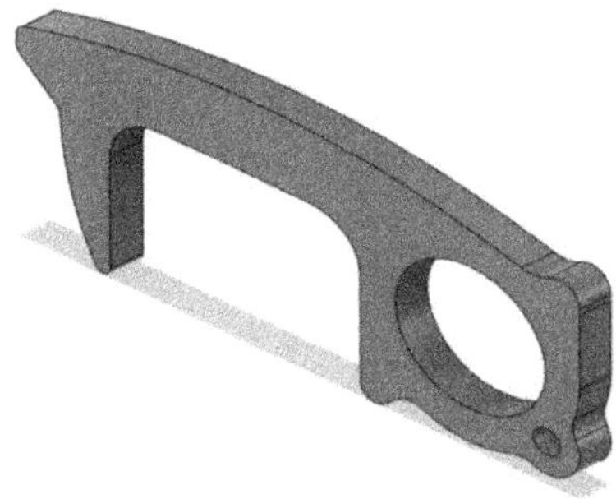

Personal protection PP5

This multipurpose hook design had been released online by the Ariane-Group (Paris, France) during the pandemic. The current design has been performed by BONE 3D based on available open-source data and technological optimisation. The rendering above represents an improvement of the initial design, which was more complex. The final model was developed the 25th of May 2020 and then systematically produced.

Date of first request	May 2020
Origin of the request	Hôpital Necker - Enfants Malades
People involved in design	Ariane Group, BONE 3D engineers
Quantity produced	1302
Destination	All Greater Paris registrars

	One hook
Layer thickness (mm)	0,33
Filling density	Sparse high density
Wall thickness	1.32
Print duration	27 min
ABS quantity (cm3)	14.5
Support quantity (cm3)	5.17
Raw material costs (€)	3.58€

Scientific publication

François PM, Bonnet X, Kosior J, Adam J, Khonsari RH. Scientific publication 3D-printed contact-free devices designed and dispatched against the COVID19 pandemic: the 3D COVID initiative. J Stom Oral Maxillofac Surg 2021;122:381-385.

7.1.6 Sheathed hook

Personal protection PP6

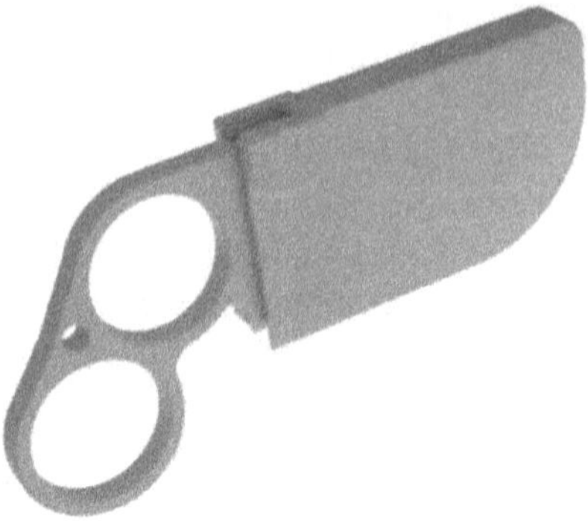

This tool, also aims to limit the spread of the virus by integrating a part allowing to press buttons as well as a hook allowing to open and close doors. A sheath is added to the device for protection and to enclose the part in contact with potential contaminated surfaces.

Date of first request	May 2020
Origin of the request	All services
People involved in design	BONE 3D engineers
Quantity produced	16
Destination	Arbalète elementary school (75005)

	One hook	One sheath
Layer thickness (mm)	0,33	0.33
Filling density	100%	100%
Wall thickness	1.32	1.32
Print duration	25 min	33 min
ABS quantity (cm3)	8.07	9.60
Support quantity (cm3)	3.84	9.27
Raw material costs (€)	2.17€	3.43€

7.1.7 Hook & Push

Personal protection PP7

This device, inspired by the button pusher, consists in limiting the spread of the virus by integrating a retractable part allowing to press any type of buttons, as well as a hook part allowing to open and close doors without contact. This device was not produced, but given its architecture, it should be printed in Polyjet so that the retractable part can slide inside the envelope.

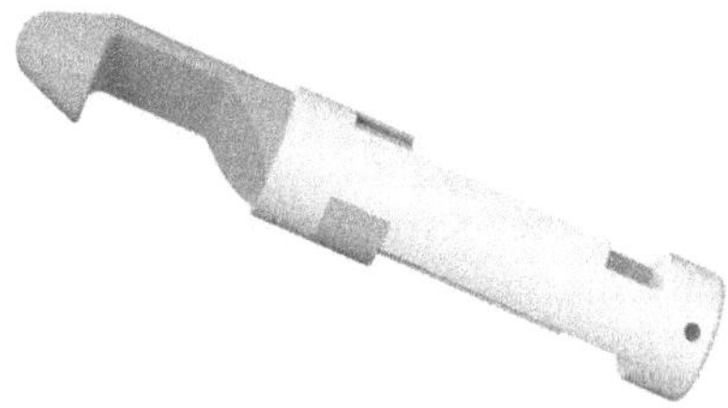

Date of first request	May 2020
Origin of the request	All services
People involved in design	Design student from Estienne school
Quantity produced	0
Destination	Not distributed

	One pusher	
Layer thickness (mm)	Printing with Polyjet	-
Filling density		-
Wall thickness		-
Print duration		-
Resin quantity (g)	Verocyan Vivid	-
	Veropure White	-
	Total (+ purge)	-
Support quantity (g)		-
Raw material costs (€)		-

7.1.8 Google frames

Personal protection PP8

Google frames were the first design formally requested by AGEPS. Large quantities were produced but were never distributed within the AP-HP network due to defective logistics: 90% of the devices produced were not requested by the structures that had initially ordered them. This case emphasizes the importance of a dedicated logistic service for emergency platforms in large structures such as AP-HP in order to follow-up the distribution of the production.
Technically, in order to minimise support use, google frames were initially printed vertically with minimal use of support but this solution raised technical problems (vibrations of the branches leading to ABS spill). The production was then performed based on horizontal stacks, requiring extensive post-treatment.

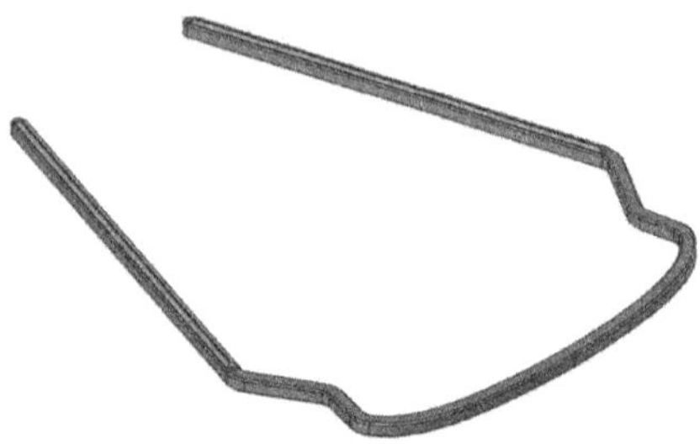

Date of first request	April 2020
Origin of the request	AGEPS
People involved in design	BONE 3D engineers
Quantity produced	1500
Destination	Pitié (approx. 150 pieces) + not distributed

	One frame	40 frames
Layer thickness (mm)	0,33	0.33
Filling density	32%	32%
Wall thickness	1.98	1.98
Print duration	24 min	18 h 46 min
ABS quantity (cm3)	8.20	993.31
Support quantity (cm3)	7.32	305.70
Raw material costs (€)	2.82€	108.77€

7.1.9 Face shield

Personal protection PP9

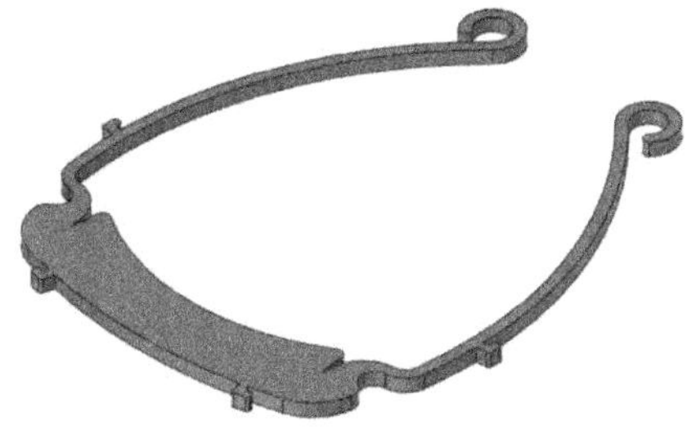

The initial design of the head-shield frame was provided by Mako Conception[1] and was secondarily optimized by BONE 3D engineers thanks to a review of all available designs. A total number of 12900 transparent plastic sheets were offered to 3D COVID by JPG (via its relationship director and customer experience)[2] and were distributed to the various recipients of the frames.

1 https://mako.paris
2 JPG, Survilliers, France: https://www.jpg.fr

Date of first request	April 2020
Origin of the request	All AP-HP hospitals
People involved in design	BONE 3D engineers + ENSAM
Quantity produced	3751
Destination	All services

	One frame	90 frames[3]
Layer thickness (mm)	0,33	0.33
Filling density	Sparse high density	Sparse high density
Wall thickness	1.32	1.32
Print duration	44 min	76 h 56 min
ABS quantity (cm3)	22.15	1860.26
Support quantity (cm3)	7.30	737.30
Raw material costs (€)	5.35€	471.64€

3. Only F370 printers allow printing 90 frames at once.

Destination	Number distributed
Vth district city hall	600
Hôpital Necker - Enfants Malades	165
SAMU 60	50
Fondation des 'Gueules Cassées'	25
Internal Medicine (Hôpital Cochin)	50
Emergency department (Hôpital Robert Debré)	120
Centre Cardiologique du Nord	100
Pharmacy (Hôpital Cochin)	10
Radiology (Hôpital Hôtel-Dieu)	100
Economat (Hôpital Cochin)	30
Bulle (Hôpital Cochin)	10
Palliative care (Hôpital Cochin)	20
Security (Hôpital Cochin)	15
Direction of Research (Hôpital Cochin)	15
IT support department (Hôpital Cochin)	50
Central kitchen (Hôpital Cochin)	100
Social services (Hôpital Cochin)	10
Virology department (Hôpital Cochin)	25
Biochemistry department (Hôpital Cochin)	25
Not targeted (maintenance, security and administration)	2251
TOTAL	3751

7.1.10 Baby face shield

Personal protection PP10

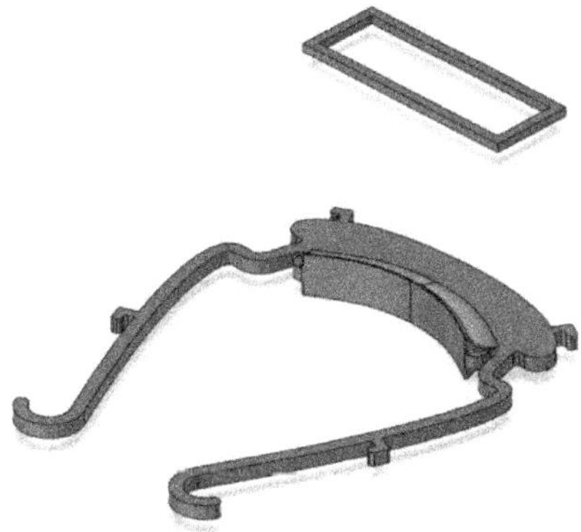

This smaller-sized frame was developed secondarily to fit baby heads. The device did not go beyond the prototyping stage.

Date of first request	May 2020
Origin of the request	AP-HP physician (nuclear medicine)
People involved in design	BONE 3D engineers
Quantity produced	15
Destination	Prototyping

	One frame	90 frames[2]
Layer thickness (mm)	0,33	0.33
Filling density	Sparse high density	Sparse high density
Wall thickness	1.32	1.32
Print duration	44 min	76 h 56 min
ABS quantity (cm3)	22.15	1860.26
Support quantity (cm3)	7.30	737.30
Raw material costs (€)	5.35€	471.64€

2 Only F370 allow printing 90 frames at once.

7.1.11 Nasal protection

Personal protection PP11

Silicon nasal protections were designed based on ABS-printed moulds. The silicon used for injections was DROPSTIL F556 20 shore A 1:1 (Prevent Transformation, Châteauneuf-sur-Isère, France), which is biocompatible and approved for skin contact. After several injection trials, it was decided to have the injections performed by the silicon provider (Prevent Transformation).

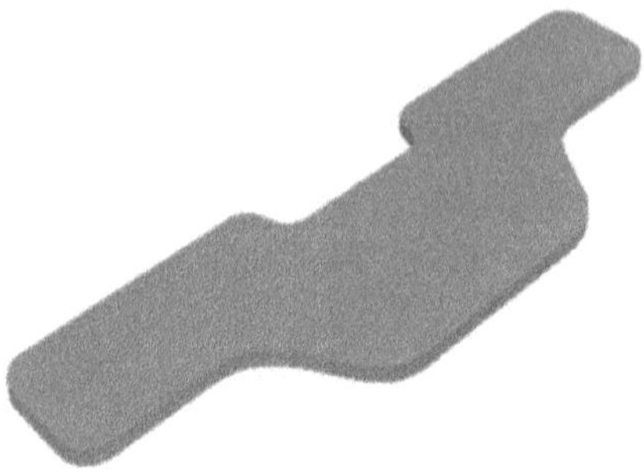

Date of first request	May 2020
Origin of the request	All services
People involved in design	BONE 3D engineers + AP-HP surgery trainee
Quantity produced	1000
Destination	Hôpital Necker - Enfants Malades

	Mould	Protection
Layer thickness (mm)	0,33	NA
Filling density	100%	NA
Wall thickness	1.32	NA
Print duration	40 min for 1 mould	24 h for 1000
Raw material quantity (cm3)	22.15 (ABS)	3mL (silicon)
Support quantity (cm3)	7.30	NA
Raw material costs (€)	5.35€	1.02€

Scientific publication

Kogane N, Adam J, Perrin B, Khonsari RH. Silicon nasal protection for FFP2 masks users: the 3D COVID initiative. J Stom Oral Maxillofac Surg (in preparation).

7.1.12 Contactless door handles

Personal protection PP12

Contactless door handles were designed before the 3D COVID project by BONE 3D and Hôpital Necker - Enfants Malades for internal distribution (see section 0). This object allows users to open and close doors with their forearms to limit the spread of the virus.

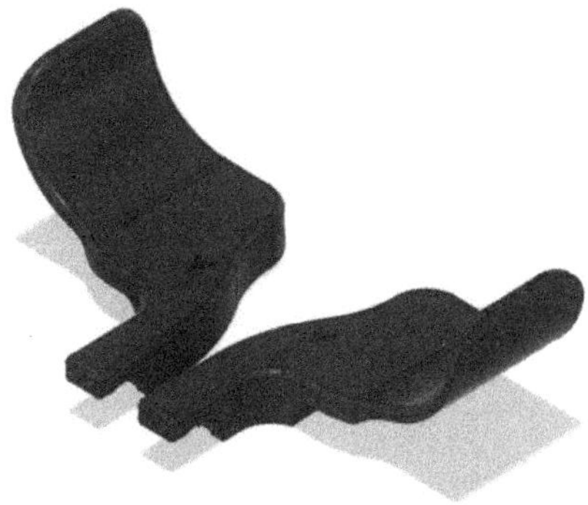

Door opener type №1 diameter 19 / diameter 20 / type 2

Date of first request	May 2020
Origin of the request	All services
People involved in design	BONE 3D engineers + ENSAM
Quantity produced	3882
Destination	Pitié/Necker/Imagine/AGEPS/Cochin and many AP-HP hospitals + administrations

	One door handle
Layer thickness (mm)	Depending of each door handle (over 18 different types available)
Filling density	
Wall thickness	
Print duration	
ABS quantity (cm3)	
Support quantity (cm3)	
Raw material costs (€)	5-8 €

Scientific publication

François PM, Bonnet X, Kosior J, Adam J, Khonsari RH. Scientific publication 3D-printed contact-free devices designed and dispatched against the COVID19 pandemic: the 3D COVID initiative. J Stom Oral Maxillofac Surg 2020;122:381-385

7.1.13 Anti-fogging device for face masks

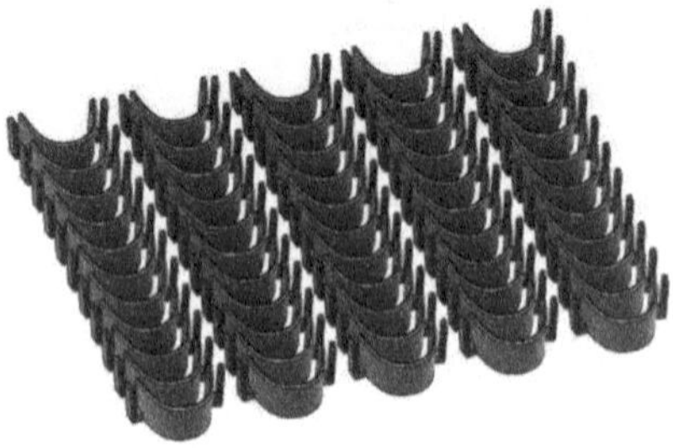

Personal protection PP13

This is an anti-fogging device to be fixed to face masks in contact with the nasal dorsum.

Date of first request	September 2020
Origin of the request	Hôpital Cochin
People involved in design	BONE 3D engineers
Quantity produced	550
Destination	Hôpital Cochin + Hôpital Necker - Enfants Malades

	Anti-fogging device for 55 devices
Layer thickness (mm)	0,33
Filling density	100%
Wall thickness	1.98
Print duration	8 h 39 min
ABS quantity (cm3)	189.75
Support quantity (cm3)	231.165
Raw material costs (€)	69.30€

7.1.14 Face mask armature

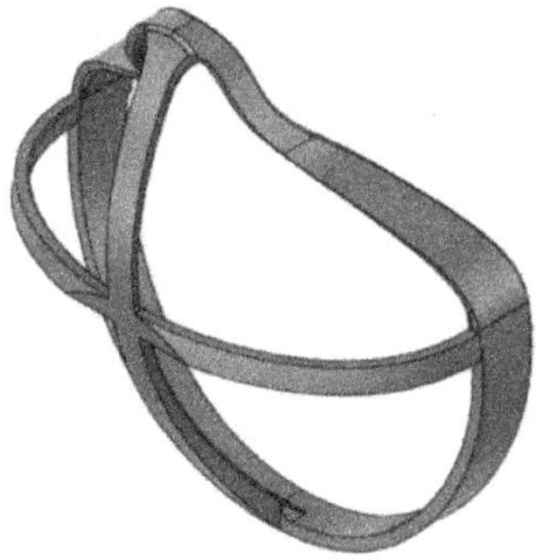

Personal protection PP14

This is a support placed under face masks in order to increase comfort of use, specially when speaking. Only two prototypes were produced.

Date of first request	September 2020
Origin of the request	Hôpital Cochin
People involved in design	BONE 3D engineers
Quantity produced	2
Destination	Hôpital Cochin

	One mask armature
Layer thickness (mm)	0,33
Filling density	100%
Wall thickness	1.98
Print duration	1 h 42 min
ABS quantity (cm3)	7.697
Support quantity (cm3)	21.44
Raw material costs (€)	4.62€

7.2 Medical equipment

7.2.1 Medical devices

7.2.1.1 Intensive care joints: from ABS to polyjet

Medical device MD1

A series of various intensive care joints were reproduced, initially in ABS. The first set of joints we produced had 0.18 of layer thickness, 100% filling density and 0.7 wall thickness. This first set had significant parietal leaks, revealed by tests performed at an intensive care unit at Pitié-Salpêtrière Hospital.

A second set with 0.33 of layer thickness, 100% filling density, 2.6 wall thickness and surface coating[1] was then tested, and no leaks were reported along their bodies. Nevertheless, the junction of the joints showed significant leaks, most probably due to the irregular surface of ABS-printed devices with added coating. We then decided to produce these joints using polyjet technology and a biocompatible resin (MED610 from Stratasys)[2].

In collaboration with an intensive care unit at Pitié-Salpêtrière hospital (Paris), we have compared the characteristics in terms of leakage of joints printed in ABS (0.7 mm and 2.6 mm wall thicknesses), with and without coating, with the characteristics of polyjet-printed MED610 joints. Additional biomechanical investigations on the joints have been performed at Ecole nationale supérieure des techniques appliquées (Palaiseau, France), an engineering of the Greater Paris region. Altogether, these results, have determined the optimal 3D-printing technique for ventilation joints in terms of reliability and cost, and confirmed that FDM with coating can be used for this purpose.

1 Nano Seal 180W+ (JELN Imprägnierung, Schwalmtal, Germany)

2 All tests were performed by intensivists from Pitié-Salpêtrière Hospital and technicians from ASV Santé (www.asvsante.fr).

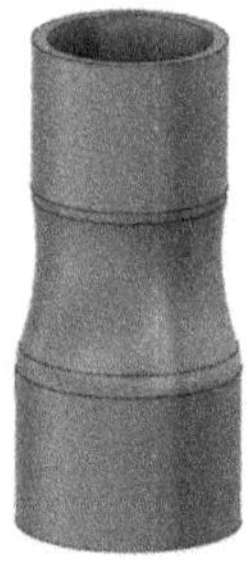

An F18-F22 joint

Date of first request	May 2020
Origin of the request	Intensive care unit, Pitié-Salpêtrière Hospital
People involved in design	BONE 3D engineers + ENSAM
Quantity produced	188
Destination	Not distributed

Scientific publication

Khonsari RH, Oranger M, François PM, Mendoza-Ruiz A, Leroux K, Boussaid G, Prieur D, Hodge JP, Belle A, Midler V, Morelot-Panzini C, Patout M, Gonzalez-Bermejo J. Quality versus emergency: How good were ventilation fittings produced by additive manufacturing to address shortages during the COVID19 pandemic? PLoS One 2022;17:e0263808.

Device	Time	MED610 (g)	Support (g)	3D rendering
F18F22	4h27	26	52	
F22F22 short	1h46	24	45	
F22F22 long	4h24	31	49	
F22	2h40	23	30	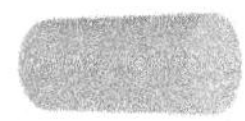
F22M22 short	2h40	19	32	
F22M22 T	4h23	34	60	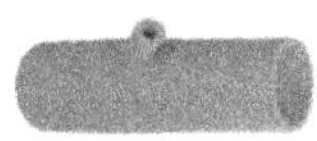
F22M22 long	4h23	33	54	
F21M22 long	4h26	39	74	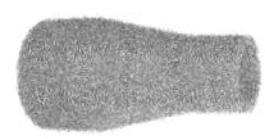
M22M22 court	2h39	18	26	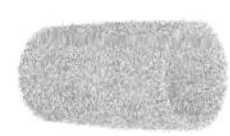
F22M22F22	4h30	42	89	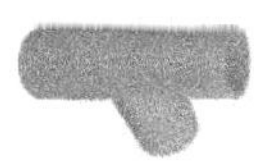
F22M22 T	4h21	33	65	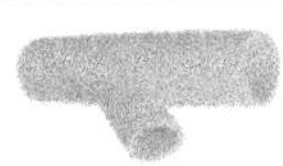
M22M22 long	4h21	29	41	
M22M22M22	4h29	39	82	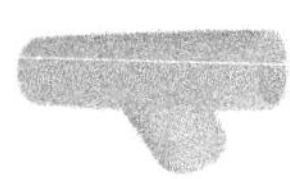
M31M22	4h25	36	64	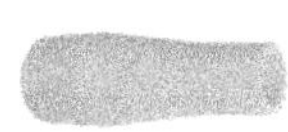
F18F20 T	4h53	25	73	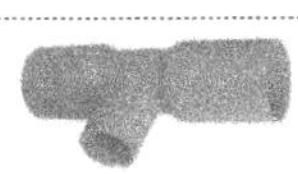

7.2.1.2 Pediatric intensive care joint

Medical device MD2

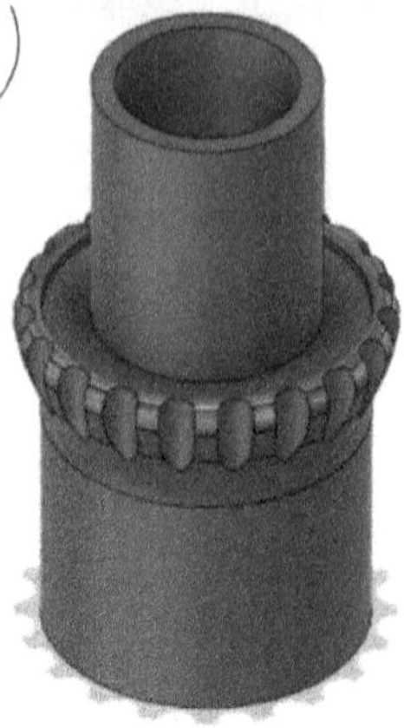

This specific joint was requested by the neonatology department of Hôpital Cochin. This joint was out of order at the beginning of the crisis and was used to connect specific filters on paediatric ventilators. Intensive care specialists provided the team with one sample of the joint, which was reproduced by the 3D COVID team. This joint was the first medical device produced by the team and did not go through formal validation procedures. 20 pieces were printed and delivered to neonatal intensivists for testing, who did not request for more pieces or modifications. These devices were produced before the extensive leakage testing performed on other ventilation connectors (see section 7.2.1.1) and we had no precise idea of their quality when they were delivered to users: this case underlines the importance of strict quality control when producing 3D-printed medical devices, even in emergency conditions, specially knowing what leakage represents in conditions with risks of viral spread.

Date of first request	April 2020
Origin of the request	Neonatal intensive care unit (Hôpital Cochin)
People involved in design	BONE 3D engineers
Quantity produced	20
Destination	Neonatal intensive care unit (Hôpital Cochin)

	One joint
Layer thickness (mm)	0,18
Filling density	100%
Wall thickness	0.36
Print duration	1 h 39 min
ABS quantity (cm3)	9.01
Support quantity (cm3)	2.96
Raw material costs (€)	2.18€

7.2.1.3 Prone head holder for intensive care

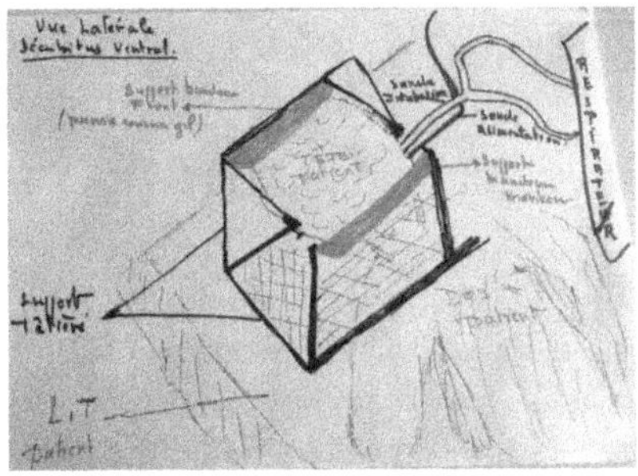

Medical device MD3

An initial sketch was sent by SMS by an intensive care head nurse to the 3D COVID team in order to describe her needs in terms of prone head holder. This device was engineered in order to avoid bedsores, due to the ventral position required to treat COVID-19 patients. The design allowed putting the head of the patient in a safe position while assuring enough space for tubes. Secondarily it was also used by radiologists as a stable head holder during radiologic exams. Contact was secured using medical gel cushions from the operating room.

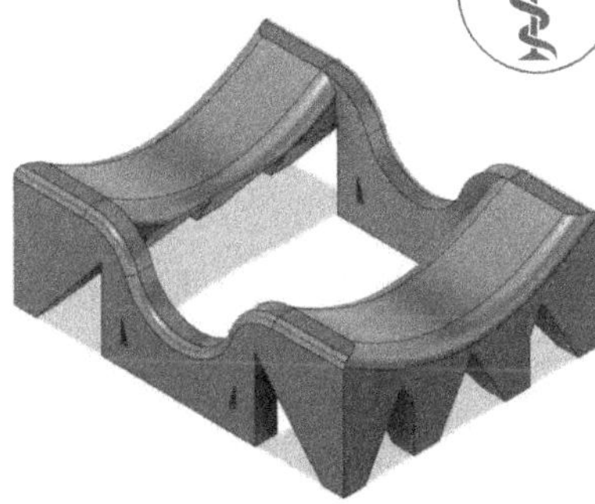

Date of first request	April 2020
Origin of the request	Head intensive care nurse (Hôpital Bichat)
People involved in design	BONE 3D engineers
Quantity produced	23
Destination	Head intensive care nurse (Hôpital Bichat)

	One holder
Layer thickness (mm)	0,22
Filling density	12%
Wall thickness	1.98
Print duration	10 h 02 min
ABS quantity (cm3)	298.54
Support quantity (cm3)	9.48
Raw material costs (€)	55.93€

7.2.1.4 Snorkeling mask - ventilation

Medical device MD4

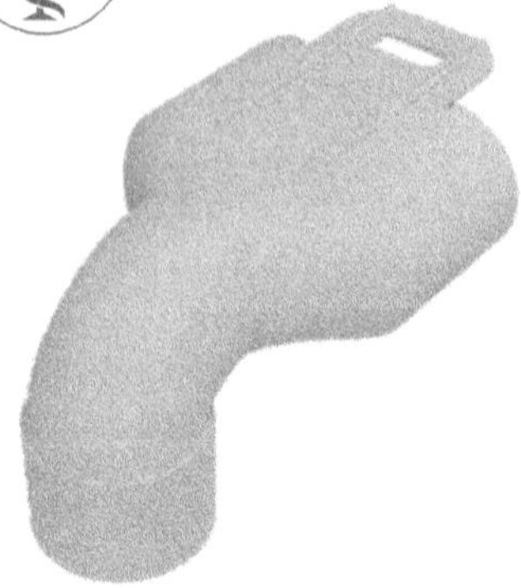

This adapter was used with a Decathlon EasyBreath snorkeling mask in order to transform it into a ventilation device. The story behind its design has been reported in a publication from our team (Thierry et al. 2020, see below). Snorkeling masks were finally never used as ventilation devices at AP-HP.

Date of first request	April 2020
Origin of the request	Online demand
People involved in design	BONE 3D engineers
Quantity produced	199
Destination	Not used

	Snorkeling - ventilation connector
Layer thickness (mm)	0,25
Filling density	Sparse high density
Wall thickness	1.016
Print duration	2 h 11 min
ABS quantity (cm3)	17.68
Support quantity (cm3)	12.45
Raw material costs (€)	5.48€

Scientific publication

Thierry B, Célérier C, Simon F, Lacroix C, Khonsari RH. How and Why Use the EasyBreath® Decathlon Surface Snorkeling Mask as a Personal Protective Equipment During the COVID-19 Pandemic? Eur Ann Otorhinolaryngol Head Neck Dis 2020;137;329-331.

7.2.1.5 Snorkeling mask - protection

Medical device MD5

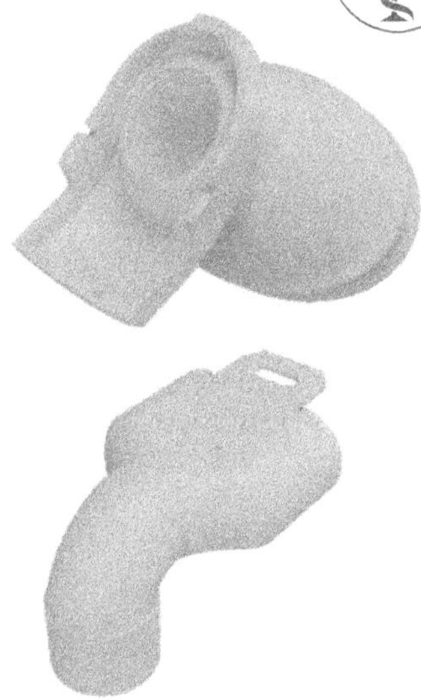

Snorkeling masks could also be used as protection devices (see Thierry et al. 2020). A polyjet-printed joint in Agilus (on J735) was added to the lower connector (upper device) in order to minimize leaks. Nevetheless, the parietal leaks of the two FDM-printed components were not evaluated professionally as for ventilation connectors (section 7.2.1.1) and could potentially have been responsible for viral dissemination.

Date of first request	07/04/2020
Origin of the request	Online demand
People involved in design	Sylvain Persohn, Juliette Prébot
Quantity produced	199
Destination	Not used

	Upper valve	Lower valve
Layer thickness (mm)	0,25	0.25
Filling density	Sparse high density	Sparse high density
Wall thickness	1.16	1.16
Print duration	2 h 08 min	2 h 22 min
ABS quantity (cm3)	26.31	16.67
Support quantity (cm3)	9.53	13.60
Raw material costs (€)	6.51€	5.50€

Scientific publication

Thierry B, Célérier C, Simon F, Lacroix C, Khonsari RH. How and Why Use the EasyBreath® Decathlon Surface Snorkeling Mask as a Personal Protective Equipment During the COVID-19 Pandemic? Eur Ann Otorhinolaryngol Head Neck Dis 2020;137;329-331.

7.2.1.6 Large mucus sucker

Medical device MD6

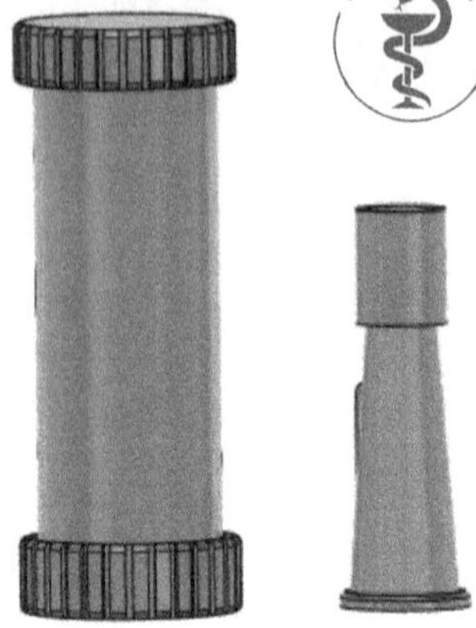

This device was designed after an early request from AGEPS but was never tested because its lack of transparency was considered as a non-negotiable issue. Transparent or semi-transparent suckers could have been produced using polyjet printing.

Date of first request	April 2020
Origin of the request	AGEPS
People involved in design	BONE 3D engineers
Quantity produced	20
Destination	Not distributed

	One sucker	4 suckers
Layer thickness (mm)	0,33	0.33
Filling density	100%	100%
Wall thickness	0.66	1.32
Print duration	1 h 30 min	4 h 41 min
ABS quantity (cm3)	18.23	55.40
Support quantity (cm3)	10.30	58.38
Raw material costs (€)	5.19€	20.66€

7.2.1.7 Fibroscopic mucus sucker

Medical device MD7

This device was similar to 7.2.1.6.

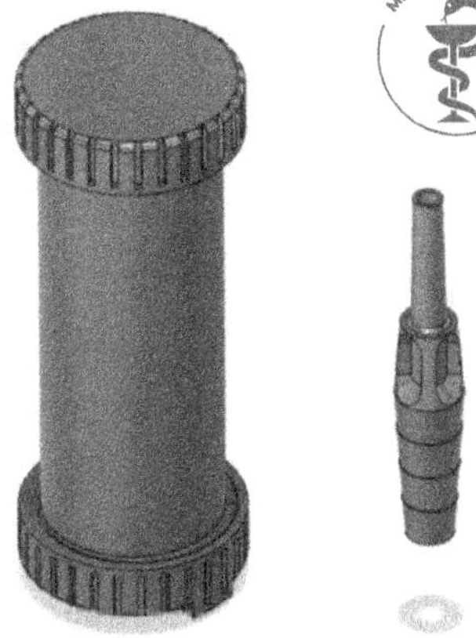

Date of first request	April 2020
Origin of the request	AGEPS
People involved in design	BONE 3D engineers
Quantity produced	20
Destination	Not distributed

	One sucker	4 suckers
Layer thickness (mm)	0,33	0.33
Filling density	100%	100%
Wall thickness	0.66	1.32
Print duration	1 h 30 min	4 h 41 min
ABS quantity (cm3)	18.23	55.40
Support quantity (cm3)	10.30	58.38
Raw material costs (€)	5.19€	20.66€

2.7.1.8 Intubation fixator

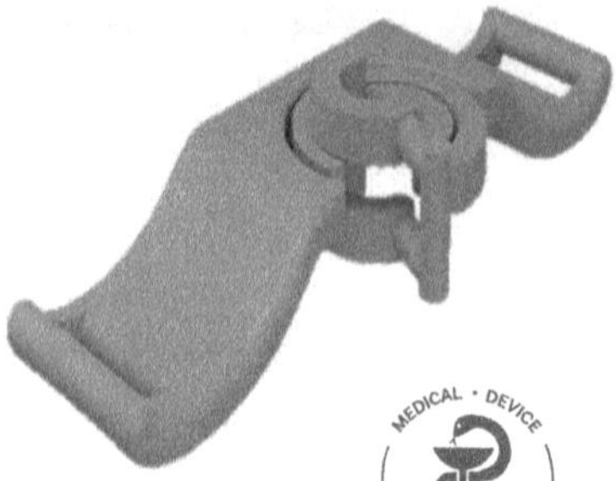

Medical device MD8

This device was intended to secure intubation tubes when endotracheal tubes were used as tracheostomy cannula due to shortages. Its design was not finalized.

Date of first request	NA
Origin of the request	Pitié Salpétrière hospital
People involved in design	AP-HP surgery trainee
Quantity produced	5
Destination	Not distributed

	One fixator
Layer thickness (mm)	0,33
Filling density	100%
Wall thickness	1.32
Print duration	1 h 06 min
ABS quantity (cm3)	16.37
Support quantity (cm3)	14.37
Raw material costs (€)	5.59€

2.7.1.9 Non-invasive ventilation mask

Medical device MD9

The core of the mask frame was printed in 3D and a silicone component was added to guarantee the seal and comfort of the patient in the contact zone with the skin. The device was attached to the patient face with elastic bands that were placed around the head. The testing of this mask was organised unilaterally by AGEPS (see section 3.14) and it was rejected at once by the chosen medical experts because the 3D printed core was not transparent. Development was then stopped.

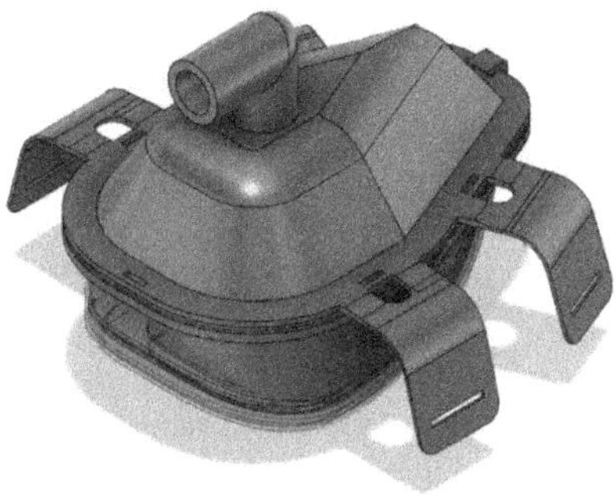

Date of first request	April 2020
Origin of the request	AGEPS
People involved in design	BONE 3D engineers
Quantity produced	35
Destination	ANSM

	One mask frame	One mould	Silicon part
Layer thickness (mm)	0,33	0.33	NA
Filling density	100%	Polyjet 28 microns	100%
Wall thickness	1.32		1.1
Print duration	6 h 04 min	18 h 58 min	5-10 min (reticulation)
Raw material Quantity (cm3)	72.77 (ABS)	1739g (Vero Magenta)	37.7 mL
Support quantity (cm3)	84.31	600g (SUP706B)	NA
Raw material costs (€)	28.53€	574.22€	12.75€

2.2.1.10 High-concentration ventilation masks

Medical device MD10

This mask allowed an increase in oxygen concentration (from 60 to 80%). For issues due to its transparency, developed was stopped after the production of the first prototypes (see section 3.14).

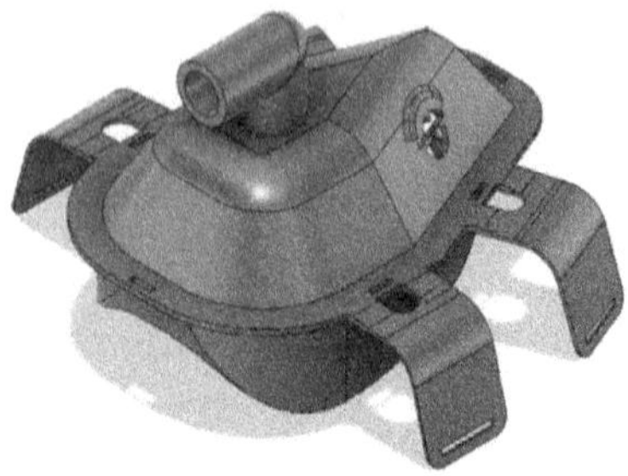

Date of first request	April 2020
Origin of the request	AGEPS
People involved in design	BONE 3D engineers
Quantity produced	35
Destination	ANSM

	One mask frame	One mould	Silicon part
Layer thickness (mm)	0,33	0.33	NA
Filling density	100%	Polyjet 28 microns	100%
Wall thickness	1.32		1.1
Print duration	5 h 22 min	18 h 58 min	5-10 min (reticulation)
Raw material Quantity (cm3)	72.27 (ABS)	1739g (Vero Magenta)	37.7 mL
Support quantity (cm3)	85.95	600g (SUP706B)	NA
Raw material costs (€)	28.73€	574.22€	12.75€

7.2.1.11 Single-use intubation blade

Medical device MD11

This single-use blade was intended for McGrath glottiscopes. This device was designed to be printed using MED610 polyjet resin, according to ISO 10993. The development was stopped after the first wave.

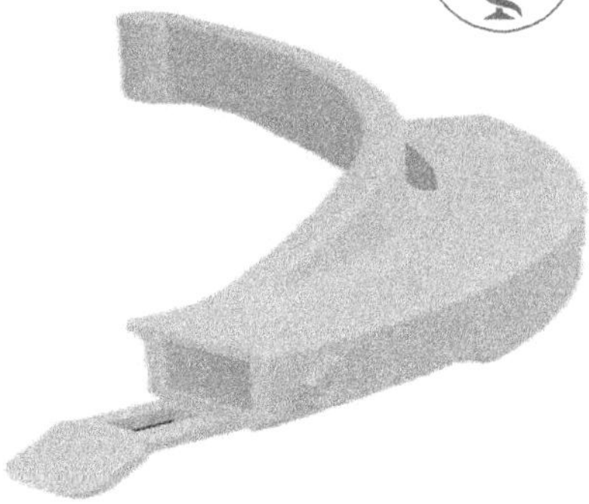

Date of first request	March 2020
Origin of the request	Hôpital Necker - Enfants Malades
People involved in design	ENSTA engineer
Quantity produced	2
Destination	Not distributed

	One glotticope blade
Layer thickness (mm)	NA
Filling density	NA
Wall thickness	NA
Print duration	3 h 19 min (high mix)
ABS quantity (cm3)	53
Support quantity (cm3)	83
Raw material costs (€)	29.19€

7.2.1.12 AirTraq protection

Medical device MD12

This design was not completed, and development was abandoned after the first wave. The point of the design was to provide protection for users when performing at risk procedures on airways of COVID patients.

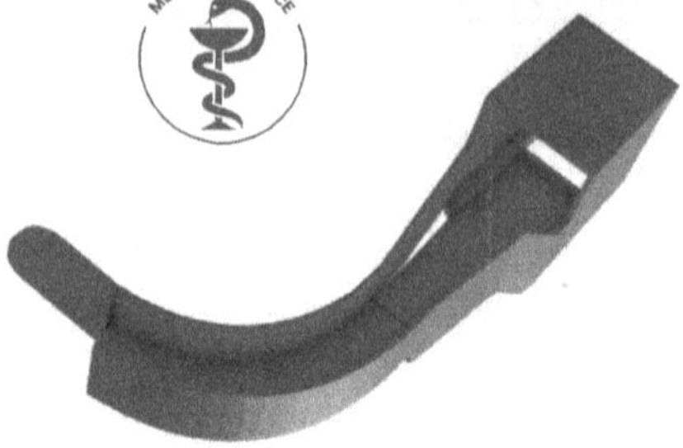

Date of first request	March 2020
Origin of the request	Bicêtre hospital
People involved in design	ENSTA engineer
Quantity produced	0
Destination	Not distributed

	One protection device
Layer thickness (mm)	NA
Filling density	NA
Wall thickness	NA
Print duration	8 h 41 min (high mix)
ABS quantity (cm3)	147
Support quantity (cm3)	283
Raw material costs (€)	86.89€

7.2.1.13 Suture holder for heart valve surgery

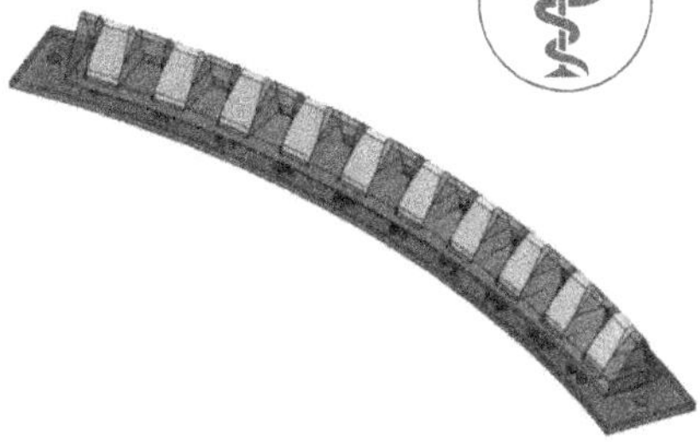

Medical device MD13

This device allowed the sutures to be stretched around the surgical field during thoracotomies in cardiovascular surgery. It was missing during the first wave of the pandemic due to difficult imports from the United States. The device consisted in a medical silicone part produced using a 3D printed mold, and in an ABS 3D-printed main component. The printed ABS part had to be sterilized using Sterrad while the silicone part could be sterilized using autoclave. The ABS part and the silicone part were thus sterilized separately and then assembled directly in the operating room. This device was chosen as the first device to be preferentially approved as a medical device with submission of an application to ANSM, but the process was not supported by AGEPS and was never completed.

Date of first request	April 2020
Origin of the request	Cardiovascular surgeon (Bichat Hospital)
People involved in design	BONE 3D engineers
Quantity produced	40
Destination	AGEPS

	One mask frame	One mould	Silicon part
Layer thickness (mm)	0,33	0.33	NA
Filling density	100%	100%	NA
Wall thickness	1.32	1.32	NA
Print duration	1 h 32 min	2 h 05 min	5-10 min (reticulation)
Raw material Quantity (cm3)	31.79 (ABS)	68.93 (ABS)	50 mL
Support quantity (cm3)	15.92	7.19	NA
Raw material costs (€)	8.67€	13.83€	16.90€

Scientific publication

Laliève L, Adam J, Nataf P, Khonsari RH. 3D-printed suture guide for thoracic and cardiovascular surgery produced during the COVID19 pandemic. Ann 3D Printed Med 2021;1:100005.

7.2.1.14 Boussignac valve

Medical device MD14

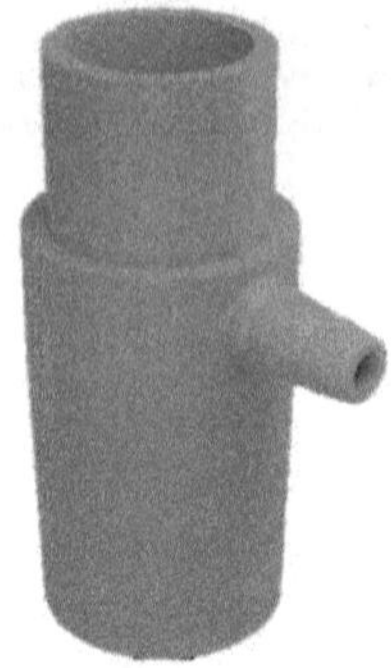

The Continuous Positive Airway Pressure (CPAP) Breathing Device is a breathing aid for patients to maintain a pressure in the airway above atmospheric pressure at the end of exhalation. Georges Boussignac, the creator of this method, worked with the 3D COVID team for its optimization for 3D printing. First prototyped in ABS, this valve was then printed in polyjet with biocompatible MED610 resin. The design was conducted by an independent engineer, who did not wish to pursue his work for validation of the device after the first two waves, and the project was consequently paused.

Date of first request	April 2020
Origin of the request	AGEPS
People involved in design	Independent engineer
Quantity produced	5
Destination	Biomechanical testing initiated

	One valve
Layer thickness (mm)	NA
Filling density	NA
Wall thickness	NA
Print duration	3 h 40 min (high mix)
ABS quantity (cm3)	48
Support quantity (cm3)	65
Raw material costs (€)	25.30€

7.2.1.15 Tulip OR tube holder

Medical device MD15

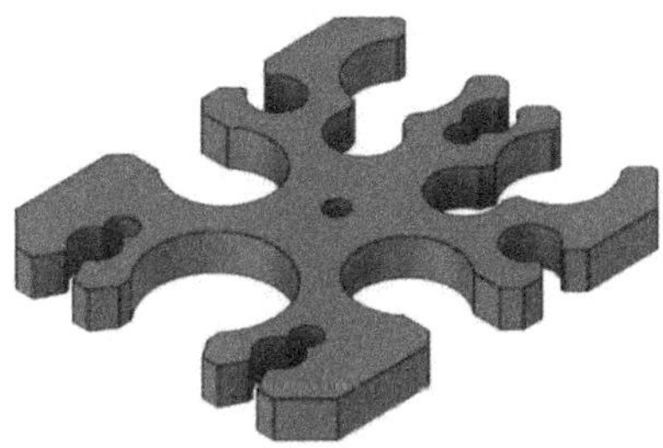

This device used in anaesthesia departments allows fixing tubes around the patient bed. The different sizes of the branches allow adaptation to different diameters of tubes. This device was considered for validation as a medical device by ANSM but the process was not initiated.

Date of first request	May 2020
Origin of the request	Operating room nurse (Hôpital Necker - Enfants Malades)
People involved in design	BONE 3D engineer
Quantity produced	5
Destination	ANSM assessment considered

	One glotticope blade
Layer thickness (mm)	0.33
Filling density	100%
Wall thickness	1.32
Print duration	53 min
ABS quantity (cm3)	30.63
Support quantity (cm3)	7.71
Raw material costs (€)	6.97€

7.2.1.16 Syringe elongator

Medical device MD16

This is a connector device for specific syringes.

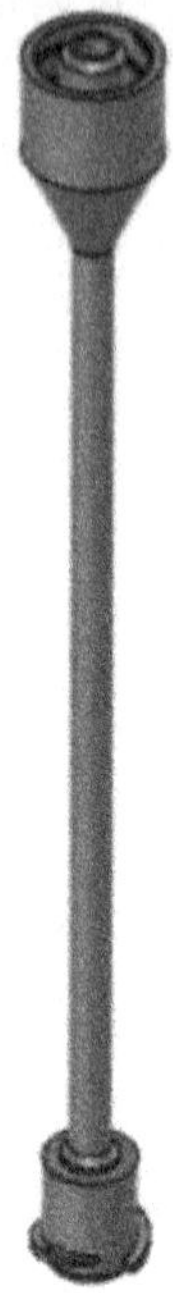

Date of first request	Septembre 2020
Origin of the request	Pharmacy (Hôpital Cochin)
People involved in design	BONE 3D engineer
Quantity produced	0
Destination	Hôpital Cochin

	One syringe
Layer thickness (mm)	0.1
Print duration	3 h 19 min
Resin quantity (mL)	2.87
Resin	Surgical Guide
Raw material costs (€)	0.65€

7.2.1.17 Connector for compressor

Medical device MD17

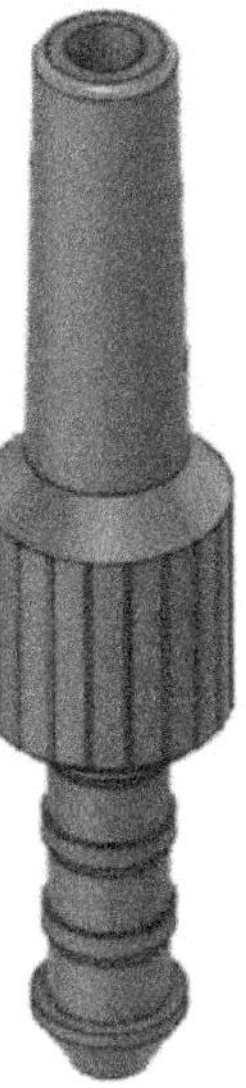

This is piece is a compressor connection component.

Date of first request	July 2020
Origin of the request	Intensive care unit (Hôpital Cochin)
People involved in design	BONE 3D engineer
Quantity produced	2
Destination	Hôpital Cochin

	One compressor
Layer thickness (mm)	0.33
Filling density	100%
Wall thickness	1.98
Print duration	13 min
ABS quantity (cm3)	2.496
Support quantity (cm3)	2.314
Raw material costs (€)	0.79€

7.2.2 Devices for physical therapy

For a significant number of physical therapy devices, the status of medical device is not clear. Most of these devices are currently manufactured without specific regulatory background by physiotherapists themselves. All designs were conceived by occupational therapist + engineer duos based on existing hand-made devices and analyses of needs.

7.2.2.1 Laser helmet

Rehabilitation device RD1

This device is a laser holder for patients with proprioception disorders. It is designed as a helmet on which a laser pointer can be clipped.

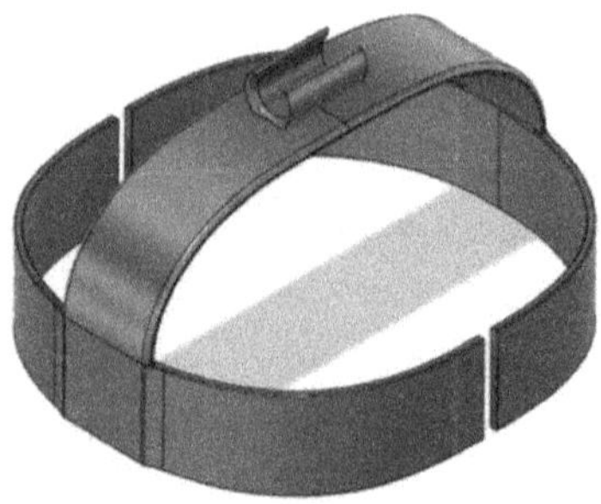

Date of first request	June 2020
Origin of the request	Occupational therapy (Hôpital Cochin)
People involved in design	BONE 3D engineer
Quantity produced	5
Destination	Hôpital Cochin

	One laser helmet
Layer thickness (mm)	0.33
Filling density	100%
Wall thickness	1.32
Print duration	4 h 58 min
ABS quantity (cm3)	96.16
Support quantity (cm3)	63.53
Raw material costs (€)	29€

7.2.2.2 Zipper opener

Rehabilitation device RD2

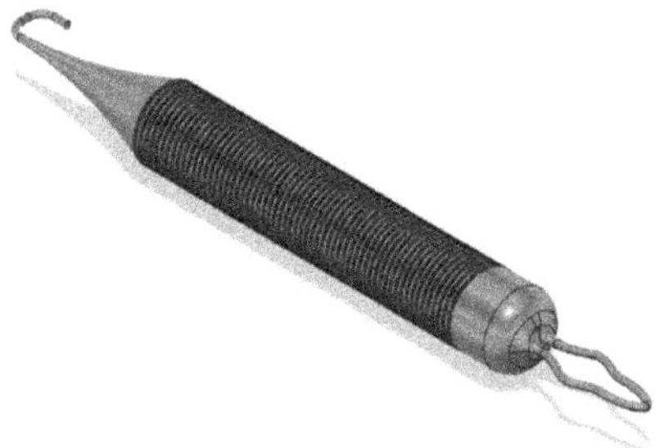

This device intends to help patients with motor impairment to handle buttons and zippers. Initial ABS prototypes would break easily, and the design requires improvement.

Date of first request	June 2020
Origin of the request	Occupational Therapy (Hôpital Cochin)
People involved in design	BONE 3D engineer
Quantity produced	5
Destination	Hôpital Cochin

	One unzipper and hook
Layer thickness (mm)	0.25
Filling density	32%
Wall thickness	1.98
Print duration	2 h 32 min
ABS quantity (cm3)	37.66
Support quantity (cm3)	15.19
Raw material costs (€)	9.60€

7.2.2.3 Single-sided bottle opener

Rehabilitation device RD3

The universal opener adapts to the main types of bottles and objects to unscrew. This product allows people suffering from arthritis or muscular disorders to screw and unscrew with ease.

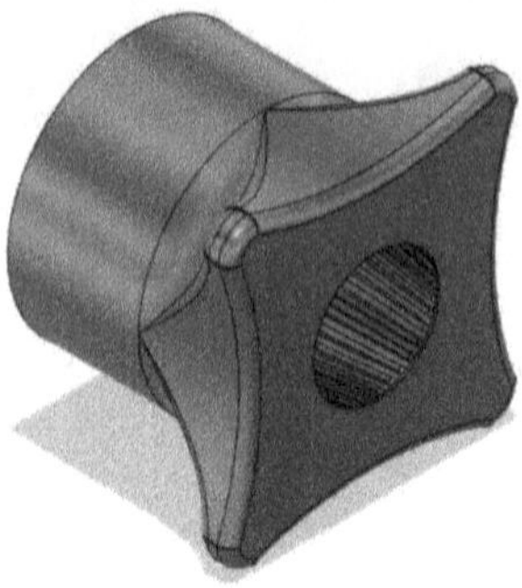

Date of first request	June 2020
Origin of the request	Occupational Therapy (Hôpital Cochin)
People involved in design	BONE 3D engineer
Quantity produced	5
Destination	Hôpital Cochin

	One universal opener
Layer thickness (mm)	0.25
Filling density	100%
Wall thickness	0.81
Print duration	6 h 06 min
ABS quantity (cm3)	33.87
Support quantity (cm3)	4.3
Raw material costs (€)	6.94€

7.2.2.4 Double-sided bottle opener

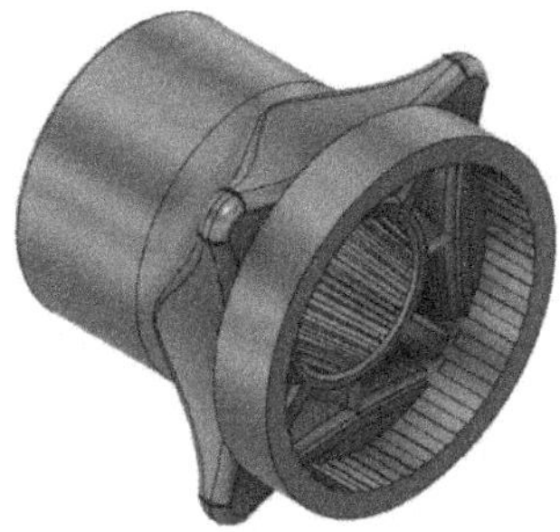

Rehabilitation device RD4

This device is a universal opener for occupational therapy.

Date of first request	September 2020
Origin of the request	Occupational Therapy (Hôpital Cochin)
People involved in design	BONE 3D engineer
Quantity produced	10
Destination	Hôpital Cochin

	Double-sided opener
Layer thickness (mm)	0.25
Filling density	100%
Wall thickness	0.81
Print duration	8 h 54 min
ABS quantity (cm3)	38.361
Support quantity (cm3)	33.283
Raw material costs (€)	11.72€

7.2.2.5 Double-sided bottle opener (variant)

Rehabilitation device RD5

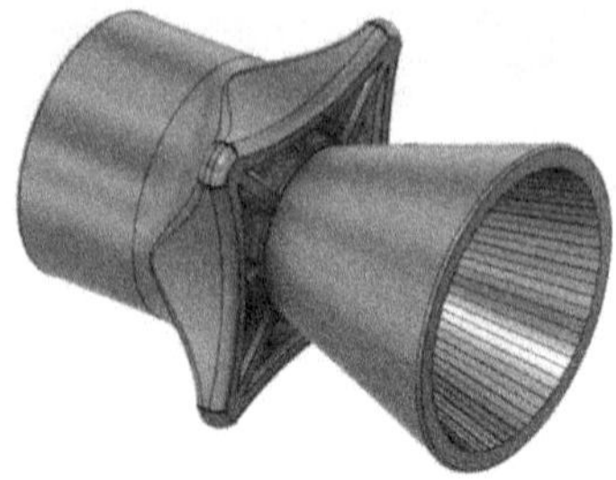

This is a double-sided universal opener for patient in occupational therapy. Devices RD3, RD4 and RD5 were also prototyped using TPU with promising results.

Date of first request	September 2020
Origin of the request	Occupational Therapy (Hôpital Cochin)
People involved in design	BONE 3D engineer
Quantity produced	10
Destination	Hôpital Cochin

	Double-sided opener
Layer thickness (mm)	0.25
Filling density	100%
Wall thickness	0.81
Print duration	10 h 33 min
ABS quantity (cm3)	47.007
Support quantity (cm3)	44.443
Raw material costs (€)	15.02€

7.2.2.6 Rehabilitation pliers

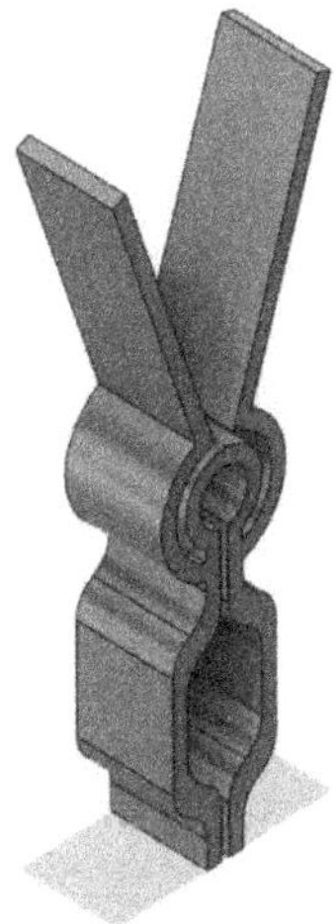

Rehabilitation device RD6

This device is a rehabilitation forceps for patients with osteoarthritis or who have undergone surgery. This device is often used to open yoghurt pots or similar packages.

Date of first request	June 2020
Origin of the request	Occupational Therapy (Hôpital Cochin)
People involved in design	BONE 3D engineer
Quantity produced	5
Destination	Hôpital Cochin

	One reeducation pliers
Layer thickness (mm)	0.33
Filling density	100%
Wall thickness	1.32
Print duration	14 min
ABS quantity (cm3)	3.65
Support quantity (cm3)	1.5
Raw material costs (€)	0.94€

7.2.2.7 Crutch holder

Rehabilitation device RD7

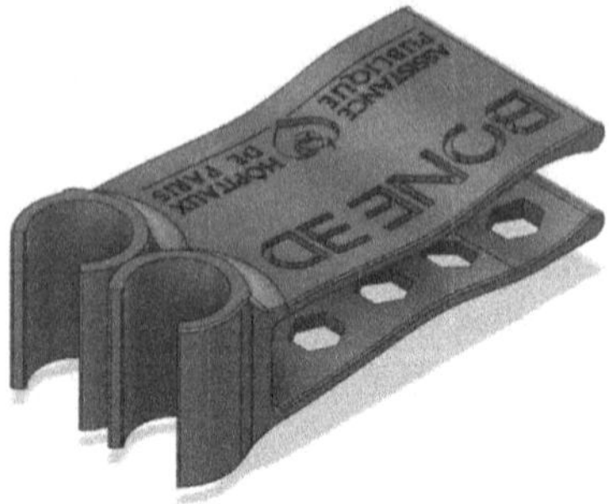

This device allows wedging crutches on table borders. 3D-printing offers unique potentialities to physical and occupational therapists by enabling the production of larger quantities of devices that were otherwise assembled manually (see figure below, comparing the hand-made crutch holder with the 3D-printed version). This device has also been successfully prototyped using TPU.

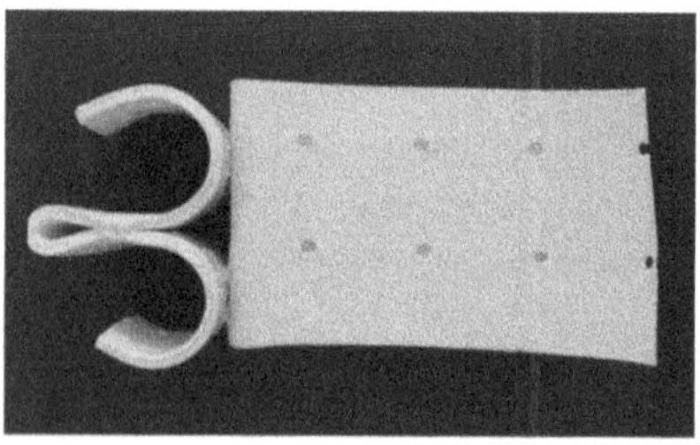

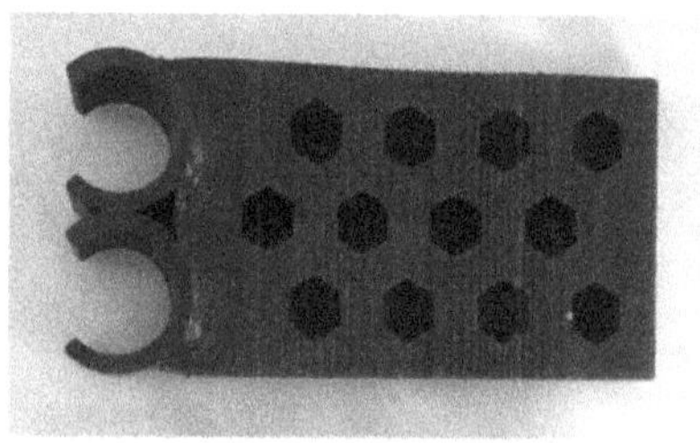

Date of first request	June 2020
Origin of the request	Occupational therapy (Hôpital Cochin)
People involved in design	BONE 3D engineer
Quantity produced	5
Destination	Hôpital Cochin

	One crutch holder
Layer thickness (mm)	0.25
Filling density	100%
Wall thickness	0.81
Print duration	9 h 42 min
ABS quantity (cm3)	57.88
Support quantity (cm3)	35.63
Raw material costs (€)	16.98€

7.2.2.8 Single-sided vial-opener

Rehabilitation device RD8

This device is a vial-opener for occupational therapy that can also be of help in various biology, pharmacy or research laboratories.

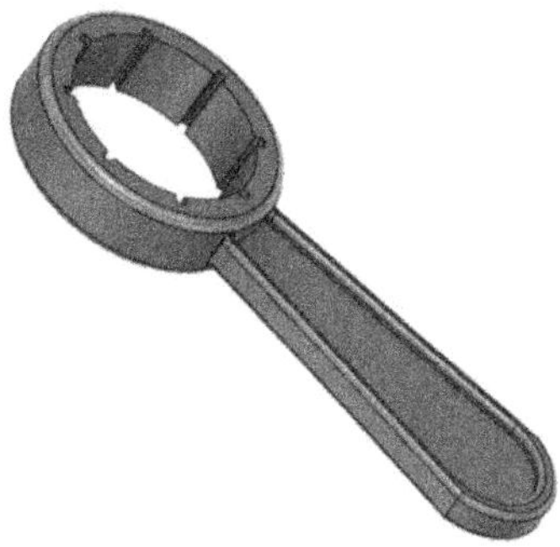

Date of first request	September 2020
Origin of the request	Occupational Therapy (Hôpital Cochin)
People involved in design	BONE 3D engineer
Quantity produced	5
Destination	Hôpital Cochin

	One bottle-opener
Layer thickness (mm)	0.33
Filling density	100%
Wall thickness	1.98
Print duration	1 h 26 min
ABS quantity (cm3)	34.601
Support quantity (cm3)	15.563
Raw material costs (€)	8.09€

7.2.2.9 Double-sided vial-opener

Rehabilitation device RD9

This device is a double-sided variant of the RD8 vial-opener for occupational therapy.

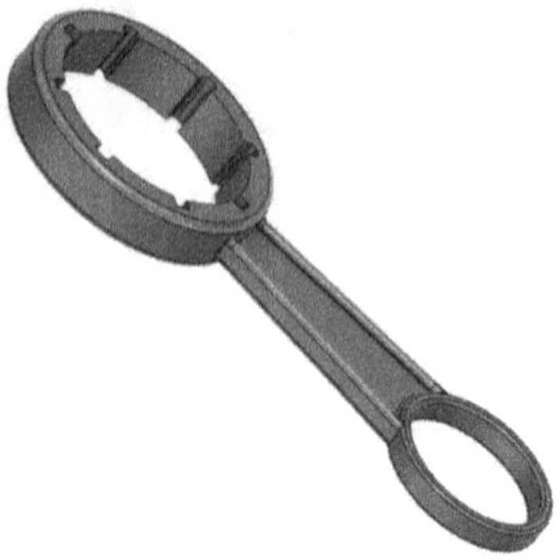

Date of first request	September 2020
Origin of the request	Occupational Therapy (Hôpital Cochin)
People involved in design	BONE 3D engineer
Quantity produced	2
Destination	Hôpital Cochin

	One vial-opener
Layer thickness (mm)	0.33
Filling density	100%
Wall thickness	1.98
Print duration	1 h 42 min
ABS quantity (cm3)	40.858
Support quantity (cm3)	19.901
Raw material costs (€)	9.74€

7.2.2.10 Diplopia glasses

Rehabilitation device RD10

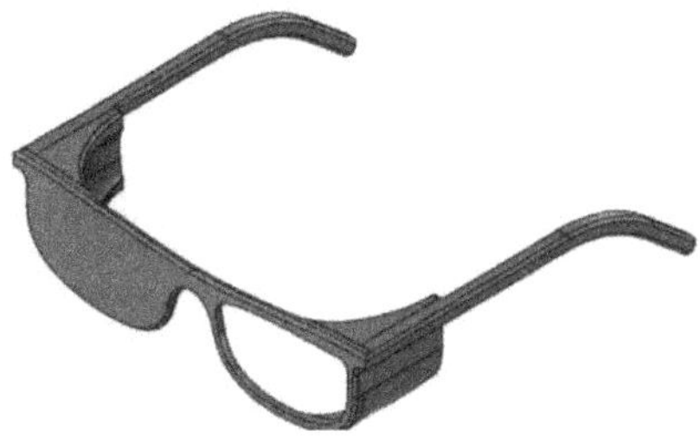

This device is used for instance in age-related macular degeneration. The device is available with a cache on the left or right sides.

Date of first request	September 2020
Origin of the request	Virology (Hôpital Cochin)
People involved in design	BONE 3D engineer
Quantity produced	2
Destination	Hôpital Cochin

	One pair of spectacles
Layer thickness (mm)	0.33
Filling density	100%
Wall thickness	1.98
Print duration	1 h 49 min
ABS quantity (cm3)	19.152
Support quantity (cm3)	16.021
Raw material costs (€)	5.78€

7.2.2.11 Infusion pole holder

Rehabilitation device RD11

This is a support for wheelchairs that allows the patient to have infusions pole hooked up, which will allow moving around with poles while sitting in a wheelchair.

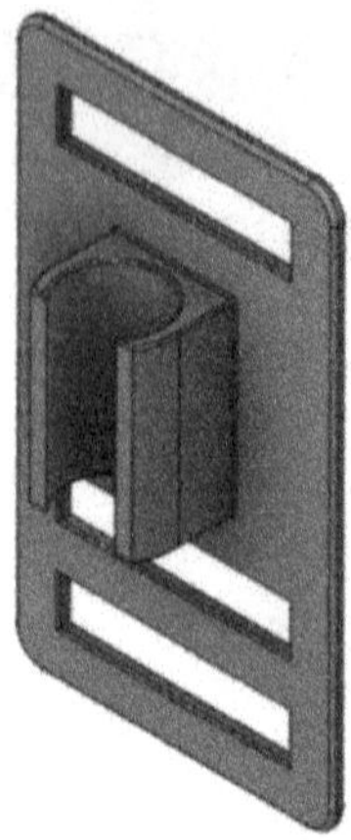

Date of first request	September 2020
Origin of the request	Occupational therapy (Hôpital Cochin)
People involved in design	BONE 3D engineer
Quantity produced	3
Destination	Hôpital Cochin

	One pole holder
Layer thickness (mm)	0.25
Filling density	100%
Wall thickness	0.81
Print duration	4 h 41 min
ABS quantity (cm3)	30.544
Support quantity (cm3)	14.728
Raw material costs (€)	7.26€

7.2.2.12 Board game coins

Rehabilitation device RD12

These coins are used in occupational therapy for various board games designed for patient rehabilitation.

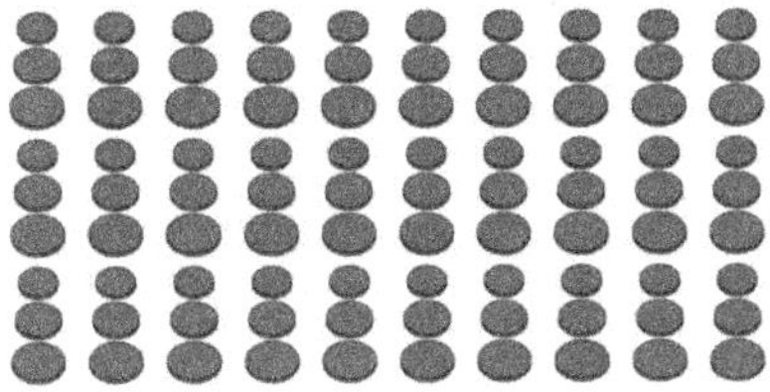

Date of first request	September 2020
Origin of the request	Occupational therapy (Hôpital Cochin)
People involved in design	BONE 3D engineer
Quantity produced	180
Destination	Hôpital Cochin

	One set of coins (90)
Layer thickness (mm)	0.33
Filling density	100%
Wall thickness	1.98
Print duration	2 h 48 min
ABS quantity (cm3)	61.785
Support quantity (cm3)	50.279
Raw material costs (€)	18.32€

7.2.2.13 Wheelchair brake

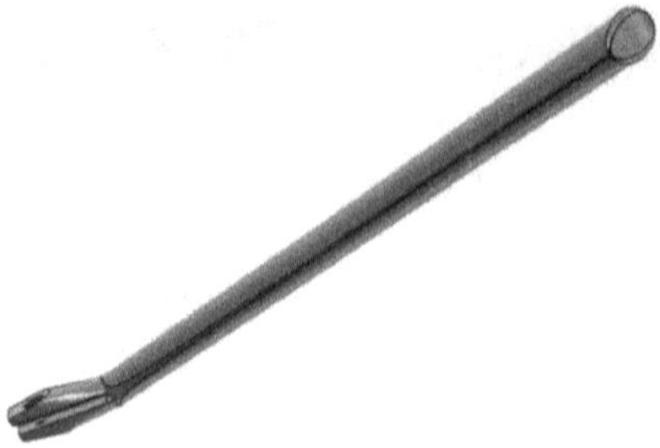

Rehabilitation device RD13

This is a wheelchair brake used in occupational therapy.

Date of first request	September 2020
Origin of the request	Occupational therapy (Hôpital Cochin)
People involved in design	BONE 3D engineer
Quantity produced	1
Destination	Hôpital Cochin

	One brake
Layer thickness (mm)	0.33
Filling density	100%
Wall thickness	1.98
Print duration	2 h 08 min
ABS quantity (cm3)	44.666
Support quantity (cm3)	21.827
Raw material costs (€)	10.73€

7.2.2.14 Large-grip screw-driver

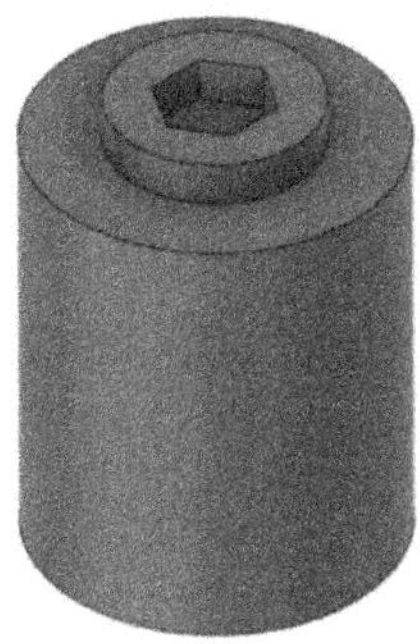

Rehabilitation device RD14

This piece is to help people unscrew or screw with a large grip.

Date of first request	September 2020
Origin of the request	Occupational therapy (Hôpital Cochin)
People involved in design	BONE 3D engineer
Quantity produced	1
Destination	Hôpital Cochin

	One screw holder
Layer thickness (mm)	0.33
Filling density	100%
Wall thickness	1.98
Print duration	48 min
ABS quantity (cm3)	23.403
Support quantity (cm3)	1.864
Raw material costs (€)	4.10€

7.2.2.15 Large-grip bottle-opener

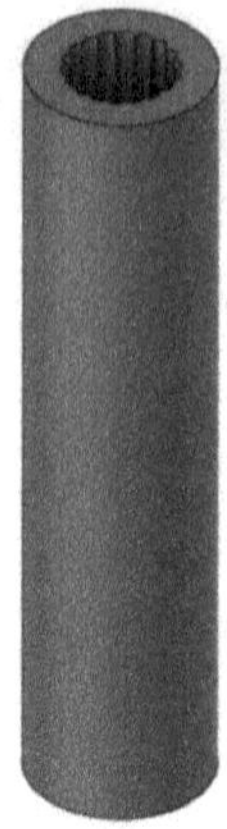

Rehabilitation device RD15

This piece is to help open bottles with a large grip.

Date of first request	September 2020
Origin of the request	Occupational therapy (Hôpital Cochin)
People involved in design	BONE 3D engineer
Quantity produced	1
Destination	Hôpital Cochin

	One handle
Layer thickness (mm)	0.33
Filling density	100%
Wall thickness	1.98
Print duration	1 h 51 min
ABS quantity (cm3)	47.334
Support quantity (cm3)	13.399
Raw material costs (€)	9.90€

7.2.3 General medical equipment

In this category, the medical device status of a significant number of objects is not clear, as they could be reasonably registered as class I devices, in a similar manner as for devices designed for physical therapy. Nevertheless, none of these devices is formally, to our best knowledge, considered as a medical device.

7.2.3.1 Armrest for CT-scan

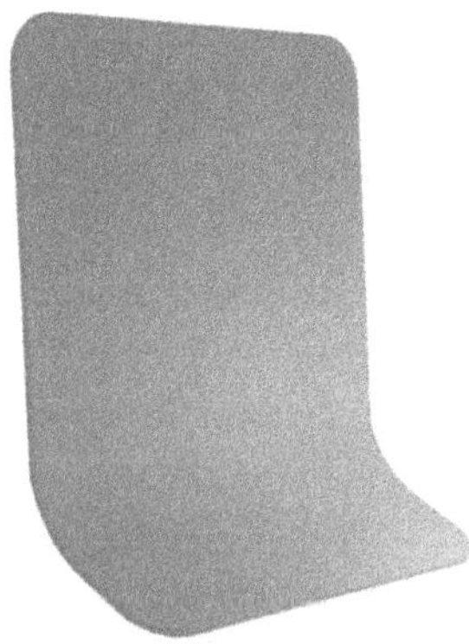

General medical equipment GME1

This device is placed under the trunk of patients undergoing a CT-scan or MRI in prone position.

Date of first request	May 2020
Origin of the request	Radiology department (Hôpital Cochin)
People involved in design	BONE 3D engineer
Quantity produced	20
Destination	Radiology department (Hôpital Cochin)

	One armrest
Layer thickness (mm)	0.33
Filling density	100%
Wall thickness	1.32
Print duration	8 h 31 min
ABS quantity (cm3)	296.80
Support quantity (cm3)	5.27
Raw material costs (€)	54.85€

7.2.3.2 Cable duct for CT-scan

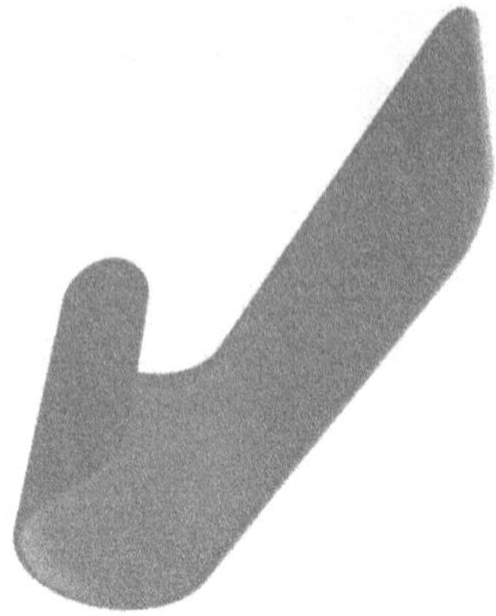

General medical equipment GME2

Date of first request	May 2020
Origin of the request	Radiology department (Hôpital Cochin)
People involved in design	BONE 3D engineer
Quantity produced	20
Destination	Radiology department (Hôpital Cochin)

	One cable duct
Layer thickness (mm)	0.66
Filling density	100%
Wall thickness	1.32
Print duration	4 h 56 min
ABS quantity (cm3)	165.79
Support quantity (cm3)	5.84
Raw material costs (€)	31.17€

7.2.3.3 Coronagrophy probe holder

General medical equipment GME3

This triple-hook allows fixing coronaropathy probes to the wall.

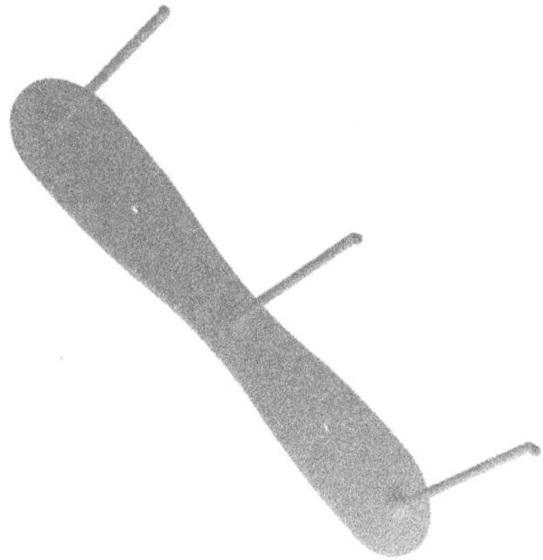

Date of first request	July 2020
Origin of the request	Intensive care unit (Hôpital Cochin)
People involved in design	BONE 3D engineer
Quantity produced	20
Destination	Intensive care unit (Hôpital Cochin)

	One probe holder
Layer thickness (mm)	0.66
Filling density	100%
Wall thickness	1.32
Print duration	3 h 08 min
ABS quantity (cm3)	46.53
Support quantity (cm3)	29.54
Raw material costs (€)	13.82€

7.2.3.4 Transfusion bag holder

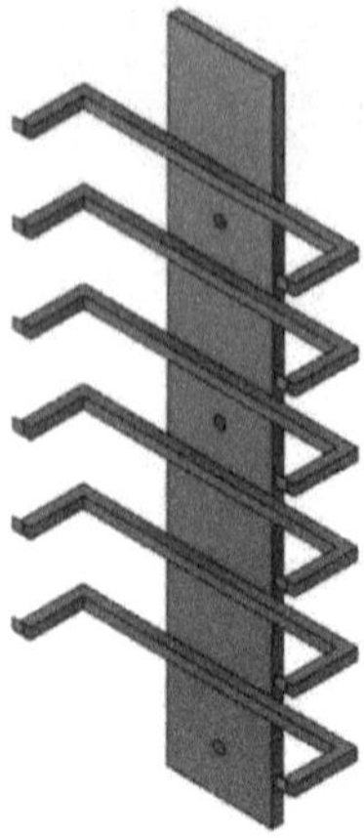

General medical equipment GME4

This device is used to hang transfusion bags.

Date of first request	September 2020
Origin of the request	Logistic department (Hôpital Cochin)
People involved in design	BONE 3D engineer
Quantity produced	2
Destination	Hôpital Cochin

	One bag holder
Layer thickness (mm)	0.33
Filling density	100%
Wall thickness	1.98
Print duration	4 h 37 min
ABS quantity (cm3)	86.002
Support quantity (cm3)	51.97
Raw material costs (€)	22.61€

7.2.3.5 MRI syringe holder

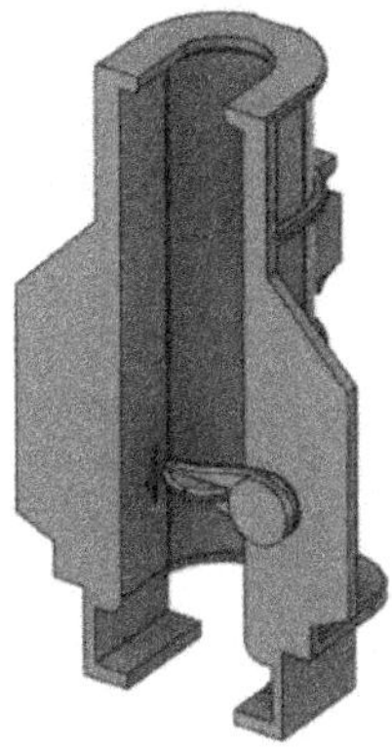

General medical equipment GME5

This is an injector holder for MRI, carrying the syringe containing the agent.

Date of first request	September 2020
Origin of the request	Radiology department (Hôpital Cochin)
People involved in design	BONE 3D engineer
Quantity produced	2
Destination	Hôpital Cochin

	One syringe holder
Layer thickness (mm)	0.33
Filling density	100%
Wall thickness	1.98
Print duration	2 h 24 min
ABS quantity (cm3)	27.19
Support quantity (cm3)	29.269
Raw material costs (€)	9.24€

7.2.3.6 Injector holrderr

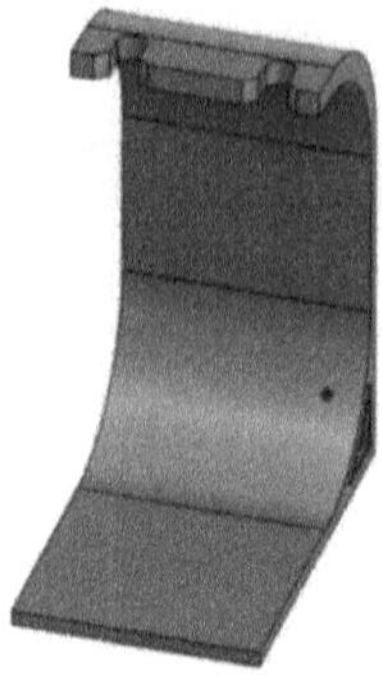

General medical equipment GME6

This is piece is designed to hold injectors.

Date of first request	April 2020
Origin of the request	Reproduction medicine (Hôpital Cochin)
People involved in design	BONE 3D engineer
Quantity produced	10
Destination	Hôpital Cochin

	One injector
Layer thickness (mm)	0.33
Filling density	100%
Wall thickness	1.98
Print duration	9 h 42 min
ABS quantity (cm3)	235.231
Support quantity (cm3)	90.409
Raw material costs (€)	53.63€

7.2.3.7 Salt spoon

General medical equipment GME7

This is a 1 g salt spoon, for patients requiring a strict diet control.

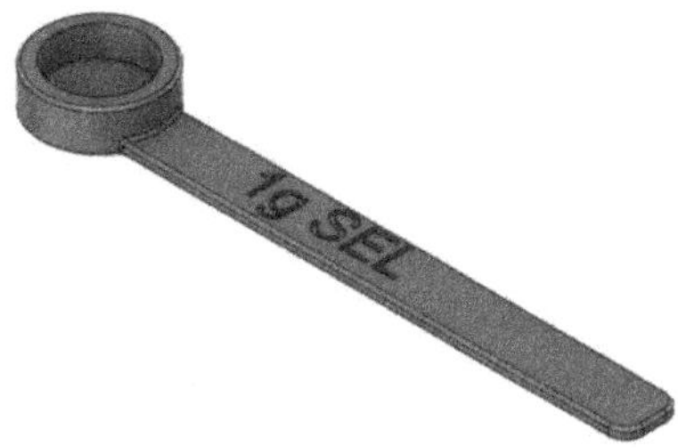

Date of first request	Septembre 2020
Origin of the request	Hôpital Cochin
People involved in design	BONE 3D engineer
Quantity produced	2000
Destination	Hôpital Cochin

	One injector
Layer thickness (mm)	0.33
Filling density	100%
Wall thickness	1.98
Print duration	31 min
ABS quantity (cm3)	4.314
Support quantity (cm3)	4.814
Raw material costs (€)	1.32€

7.2.3.8 Wrist band

General medical equipment GME8

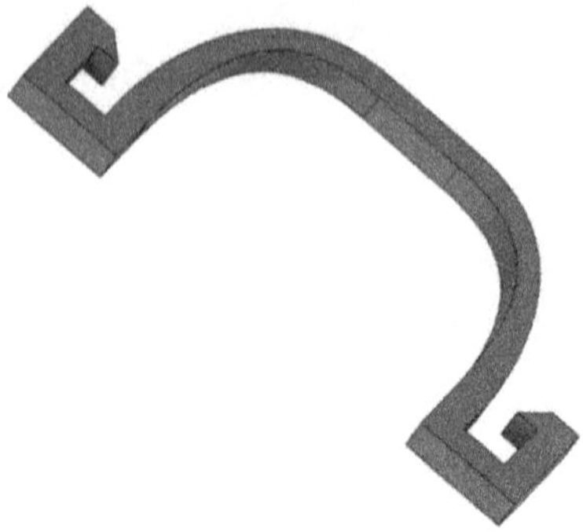

This is a device used in sleep medicine to attach various captors to the wrist of patients.

Date of first request	Septembre 2020
Origin of the request	Sleep medicine (Hôpital Cochin)
People involved in design	BONE 3D engineer
Quantity produced	10
Destination	Hôpital Cochin

	One wrist band
Layer thickness (mm)	0.33
Filling density	100%
Wall thickness	1.98
Print duration	5 min
ABS quantity (cm3)	0.887
Support quantity (cm3)	1.08
Raw material costs (€)	0.30€

7.2.3.9 Polysomnography box

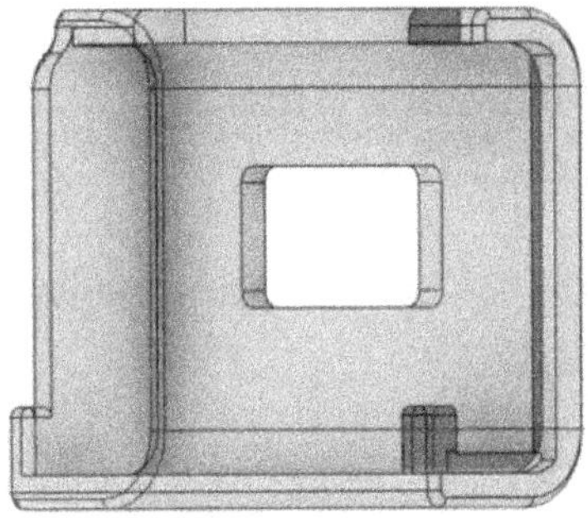

General medical equipment GME9

This is a protective box for somnography devices.

Date of first request	09/01/2020
Origin of the request	Cardiology department (Hôpital Cochin)
People involved in design	BONE 3D engineer
Quantity produced	30
Destination	Hôpital Cochin

	One box
Layer thickness (mm)	0.33
Filling density	100%
Wall thickness	1.98
Print duration	1h39 min
ABS quantity (cm3)	48.933
Support quantity (cm3)	12.864
Raw material costs (€)	9.90€

7.2.3.10 Polysomnography box (large size)

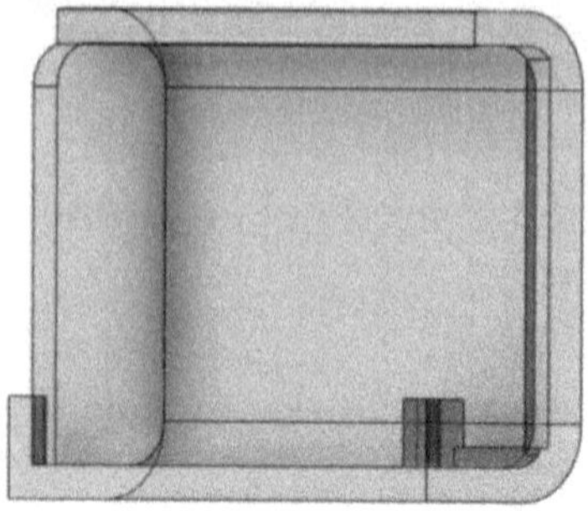

General medical equipment GME10

This is a larger protective box for somnograph devices.

Date of first request	September 2020
Origin of the request	Cardiology department (Hôpital Cochin)
People involved in design	BONE 3D engineer
Quantity produced	10
Destination	Hôpital Cochin

	One box
Layer thickness (mm)	0.33
Filling density	100%
Wall thickness	1.98
Print duration	1h46 min
ABS quantity (cm3)	52.711
Support quantity (cm3)	13.795
Raw material costs (€)	10.73€

7.2.3.11 Craddle number tags

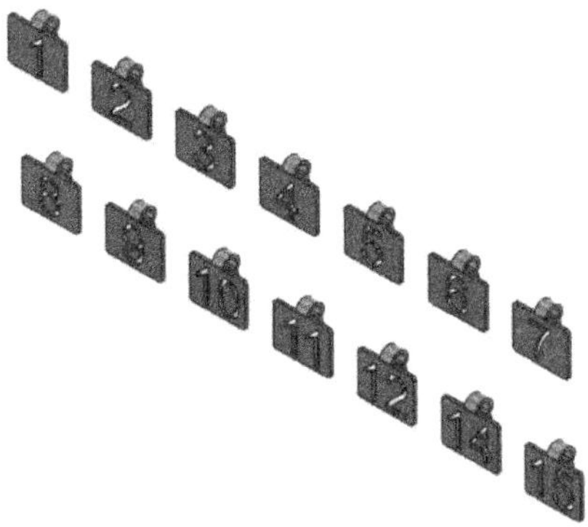

General medical equipment GME11

This device is intended to be used during the transfer of patients in cradles from the operating room to recovery, in order to avoid using name tags on beds in public areas.

Date of first request	May 2020
Origin of the request	Operating room head nurse (Hôpital Necker - Enfants Malades)
People involved in design	BONE 3D engineer
Quantity produced	30
Destination	Hôpital Necker - Enfants Malades

	One set of 14 tags
Layer thickness (mm)	0.33
Filling density	100%
Wall thickness	1.32
Print duration	1 h 20 min
ABS quantity (cm3)	34.05
Support quantity (cm3)	16.72
Raw material costs (€)	9.22€

7.2.3.12 Bed number tags

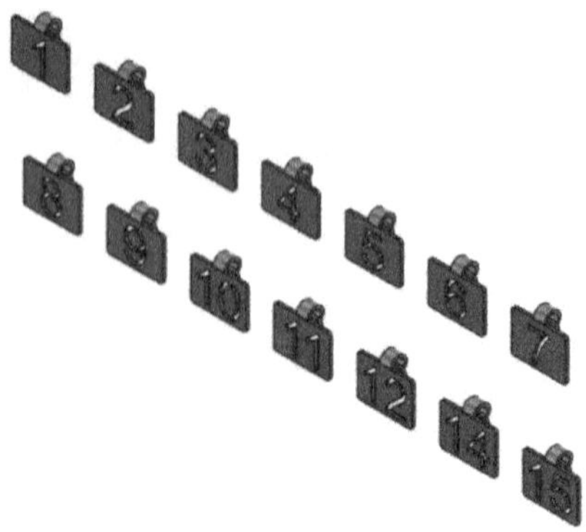

General medical equipment GME12

This device is intended to be used during the transfer of patients in beds from the operating room to recovery, in order to avoid using name tags on beds in public areas.

Date of first request	May 2020
Origin of the request	Operating room head nurse (Hôpital Necker - Enfants Malades)
People involved in design	BONE 3D engineer
Quantity produced	30
Destination	Hôpital Necker - Enfants Malades

	One set of 14 tags
Layer thickness (mm)	0.33
Filling density	100%
Wall thickness	1.32
Print duration	1 h 46 min
ABS quantity (cm3)	38.83
Support quantity (cm3)	22.85
Raw material costs (€)	11.20€

7.2.3.13 Bed cable duct

General medical equipment GME13

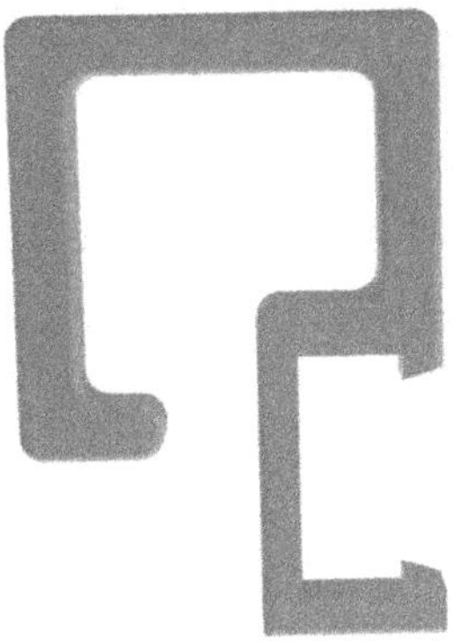

This device was designed for Phillips beds and allows the various cables to be sorted so that they do not get tangled.

Date of first request	July 2020
Origin of the request	Cardiology department (Hôpital Cochin)
People involved in design	BONE 3D engineer
Quantity produced	40
Destination	Cardiology department (Hôpital Cochin)

	One cable duct
Layer thickness (mm)	0.33
Filling density	100%
Wall thickness	1.32
Print duration	18 min
ABS quantity (cm3)	7.84
Support quantity (cm3)	3.02
Raw material costs (€)	1.98€

7.2.3.14 Anti-theft support for hand gel

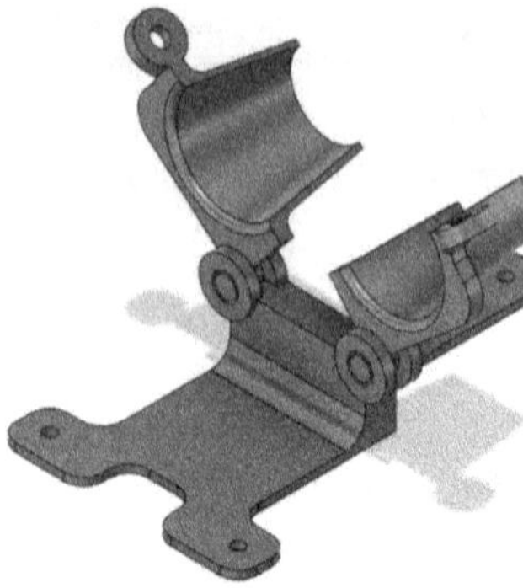

General medical equipment GME14

This wall-mounted device is equipped with an anti-theft system.

Date of first request	July 2020
Origin of the request	Occupational Therapy (Hôpital Cochin)
People involved in design	BONE 3D engineer
Quantity produced	5
Destination	Hôpital Cochin

	One support
Layer thickness (mm)	0.33
Filling density	100%
Wall thickness	1.32
Print duration	6 h 10 min
ABS quantity (cm3)	98.62
Support quantity (cm3)	55.11
Raw material costs (€)	27.92€

7.2.3.15 Standard support for hand gel

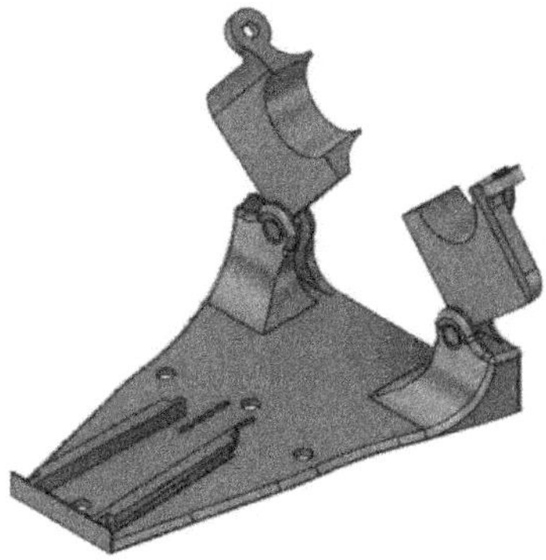

General medical equipment GME15

This piece is a support for hydrogel without the anti-theft system.

Date of first request	July 2020
Origin of the request	Occupational Therapy (Hôpital Cochin)
People involved in design	BONE 3D engineer
Quantity produced	52
Destination	Hôpital Cochin

	One hydrogel support
Layer thickness (mm)	0.33
Filling density	100%
Wall thickness	1.98
Print duration	6 h 07 min
ABS quantity (cm3)	96.636
Support quantity (cm3)	53.636
Raw material costs (€)	24.60€

7.2.3.16 Oxygen carboy support

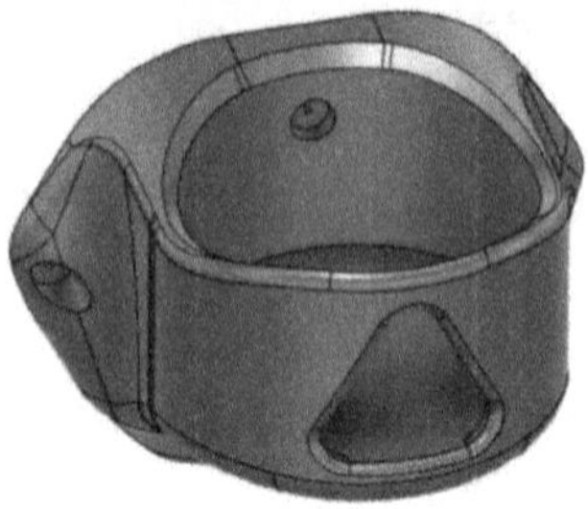

General medical equipment GME16

This is piece designed to hold an O2 carboy.

Date of first request	August 2020
Origin of the request	Intensive care (Hôpital Cochin)
People involved in design	BONE 3D engineer
Quantity produced	10
Destination	Hôpital Cochin

	One carboy
Layer thickness (mm)	0.33
Filling density	100%
Wall thickness	1.98
Print duration	2 d 3 h 23 min
ABS quantity (cm3)	1678.509
Support quantity (cm3)	413.085
Raw material costs (€)	345€

7.2.3.17 Secure briefcase for narcotics

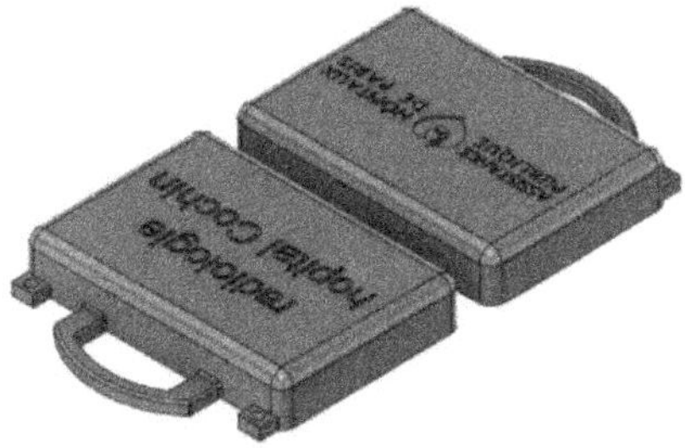

General medical equipment GME17

This briefcase was created to transport narcotic drugs within the hospital.

Date of first request	July 2020
Origin of the request	Hôpital Cochin
People involved in design	BONE 3D engineer
Quantity produced	1
Destination	Hôpital Cochin

	One briefcase
Layer thickness (mm)	0.33
Filling density	100%
Wall thickness	1.98
Print duration	1 d 13 h 18 min
ABS quantity (cm3)	650.386
Support quantity (cm3)	520.119
Raw material costs (€)	193€

7.2.4 Laboratory equipment

7.2.4.1 Radioactive storage plate

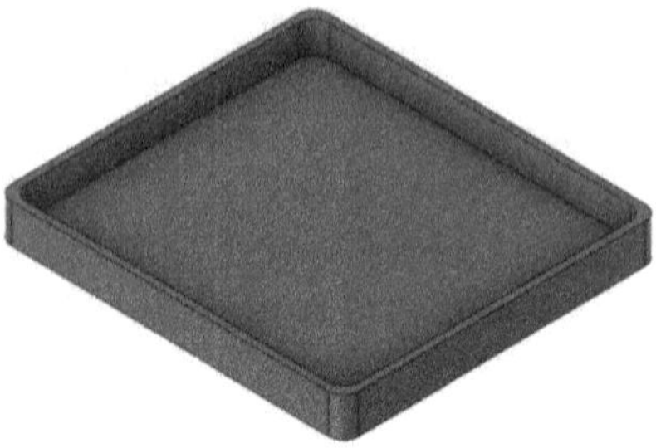

Laboratory equipment LE1

This plate is covered by a lead plate.

Date of first request	September 2020
Origin of the request	Sleep medicine (Hôpital Cochin)
People involved in design	BONE 3D engineer
Quantity produced	40
Destination	Hôpital Cochin

	One plate
Layer thickness (mm)	0.33
Filling density	100%
Wall thickness	1.98
Print duration	7 h 29 min
ABS quantity (cm3)	328.154
Support quantity (cm3)	68.446
Raw material costs (€)	65.01€

7.2.4.2 Cryotube №1

Laboratory equipment LE2

This tube is used in the Biological Resource Centre of the Hôpital Cochin to store plasma or other fluids in liquid nitrogen at -196°C.

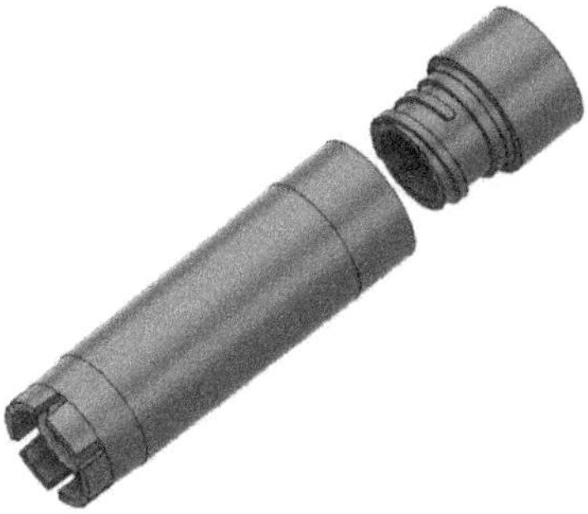

Date of first request	September 2020
Origin of the request	Hôpital Cochin
People involved in design	BONE 3D engineer
Quantity produced	1
Destination	Hôpital Cochin

	One tube
Layer thickness (mm)	0.33
Filling density	100%
Wall thickness	1.32
Print duration	50 min
ABS quantity (cm3)	5.532
Support quantity (cm3)	7.749
Raw material costs (€)	1.98€

7.2.4.3 Cryotube №2

Laboratory equipment LE3

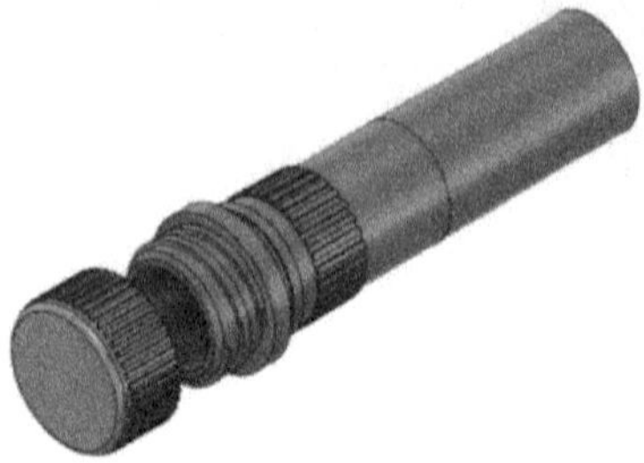

This tube is used in the Biological Resource Centre of the Hôpital Cochin to store plasma or other fluids in liquid nitrogen at -80°C.

Date of first request	September 2020
Origin of the request	Hôpital Cochin
People involved in design	BONE 3D engineer
Quantity produced	1
Destination	Hôpital Cochin

	One tube
Layer thickness (mm)	0.25
Filling density	100%
Wall thickness	1.32
Print duration	1 h 46 min
ABS quantity (cm3)	38.83
Support quantity (cm3)	22.85
Raw material costs (€)	9.90 €

7.2.4.4 Rectangular plate

Laboratory equipment LE4

This is a rectangular plastic plate for the reproduction medicine service.

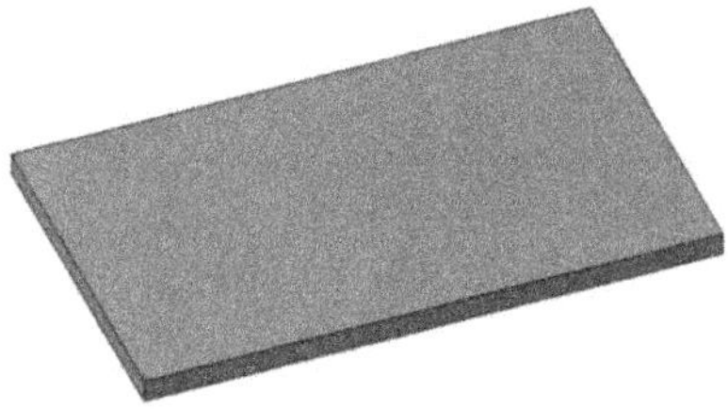

Date of first request	September 2020
Origin of the request	Hôpital Cochin
People involved in design	BONE 3D engineer
Quantity produced	2
Destination	Hôpital Cochin

	One plate
Layer thickness (mm)	0.33
Filling density	100%
Wall thickness	0.81
Print duration	1 d 20 h 33 min
ABS quantity (cm3)	356.72
Support quantity (cm3)	42.624
Raw material costs (€)	66.66 €

7.2.4.5 Vial holder №2/3

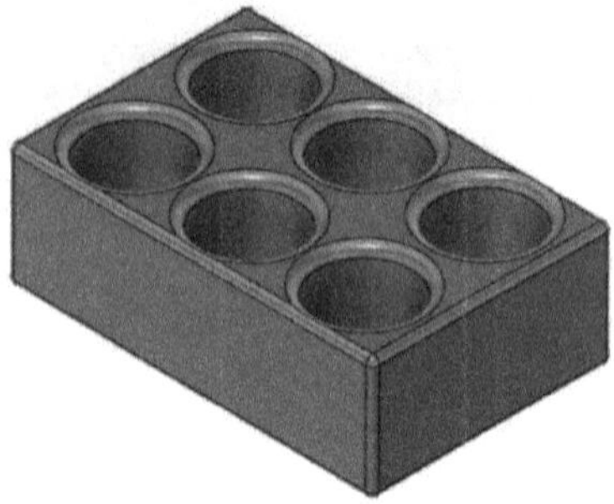

Laboratory equipment LE5

This is 2 x 3 vials holder.

Date of first request	September 2020
Origin of the request	Pharmacy (Hôpital Cochin)
People involved in design	BONE 3D engineer
Quantity produced	10
Destination	Hôpital Cochin

	One holder
Layer thickness (mm)	0.33
Filling density	100%
Wall thickness	1.98
Print duration	51 min
ABS quantity (cm3)	18.062
Support quantity (cm3)	3.191
Raw material costs (€)	3.47 €

7.2.4.6 Vial holder №2/5

Laboratory equipment LE6

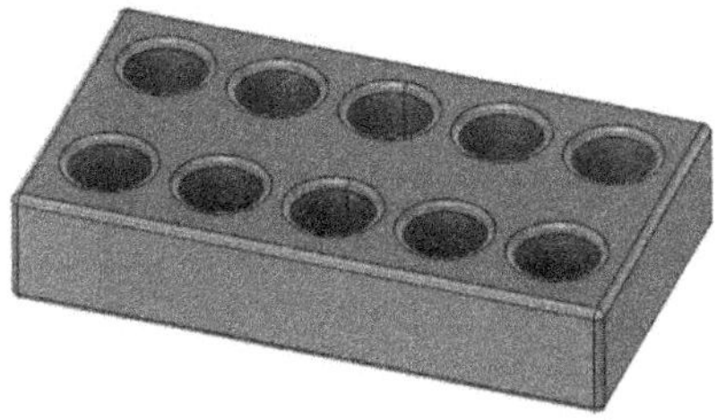

This is an Erlenmeyer holder for pharmaceutical preparations.

Date of first request	September 2020
Origin of the request	Pharmacy (Hôpital Cochin)
People involved in design	BONE 3D engineer
Quantity produced	10
Destination	Hôpital Cochin

	One holder
Layer thickness (mm)	0.33
Filling density	100%
Wall thickness	1.98
Print duration	1 h 35 min
ABS quantity (cm3)	20.365
Support quantity (cm3)	12.08
Raw material costs (€)	5.28 €

7.2.4.7 Vial holder №2/10

Laboratory equipment LE7

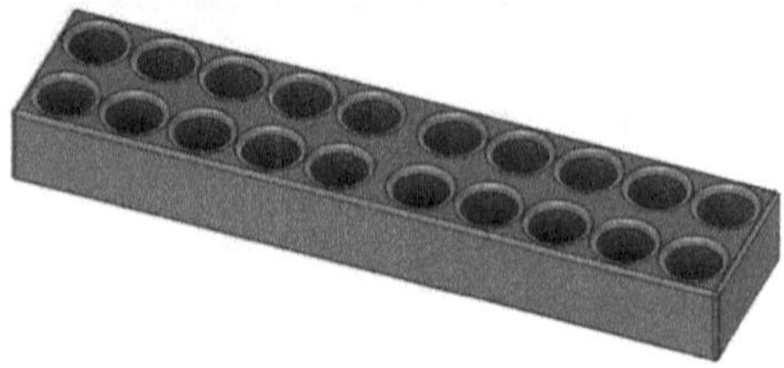

This is a 2 x 10 vial holder.

Date of first request	September 2020
Origin of the request	Pharmacy (Hôpital Cochin)
People involved in design	BONE 3D engineer
Quantity produced	10
Destination	Hôpital Cochin

	One holder
Layer thickness (mm)	0.33
Filling density	100%
Wall thickness	1.98
Print duration	2 h 29 min
ABS quantity (cm3)	50.356
Support quantity (cm3)	8.503
Raw material costs (€)	9.57 €

7.2.4.8 Mini vial holder №2/10

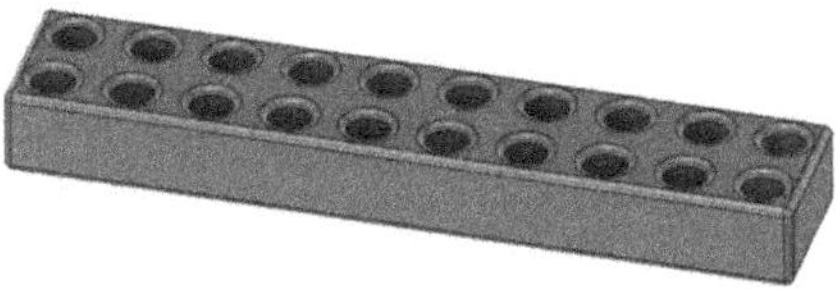

Laboratory equipment LE8

This is a 2 x 10 vial holder.

Date of first request	September 2020
Origin of the request	Pharmacy (Hôpital Cochin)
People involved in design	BONE 3D engineer
Quantity produced	10
Destination	Hôpital Cochin

	One holder
Layer thickness (mm)	0.33
Filling density	100%
Wall thickness	1.98
Print duration	2 h 29 min
ABS quantity (cm3)	50.356
Support quantity (cm3)	8.503
Raw material costs (€)	9.57 €

7.2.4.9 Vial holder №5P10/D15.6

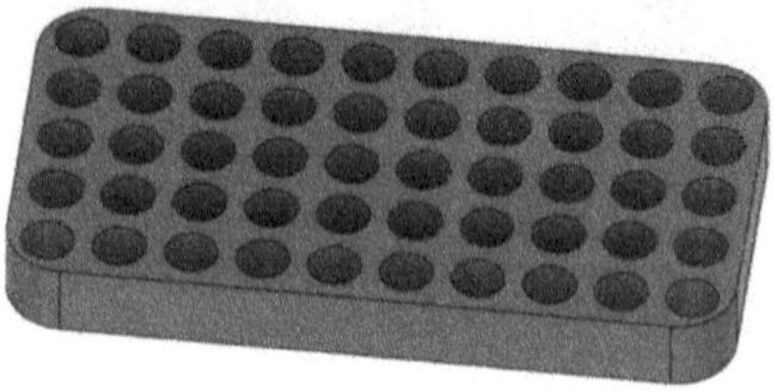

Laboratory equipment LE9

This is a 5P10 D15.6 vial holder.

Date of first request	September 2020
Origin of the request	Virology (Hôpital Cochin)
People involved in design	BONE 3D engineer
Quantity produced	10
Destination	Hôpital Cochin

	One holder
Layer thickness (mm)	0.33
Filling density	100%
Wall thickness	1.98
Print duration	9 h 13 min
ABS quantity (cm3)	234.385
Support quantity (cm3)	28.365
Raw material costs (€)	43.23 €

7.2.4.10 Vial holder №5P10 poly

Laboratory equipment LE10

This is a 5P10 poly vial holder.

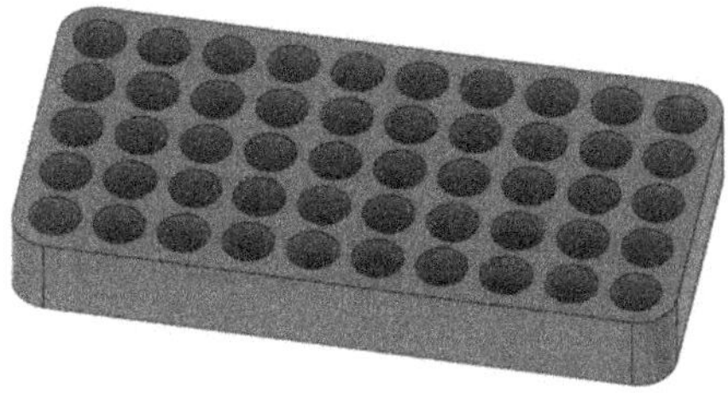

Date of first request	September 2020
Origin of the request	Virology (Hôpital Cochin)
People involved in design	BONE 3D engineer
Quantity produced	20
Destination	Hôpital Cochin

	One holder
Layer thickness (mm)	0.33
Filling density	100%
Wall thickness	1.98
Print duration	7 h 19 min
ABS quantity (cm3)	145.914
Support quantity (cm3)	18.548
Raw material costs (€)	26.90 €

7.2.4.11 Vial holder №5P10/D10

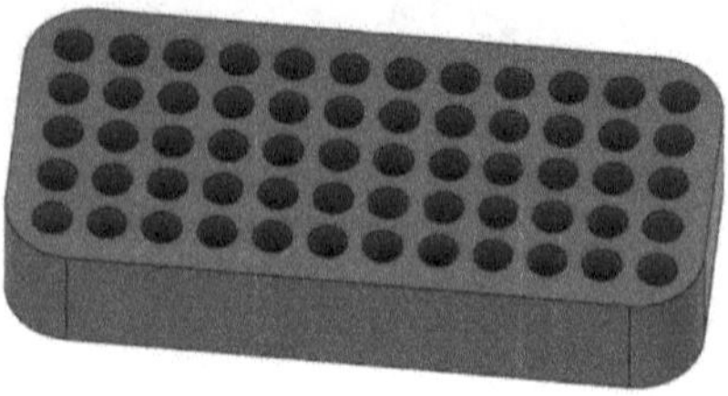

Laboratory equipment LE11

This is a 5P10 D10 vial holder.

Date of first request	September 2020
Origin of the request	Virology (Hôpital Cochin)
People involved in design	BONE 3D engineer
Quantity produced	20
Destination	Hôpital Cochin

	One holder
Layer thickness (mm)	0.33
Filling density	100%
Wall thickness	1.32
Print duration	1 h 46 min
ABS quantity (cm3)	38.83
Support quantity (cm3)	22.20
Raw material costs (€)	11.20 €

7.2.4.12 Vial holder №5P12/D10

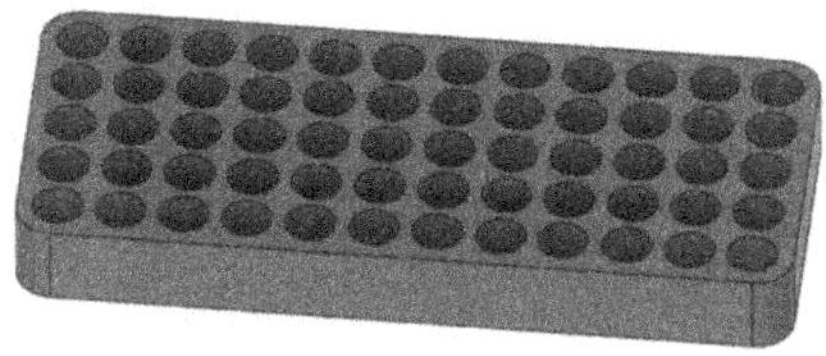

Laboratory equipment LE12

This is a 5P12 D10 vial holder.

Date of first request	September 2020
Origin of the request	Virology (Hôpital Cochin)
People involved in design	BONE 3D engineer
Quantity produced	15
Destination	Hôpital Cochin

	One holder
Layer thickness (mm)	0.33
Filling density	100%
Wall thickness	1.98
Print duration	9 h 05 min
ABS quantity (cm3)	165.568
Support quantity (cm3)	63.808
Raw material costs (€)	37.62 €

7.2.4.13 Vial holder №5P10/D10

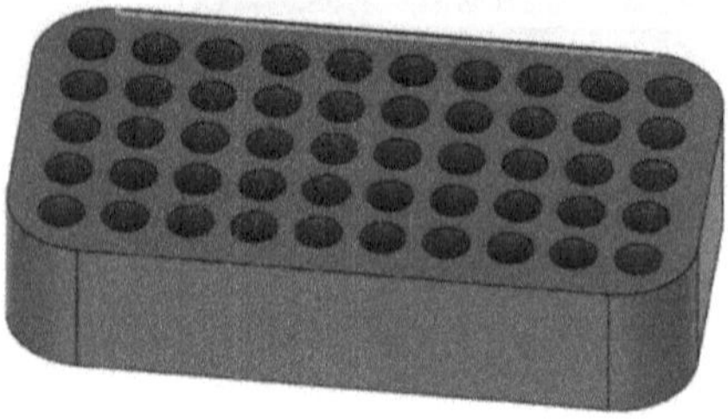

Laboratory equipment LE13

This is a 5P10 D10 vial holder.

Date of first request	September 2020
Origin of the request	Virology (Hôpital Cochin)
People involved in design	BONE 3D engineer
Quantity produced	10
Destination	Hôpital Cochin

	One holder
Layer thickness (mm)	0.33
Filling density	100%
Wall thickness	1.32
Print duration	1 h 46 min
ABS quantity (cm3)	38.83
Support quantity (cm3)	22.85
Raw material costs (€)	11.20 €

7.2.4.14 Vial holder Nº5P15

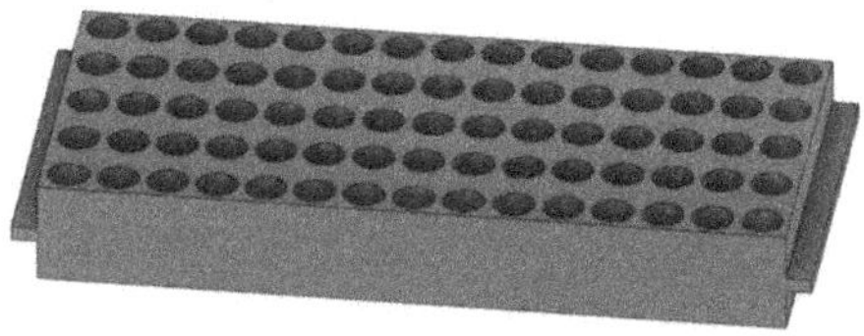

Laboratory equipment LE14

This is a 5P15 vial holder.

Date of first request	September 2020
Origin of the request	Hôpital Cochin
People involved in design	BONE 3D engineer
Quantity produced	25
Destination	Hôpital Cochin

	One holder
Layer thickness (mm)	0.33
Filling density	100%
Wall thickness	1.98
Print duration	11 h 12 min
ABS quantity (cm3)	207.634
Support quantity (cm3)	29.572
Raw material costs (€)	38.94 €

7.2.4.15 Vial holder №5P5

Laboratory equipment LE15

This is a 10P5 vial holder.

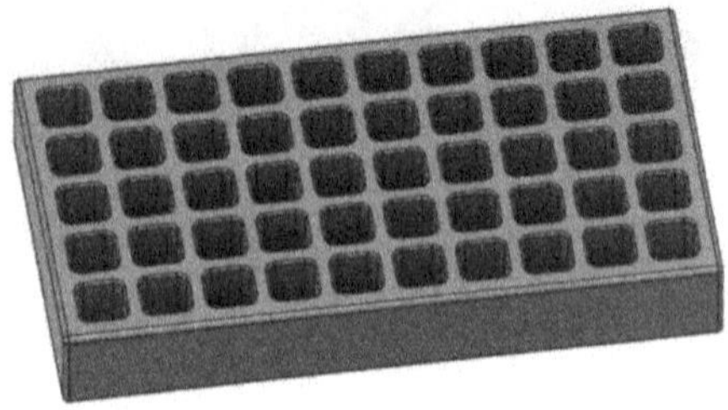

Date of first request	September 2020
Origin of the request	Virology (Hôpital Cochin)
People involved in design	BONE 3D engineer
Quantity produced	15
Destination	Hôpital Cochin

	One holder
Layer thickness (mm)	0.33
Filling density	100%
Wall thickness	1.98
Print duration	17 h 53 min
ABS quantity (cm3)	420
Support quantity (cm3)	38.596
Raw material costs (€)	75.57 €

7.2.4.16 Vial holder №12P58

Laboratory equipment LE16

This is a 12P9 vial holder.

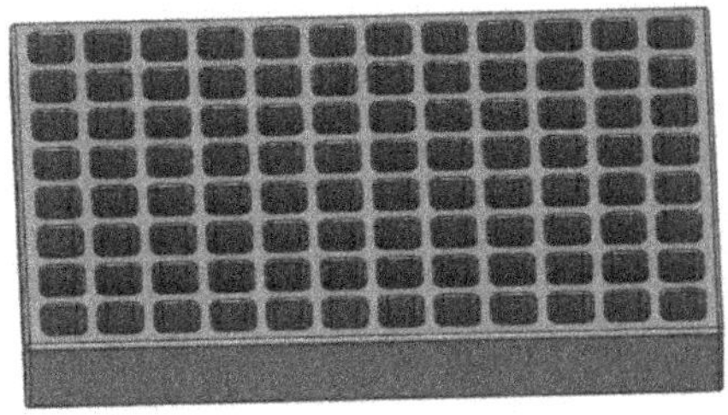

Date of first request	September 2020
Origin of the request	Hôpital Cochin
People involved in design	BONE 3D engineer
Quantity produced	1
Destination	Hôpital Cochin

	One holder
Layer thickness (mm)	0.33
Filling density	100%
Wall thickness	1.98
Print duration	1 d 10 h 12 min
ABS quantity (cm3)	752.145
Support quantity (cm3)	68.693
Raw material costs (€)	135.30 €

7.2.4.17 Vial holder №10P10
Laboratory equipment LE17

This is a 10P10 vial holder.

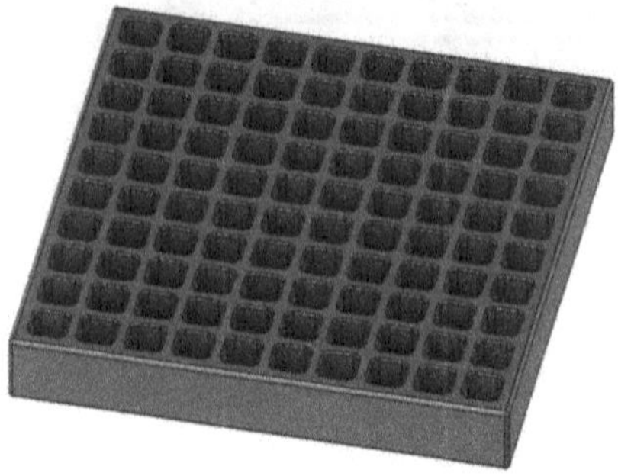

Date of first request	September 2020
Origin of the request	Hôpital Cochin
People involved in design	BONE 3D engineer
Quantity produced	50
Destination	Hôpital Cochin

	One holder
Layer thickness (mm)	0.33
Filling density	100%
Wall thickness	1.98
Print duration	16 h 36 min
ABS quantity (cm3)	412.086
Support quantity (cm3)	48.554
Raw material costs (€)	75.90 €

7.2.4.18 Erlenmeyer holder

Laboratory equipment LE18

This is an Erlenmeyer holder.

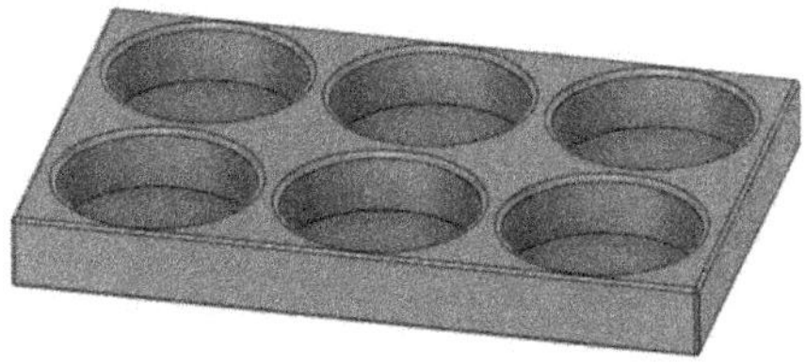

Date of first request	September 2020
Origin of the request	Pharmacy (Hôpital Cochin)
People involved in design	BONE 3D engineer
Quantity produced	15
Destination	Hôpital Cochin

	One holder
Layer thickness (mm)	0.33
Filling density	100%
Wall thickness	1.98
Print duration	3 h 33 min
ABS quantity (cm3)	121.911
Support quantity (cm3)	23.613
Raw material costs (€)	23.76 €

7.2.4.19 Centrifugation tube holder

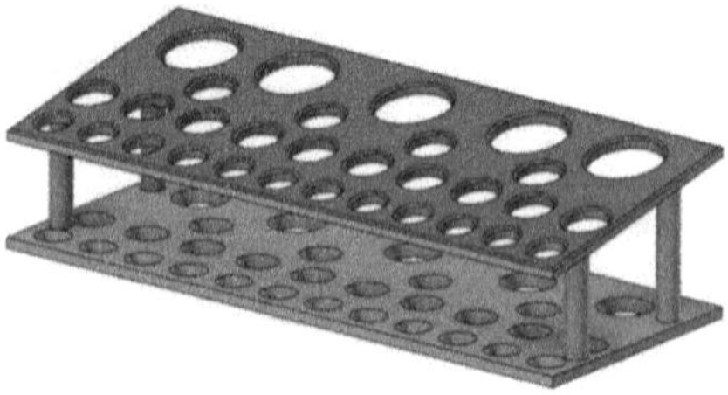

Laboratory equipment LE19

This is a centrifugation tube holder.

Date of first request	September 2020
Origin of the request	Hôpital Cochin
People involved in design	BONE 3D engineer
Quantity produced	30
Destination	Hôpital Cochin

	One holder
Layer thickness (mm)	0.33
Filling density	100%
Wall thickness	1.98
Print duration	9 h 44 min
ABS quantity (cm3)	148.037
Support quantity (cm3)	163.643
Raw material costs (€)	51.32 €

7.2.4.20 Test-tube holder

Laboratory equipment LE20

This is a rack to hold blood test-tubes.

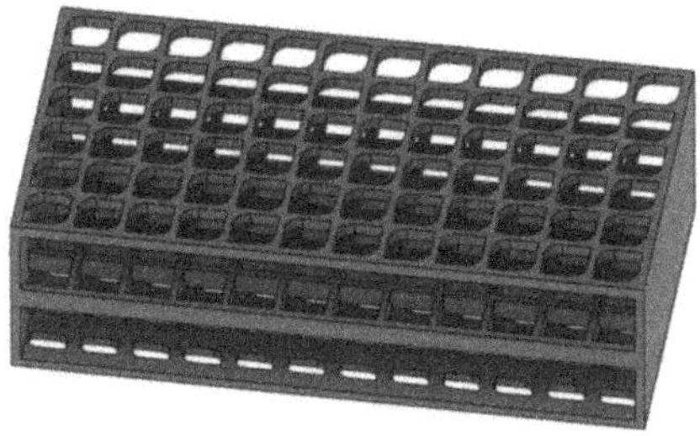

Date of first request	September 2020
Origin of the request	Pharmacy (Hôpital Cochin)
People involved in design	BONE 3D engineer
Quantity produced	20
Destination	Hôpital Cochin

	One holder
Layer thickness (mm)	0.33
Filling density	100%
Wall thickness	1.98
Print duration	9 h 58 min
ABS quantity (cm3)	129.821
Support quantity (cm3)	157.717
Raw material costs (€)	47.19 €

7.2.4.21 Tube holder №6P15

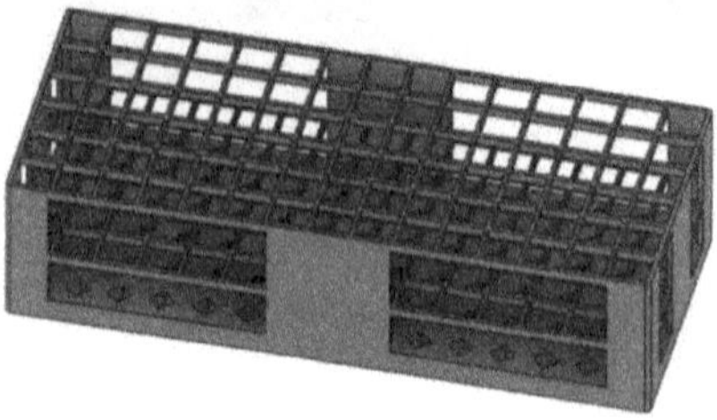

Laboratory equipment LE21

This is a 6P15 tube holder.

Date of first request	September 2020
Origin of the request	Immunology (Hôpital Cochin)
People involved in design	BONE 3D engineer
Quantity produced	1
Destination	Hôpital Cochin

	One holder
Layer thickness (mm)	0.33
Filling density	100%
Wall thickness	1.98
Print duration	16 h 52 min
ABS quantity (cm3)	188.398
Support quantity (cm3)	194.826
Raw material costs (€)	63.03 €

7.2.4.22 Cylinder pole

Laboratory equipment LE22

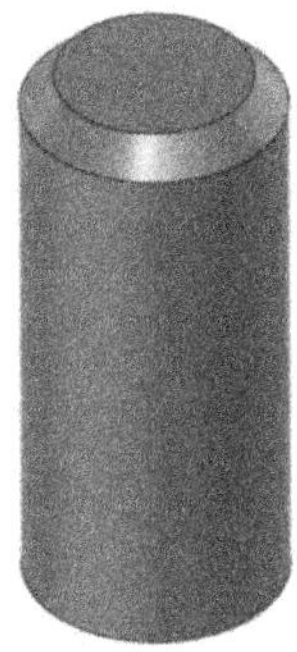

This device is a cylinder pole for pharmaceutical preparations used to calibrate the machine that labels medicine boxes.

Date of first request	September 2020
Origin of the request	Pharmacy (Hôpital Cochin)
People involved in design	BONE 3D engineer
Quantity produced	10
Destination	Hôpital Cochin

	One pole-w
Layer thickness (mm)	0.33
Filling density	100%
Wall thickness	1.98
Print duration	46 min
ABS quantity (cm3)	18.679
Support quantity (cm3)	1.173
Raw material costs (€)	3.14 €

7.2.4.23 Syringe tray

Laboratory equipment LE23

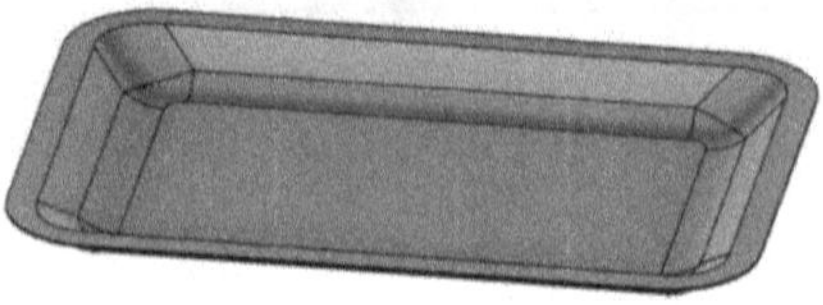

This is a syringe tray.

Date of first request	September 2020
Origin of the request	Cytogenetics (Hôpital Cochin)
People involved in design	BONE 3D engineer
Quantity produced	10
Destination	Hôpital Cochin

	One tray
Layer thickness (mm)	0.33
Filling density	100%
Wall thickness	1.98
Print duration	3 h 40 min
ABS quantity (cm3)	52.906
Support quantity (cm3)	99.746
Raw material costs (€)	24.92 €

7.2.4.24 Test-tube nitrogen rack

Laboratory equipment LE24

This device is a tray for storing the specimens in liquid nitrogen. Interestingly, developing this device allowed to show that TPU can be submitted to low temperatures. Further formal testing of this property has to be performed.

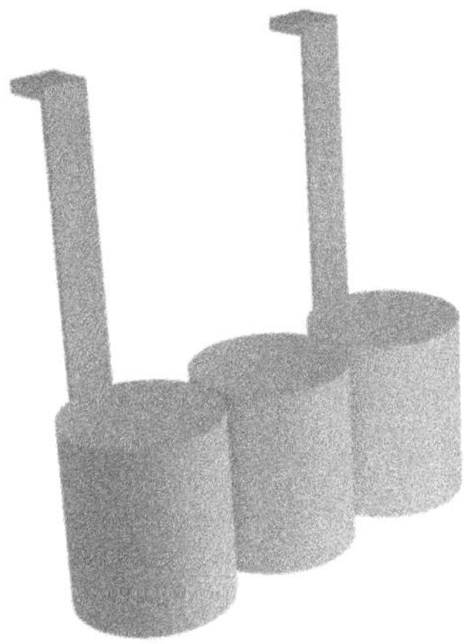

Date of first request	July 2020
Origin of the request	Reproductive medicine (Hôpital Cochin)
People involved in design	BONE 3D engineer
Quantity produced	1
Destination	Reproductive medicine (Hôpital Cochin)

	One rack
Layer thickness (mm)	0.33
Filling density	100%
Wall thickness	1.32
Print duration	30 h 52 min
TPU quantity (cm3)	52.79
Support quantity (cm3)	385.42
Raw material costs (€)	91.72 €

7.2.4.25 Cover №1

Laboratory equipment LE25

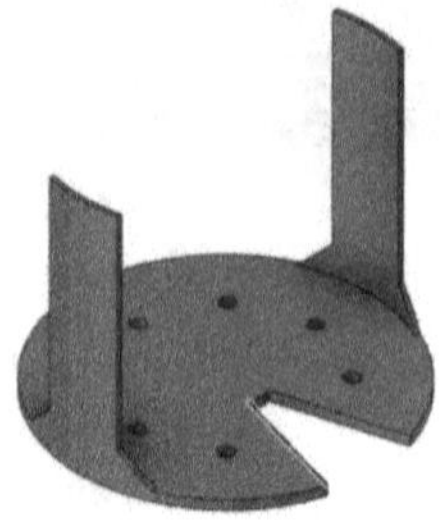

This device is a cover designed for the Reproductive medicine department.

Date of first request	September 2020
Origin of the request	Fertility medicine (Hôpital Cochin)
People involved in design	BONE 3D engineer
Quantity produced	5
Destination	Hôpital Cochin

	One cover
Layer thickness (mm)	0.33
Filling density	100%
Wall thickness	0.81
Print duration	3 h 02 min
ABS quantity (cm3)	14.162
Support quantity (cm3)	4.651
Raw material costs (€)	4.89 €

7.2.4.26 Cover №2

Laboratory equipment LE26

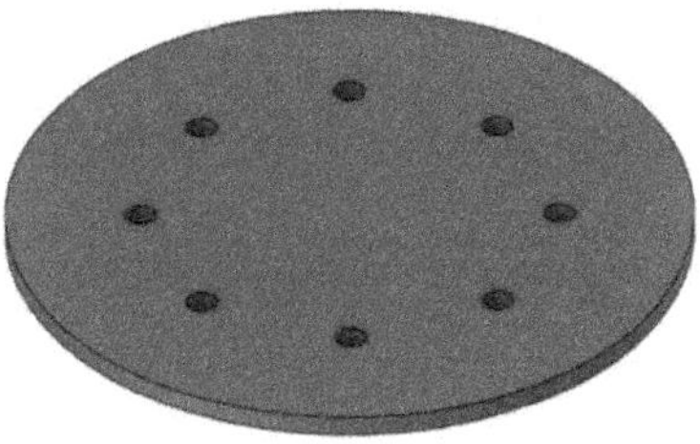

This device is another cover designed for the Reproductive medicine department.

Date of first request	July 2020
Origin of the request	Reproductive medicine (Hôpital Cochin)
People involved in design	BONE 3D engineer
Quantity produced	1
Destination	Hôpital Cochin

	One cover
Layer thickness (mm)	0.33
Filling density	100%
Wall thickness	0.81
Print duration	1 h 05 min
ABS quantity (cm3)	6.832
Support quantity (cm3)	4.862
Raw material costs (€)	2.99 €

7.2.4.27 Cover №3

Laboratory equipment LE27

This device is yet another cover designed for the Reproductive medicine department.

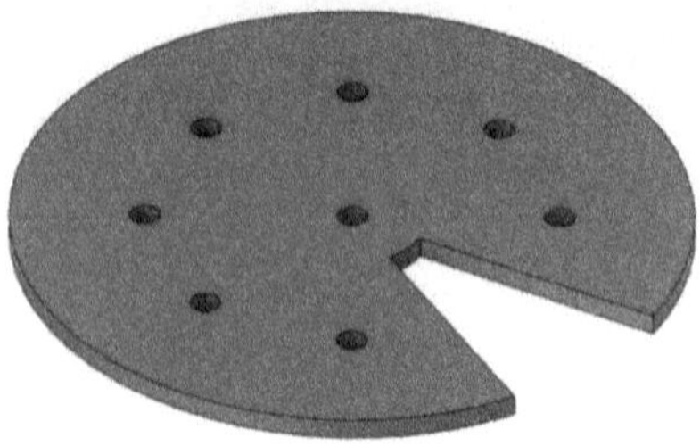

Date of first request	September 2020
Origin of the request	Reproductive medicine (Hôpital Cochin)
People involved in design	BONE 3D engineer
Quantity produced	5
Destination	Hôpital Cochin

	One cover
Layer thickness (mm)	0.33
Filling density	100%
Wall thickness	0.81
Print duration	1 h 05 min
ABS quantity (cm3)	6.732
Support quantity (cm3)	4.862
Raw material costs (€)	2.96 €

7.2.4.28 Bell for Petri dish

Laboratory equipment LE28

This piece is a bell for petri boxes.

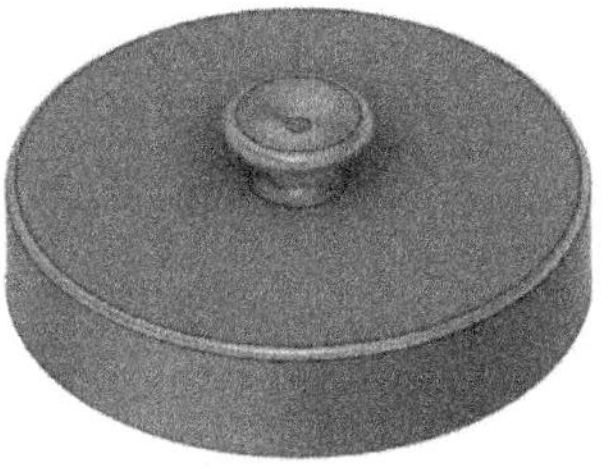

Date of first request	July 2020
Origin of the request	Reproductive medicine (Hôpital Cochin)
People involved in design	BONE 3D engineer
Quantity produced	24
Destination	Hôpital Cochin

	One Petri bell
Layer thickness (mm)	0.33
Filling density	100%
Wall thickness	1.98
Print duration	2 h 10 min
ABS quantity (cm3)	40.633
Support quantity (cm3)	46.626
Raw material costs (€)	14.20 €

7.3 General equipment

7.3.1 Large shelve support

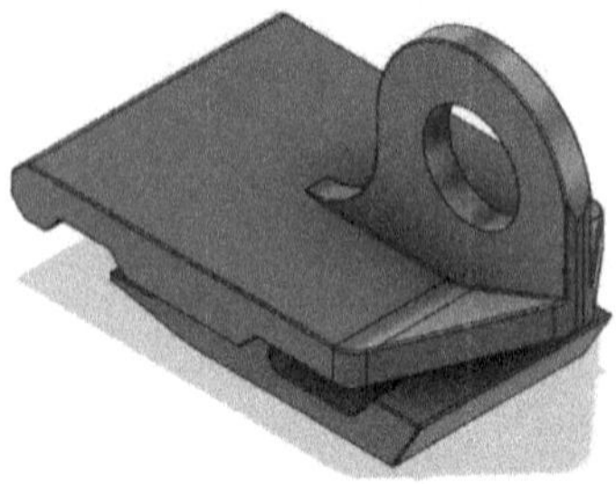

General equipment GE1

This device has been designed for a specific type of AP-HP shelf for which broken parts could not be purchased separately.

Date of first request	April 2020
Origin of the request	Logistics (Hôpital Cochin)
People involved in design	BONE 3D engineer
Quantity produced	120
Destination	Hôpital Cochin

	One shelve support (large)
Layer thickness (mm)	0.33
Filling density	100%
Wall thickness	1.32
Print duration	22 min
ABS quantity (cm3)	3.22
Support quantity (cm3)	3.18
Raw material costs (€)	1.17 €

7.3.2 Small shelve support

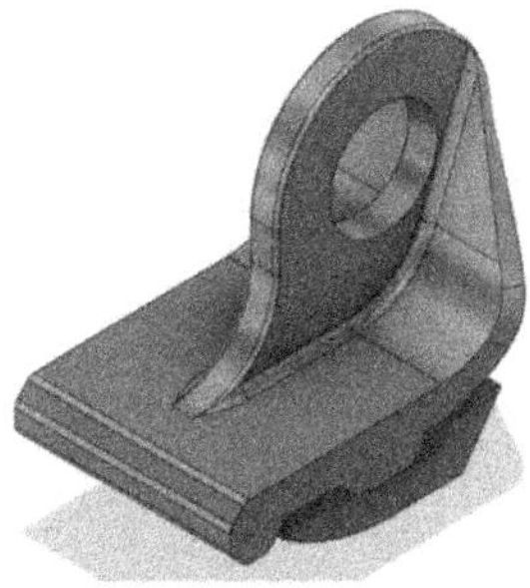

General equipment GE2

This device has been designed for another specific type of AP-HP shelf for which broken parts could not be purchased separately.

Date of first request	May 2020
Origin of the request	Logistics (Hôpital Cochin)
People involved in design	BONE 3D engineer
Quantity produced	120
Destination	Hôpital Cochin

	One shelve support (small)
Layer thickness (mm)	0.33
Filling density	100%
Wall thickness	1.32
Print duration	20 min
ABS quantity (cm3)	2.6
Support quantity (cm3)	2.67
Raw material costs (€)	0.96 €

7.3.3 Tire lever

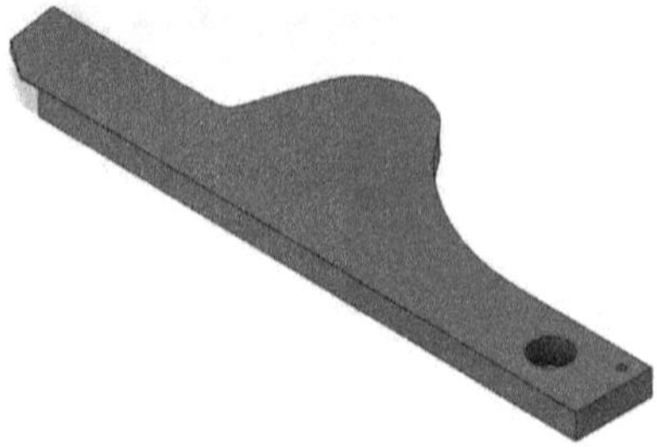

General equipment GE3

This device is a Fenwick tire lever.

Date of first request	May 2020
Origin of the request	Pneumatic services (Hôpital Cochin)
People involved in design	BONE 3D engineer
Quantity produced	5
Destination	Hôpital Cochin

	One tire lever
Layer thickness (mm)	0.33
Filling density	100%
Wall thickness	0.66
Print duration	1 h 41 min
ABS quantity (cm3)	81.58
Support quantity (cm3)	14.54
Raw material costs (€)	17.46 €

7.3.4 Reset key for fire alarm №1

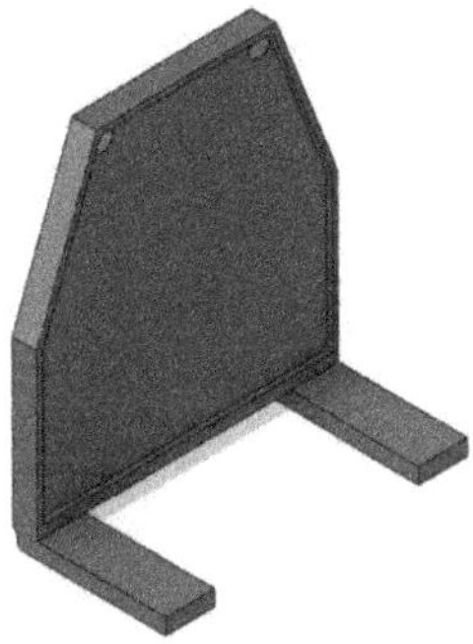

General equipment GE4

This device is yet another type of reset key for manual fire alarm triggers.

Date of first request	May 2020
Origin of the request	Fire Safety department (Hôpital Cochin)
People involved in design	BONE 3D engineer
Quantity produced	50
Destination	Hôpital Cochin

	One key
Layer thickness (mm)	0.33
Filling density	100%
Wall thickness	0.66
Print duration	1 h 09 min
ABS quantity (cm3)	10.84
Support quantity (cm3)	10.32
Raw material costs (€)	3.85 €

7.3.5 Reset key for fire alarm №2

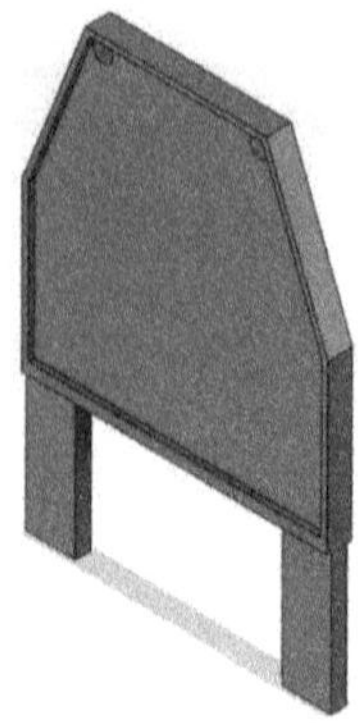

General equipment GE5

This device still another type of another type of reset key for manual fire alarm triggers.

Date of first request	May 2020
Origin of the request	Fire Safety department (Hôpital Cochin)
People involved in design	BONE 3D engineer
Quantity produced	50
Destination	Hôpital Cochin

	One key
Layer thickness (mm)	0.33
Filling density	100%
Wall thickness	0.66
Print duration	17 min
ABS quantity (cm3)	6.8
Support quantity (cm3)	6.56
Raw material costs (€)	2.43 €

7.3.6 Reset key for fire alarm №3

General equipment GE6

This device is another type of reset key for manual fire alarm triggers.

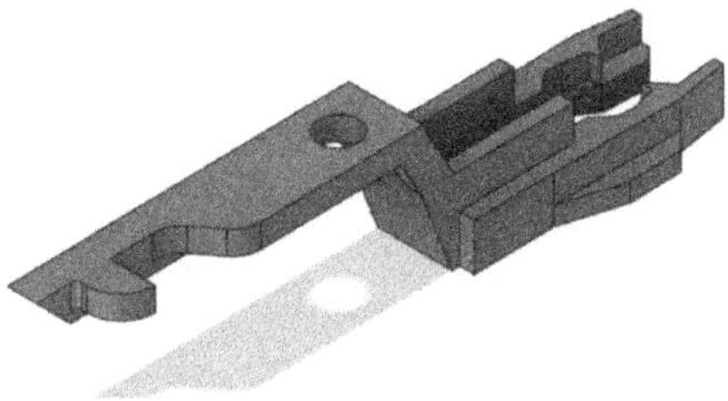

Date of first request	May 2020
Origin of the request	Fire Safety department (Hôpital Cochin)
People involved in design	BONE 3D engineer
Quantity produced	50
Destination	Hôpital Cochin

	One key
Layer thickness (mm)	0.33
Filling density	100%
Wall thickness	0.66
Print duration	16 min
ABS quantity (cm3)	2.35
Support quantity (cm3)	3.34
Raw material costs (€)	1.04 €

7.3.7 Reset key for fire alarm №4

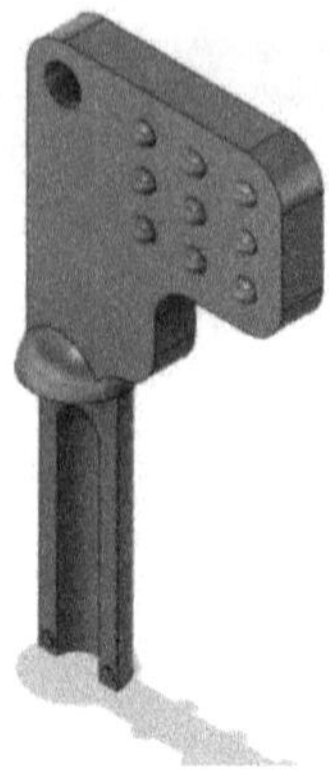

General equipment GE7

This device is a final type of reset key for manual fire alarm triggers.

Date of first request	May 2020
Origin of the request	Fire Safety department (Hôpital Cochin)
People involved in design	BONE 3D engineer
Quantity produced	50
Destination	Hôpital Cochin

	One key
Layer thickness (mm)	0.33
Filling density	100%
Wall thickness	0.66
Print duration	38 min
ABS quantity (cm3)	7.96
Support quantity (cm3)	3.79
Raw material costs (€)	2.14 €

7.3.8 Reset key for fire alarm №5

General equipment GE8

This device is a reset key for manual fire alarm triggers.

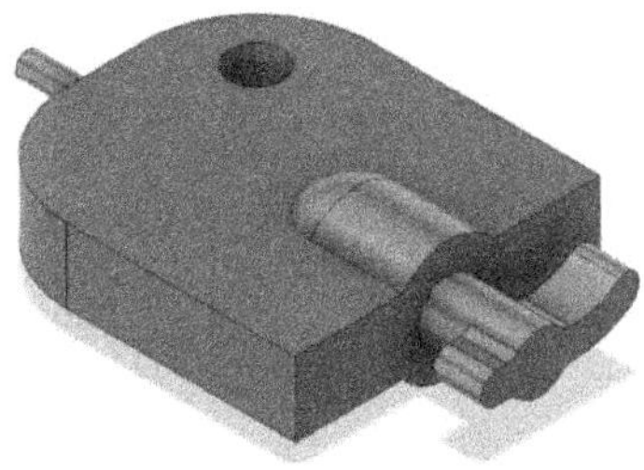

Date of first request	May 2020
Origin of the request	Fire Safety department (Hôpital Cochin)
People involved in design	BONE 3D engineer
Quantity produced	50
Destination	Hôpital Cochin

	One key
Layer thickness (mm)	0.33
Filling density	100%
Wall thickness	0.66
Print duration	19 min
ABS quantity (cm3)	4.34
Support quantity (cm3)	2.11
Raw material costs (€)	1.18 €

7.3.9 Reset key for fire alarm №6

General equipment GE9

This device is a reset key for manual fire alarm triggers.

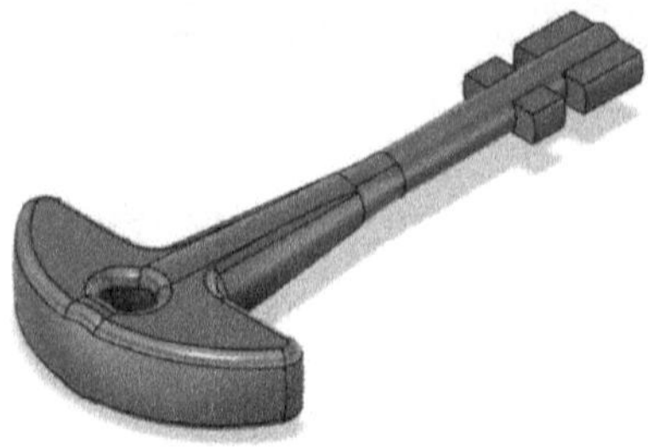

Date of first request	June 2020
Origin of the request	Occupational Therapy (Hôpital Cochin)
People involved in design	BONE 3D engineer
Quantity produced	50
Destination	Hôpital Cochin

	One key
Layer thickness (mm)	0.33
Filling density	100%
Wall thickness	0.66
Print duration	44 min
ABS quantity (cm3)	5.46
Support quantity (cm3)	7.25
Raw material costs (€)	2.31 €

7.3.10 Screw holder

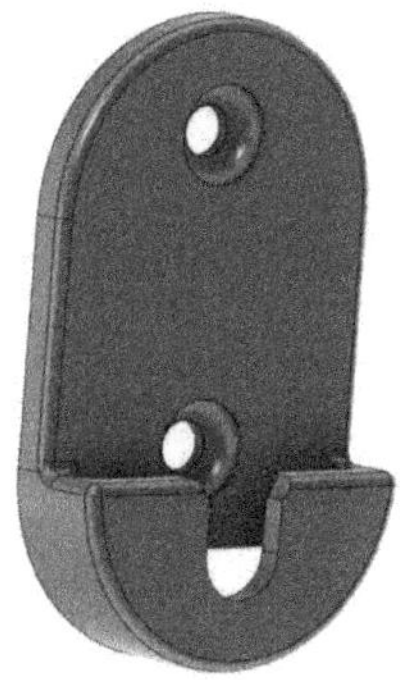

General equipment GE10

This device was intended to be used in the offices of the Security department of Hôpital Cochin.

Date of first request	May 2020
Origin of the request	Central Security department (Hôpital Cochin)
People involved in design	BONE 3D engineer
Quantity produced	10
Destination	Hôpital Cochin

	One screw holder
Layer thickness (mm)	0.33
Filling density	100%
Wall thickness	0.66
Print duration	19 min
ABS quantity (cm3)	5.72
Support quantity (cm3)	4.43
Raw material costs (€)	1.85 €

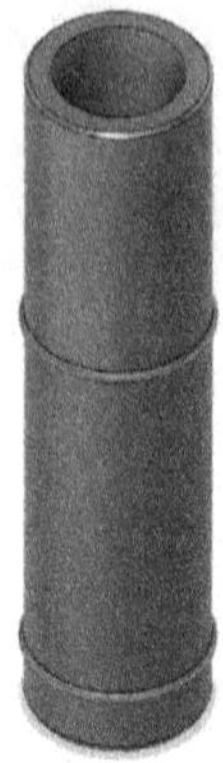

7.3.11 Overflow pipe

General equipment GE11

This device regulates the level of a liquid present in a tank by an overflow principle.

Date of first request	May 2020
Origin of the request	Maintenance Services (Hôpital Cochin)
People involved in design	BONE 3D engineer
Quantity produced	10
Destination	Hôpital Cochin

	One overflow pipe
Layer thickness (mm)	0.25
Filling density	100%
Wall thickness	0.81
Print duration	20 h 26 min
ABS quantity (cm3)	141.04
Support quantity (cm3)	25.83
Raw material costs (€)	41.82 €

7.3.12 Joint for overflow pipe

General equipment GE12

This piece is the joint for the overflow pipe.

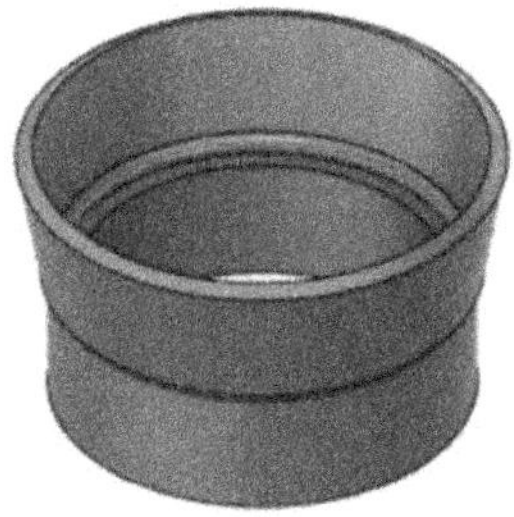

Date of first request	September 2020
Origin of the request	Cardiothoracic surgery (Hôpital Cochin)
People involved in design	BONE 3D engineer
Quantity produced	3
Destination	Hôpital Cochin

	One overflow pipe joint
Layer thickness (mm)	0.25
Filling density	100%
Wall thickness	0.81
Print duration	2 h 31 min
ABS quantity (cm3)	14.118
Support quantity (cm3)	7.872
Raw material costs (€)	5.46 €

7.3.13 Vacuum cleaner lid

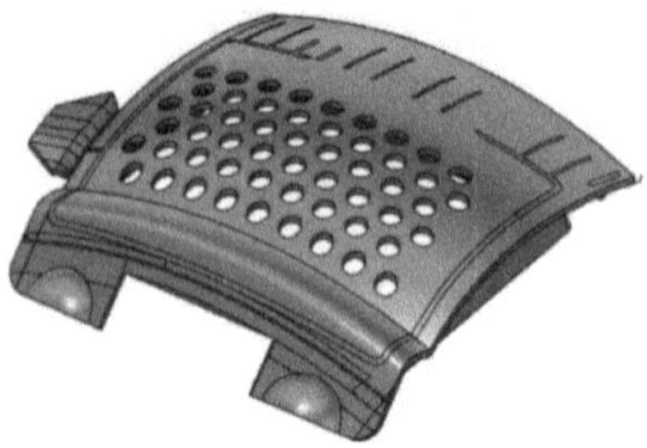

General equipment GE13

This is a vacuum cleaner lid designed from broken AP-HP equipment.

Date of first request	September 2020
Origin of the request	Hôpital Cochin
People involved in design	BONE 3D engineer
Quantity produced	3
Destination	Hôpital Cochin

	One lid
Layer thickness (mm)	0.25
Filling density	100%
Wall thickness	1.98
Print duration	9 h 57 min
ABS quantity (cm3)	79.697
Support quantity (cm3)	178.6
Raw material costs (€)	42.41 €

7.3.14 Protection for magnetic door

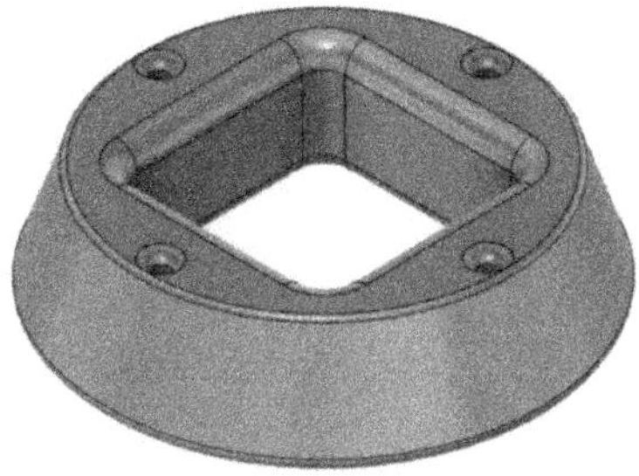

General equipment GE14

This piece is design to avoid damaging the magnet while opening a door that is maintained by such a magnet.

Date of first request	September 2020
Origin of the request	Maintenance services (Hôpital Cochin)
People involved in design	BONE 3D engineer
Quantity produced	1
Destination	Hôpital Cochin

	One protection
Layer thickness (mm)	0.25
Filling density	100%
Wall thickness	1.98
Print duration	5 h 13 min
ABS quantity (cm3)	168.668
Support quantity (cm3)	25.716
Raw material costs (€)	31.80 €

7.3.15 Salt stand

General equipment GE15

This piece is salt bottle holder.

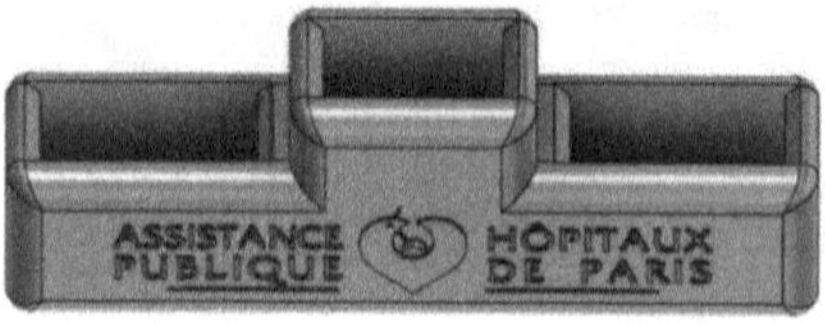

Date of first request	July 2020
Origin of the request	Maintenance services (Hôpital Cochin)
People involved in design	BONE 3D engineer
Quantity produced	4
Destination	Hôpital Cochin

	One salt stand
Layer thickness (mm)	0.25
Filling density	100%
Wall thickness	1.98
Print duration	9 h 07 min
ABS quantity (cm3)	252.067
Support quantity (cm3)	48.085
Raw material costs (€)	49.20 €

7.3.16 Silicon mould

General equipment GE16

This silicon mould was used to manufacture silicon bricks.

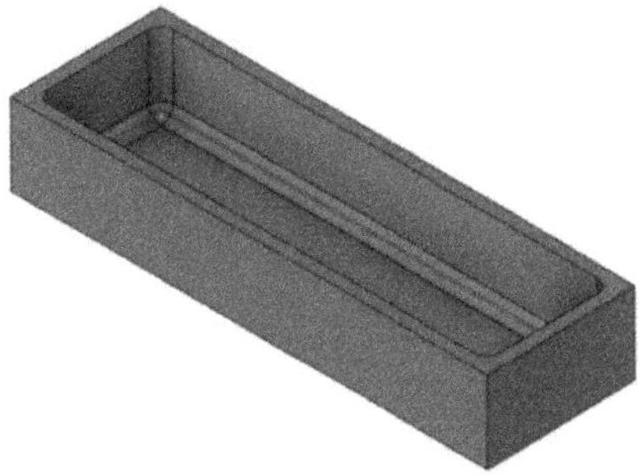

Date of first request	September 2020
Origin of the request	Hôpital Cochin
People involved in design	BONE 3D engineer
Quantity produced	1
Destination	Hôpital Cochin

	One mould
Layer thickness (mm)	0.25
Filling density	100%
Wall thickness	1.98
Print duration	2 h 44 min
ABS quantity (cm3)	90.646
Support quantity (cm3)	14.717
Raw material costs (€)	29.59 €

7.3.17 Printer spare part

General equipment GE17

This device is a printer spare part for AP-HP administration.

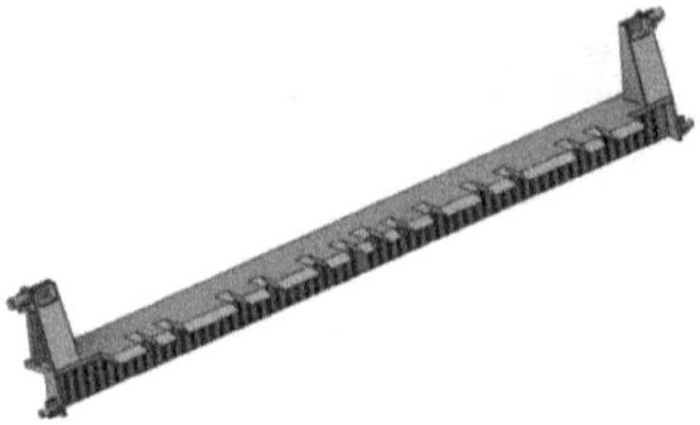

Date of first request	September 2020
Origin of the request	Hôpital Cochin
People involved in design	BONE 3D engineer
Quantity produced	1
Destination	Hôpital Cochin

	One spare part
Layer thickness (mm)	0.25
Filling density	100%
Wall thickness	1.98
Print duration	4 h 16 min
ABS quantity (cm3)	27.564
Support quantity (cm3)	54.376
Raw material costs (€)	13.37 €

7.3.18 Bolt

General equipment GE18

This device was required by occupational therapists.

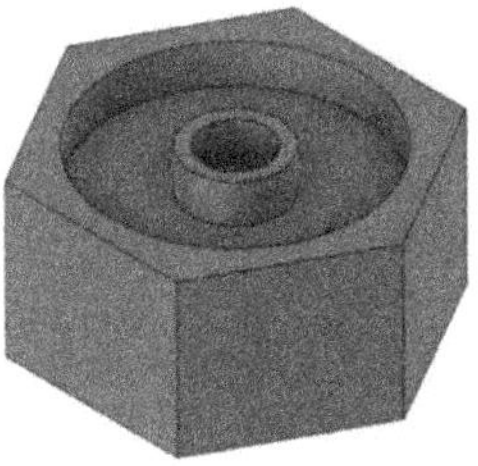

Date of first request	September 2020
Origin of the request	Occupational therapy (Hôpital Cochin)
People involved in design	BONE 3D engineer
Quantity produced	1
Destination	Hôpital Cochin

	One bolt
Layer thickness (mm)	0.33
Filling density	100%
Wall thickness	1.98
Print duration	34 min
ABS quantity (cm3)	4.223
Support quantity (cm3)	4.514
Raw material costs (€)	1.32 €

7.3.19 Document holder

General equipment GE19

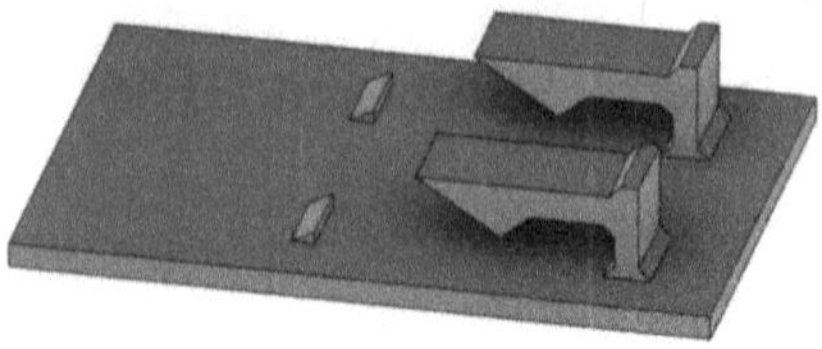

This is a document holder for occupational therapy.

Date of first request	September 2020
Origin of the request	Hôpital Cochin
People involved in design	BONE 3D engineer
Quantity produced	1
Destination	Hôpital Cochin

	One holder
Layer thickness (mm)	0.33
Filling density	100%
Wall thickness	1.98
Print duration	20 min
ABS quantity (cm3)	6.14
Support quantity (cm3)	4.775
Raw material costs (€)	1.65 €

7.3.20 Bottom plate

General equipment GE20

This is a plate to strengthen the bottom of cardboard boxes for the technical services.

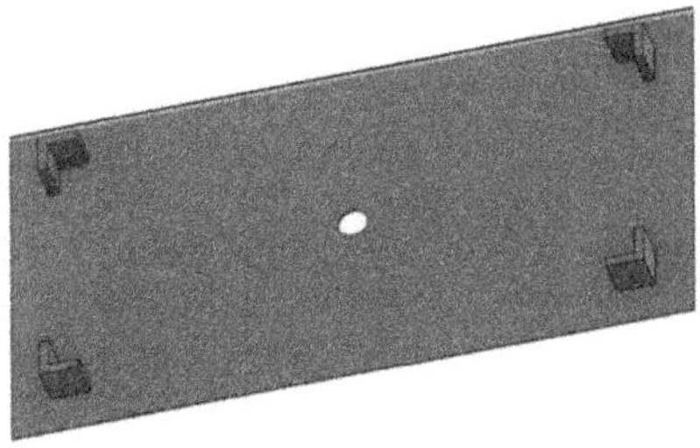

Date of first request	September 2020
Origin of the request	Hôpital Cochin
People involved in design	BONE 3D engineer
Quantity produced	2
Destination	Hôpital Cochin

	One plate
Layer thickness (mm)	0.33
Filling density	100%
Wall thickness	1.98
Print duration	2 h 08 min
ABS quantity (cm3)	43.37
Support quantity (cm3)	75.377
Raw material costs (€)	19.47 €

7.3.21 Blind holder

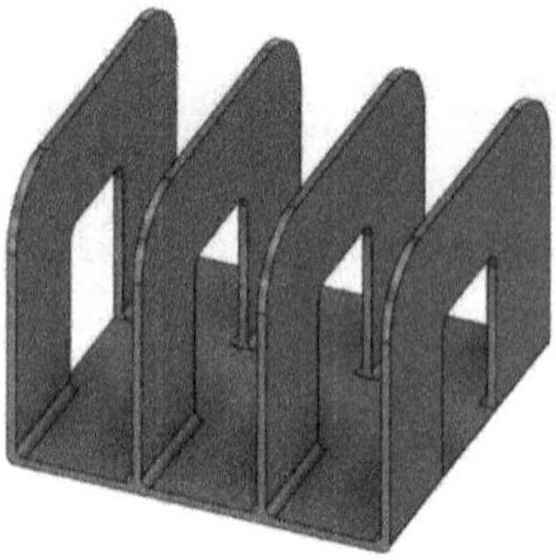

General equipment GE21

This is a blinder holder.

Date of first request	September 2020
Origin of the request	Central Administration (Hôpital Cochin)
People involved in design	BONE 3D engineer
Quantity produced	1
Destination	Central Administration (Hôpital Cochin)

	One holder
Layer thickness (mm)	0.33
Filling density	100%
Wall thickness	1.98
Print duration	20 h 04 min
ABS quantity (cm3)	671.829
Support quantity (cm3)	113.695
Raw material costs (€)	129.36 €

7.3.22 Circular joint

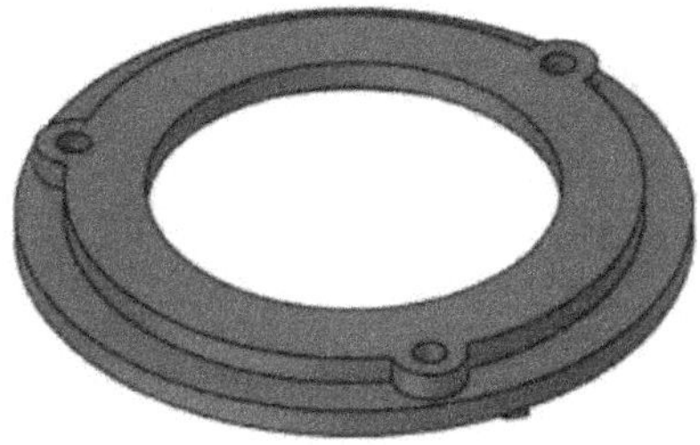

General equipment GE22

This is a specific type of joint required by AP-HP maintenance services.

Date of first request	September 2020
Origin of the request	Maintenance services (Hôpital Cochin)
People involved in design	BONE 3D engineer
Quantity produced	2
Destination	Maintenance services (Hôpital Cochin)

	One joint
Layer thickness (mm)	0.33
Filling density	100%
Wall thickness	1.98
Print duration	11 min
ABS quantity (cm3)	2.391
Support quantity (cm3)	3.413
Raw material costs (€)	0.83 €

7.3.23 U-shaped maintenance piece

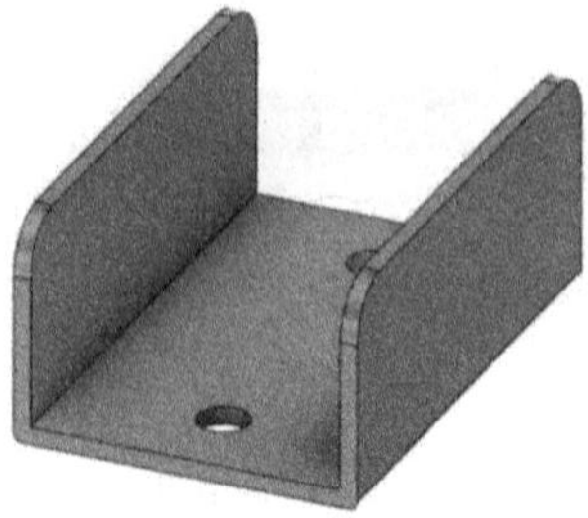

General equipment GE23

This is also a specific piece required by AP-HP maintenance.

Date of first request	September 2020
Origin of the request	Maintenance services (Hôpital Cochin)
People involved in design	BONE 3D engineer
Quantity produced	3
Destination	Maintenance services (Hôpital Cochin)

	One piece
Layer thickness (mm)	0.33
Filling density	100%
Wall thickness	1.98
Print duration	10 min
ABS quantity (cm3)	3.418
Support quantity (cm3)	1.438
Raw material costs (€)	0.66 €

7.3.24 Water-proof iPad plug

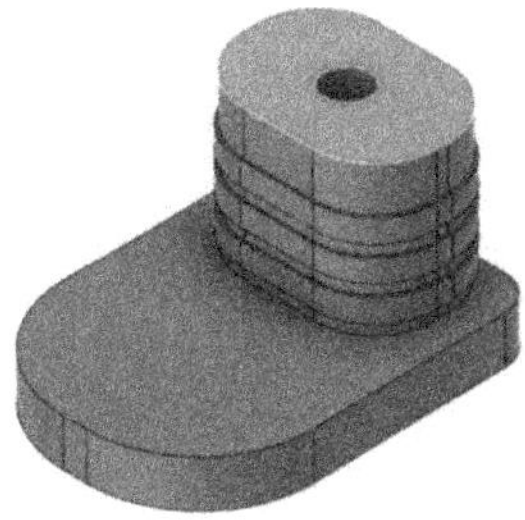

General equipment GE24

This iPad plug was requested by a paramedic from Hôpital Cochin.

Date of first request	September 2020
Origin of the request	Hôpital Cochin
People involved in design	BONE 3D engineer
Quantity produced	2
Destination	Hôpital Cochin

	One plug
Layer thickness (mm)	0.25
Filling density	100%
Wall thickness	0.81
Print duration	41 min
ABS quantity (cm3)	2.331
Support quantity (cm3)	1.118
Raw material costs (€)	0.50 €

7.3.25 iPad stand

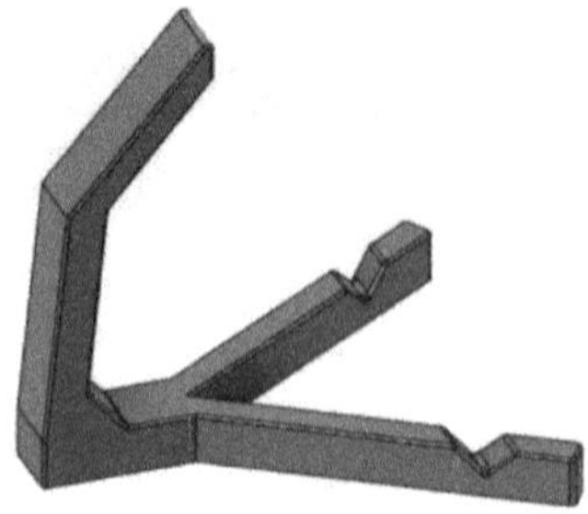

General equipment GE25

This is a iPad stant for the Reproductive medicing department.

Date of first request	September 2020
Origin of the request	Reproductive medicine (Hôpital Cochin)
People involved in design	BONE 3D engineer
Quantity produced	5
Destination	Hôpital Cochin

	One stand
Layer thickness (mm)	0.25
Filling density	100%
Wall thickness	1.98
Print duration	4 h 23 min
ABS quantity (cm3)	83.052
Support quantity (cm3)	25.993
Raw material costs (€)	17.82 €

7.3.26 iPad stand (small size)

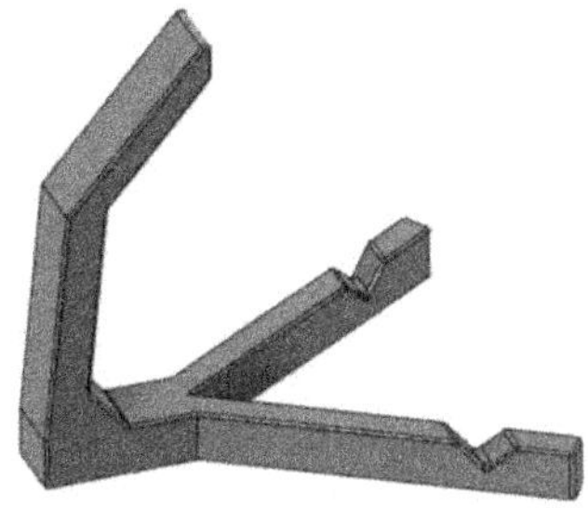

General equipment GE26

This is a iPad stant for the Reproductive medicing department.

Date of first request	September 2020
Origin of the request	Reproductive medicine (Hôpital Cochin)
People involved in design	BONE 3D engineer
Quantity produced	5
Destination	Hôpital Cochin

	One stand
Layer thickness (mm)	0.33
Filling density	100%
Wall thickness	1.98
Print duration	3 h 32 min
ABS quantity (cm3)	77.724
Support quantity (cm3)	27.14
Raw material costs (€)	17.16 €

7.3.27 Table stand

General equipment GE27

This is a specific stand for AP-HP tables.

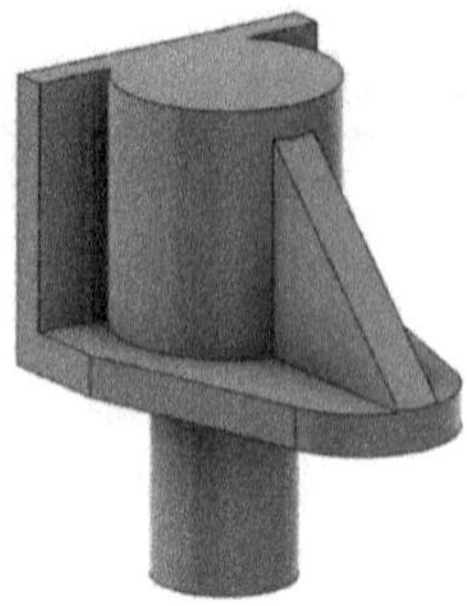

Date of first request	September 2020
Origin of the request	Logistics (Hôpital Cochin)
People involved in design	BONE 3D engineer
Quantity produced	1
Destination	Hôpital Cochin

	One stand
Layer thickness (mm)	0.33
Filling density	100%
Wall thickness	1.98
Print duration	18 min
ABS quantity (cm3)	2.141
Support quantity (cm3)	2.658
Raw material costs (€)	0.66 €

7.3.28 Box carrier

General equipment GE28

This is piece intended to help in carrying boxes.

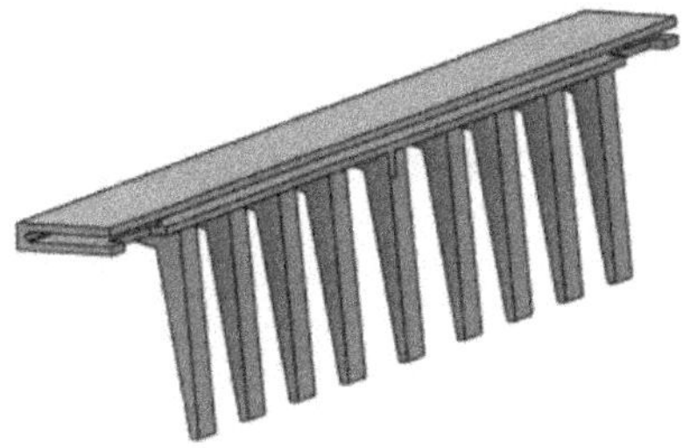

Date of first request	September 2020
Origin of the request	Radiology department (Hôpital Cochin)
People involved in design	BONE 3D engineer
Quantity produced	1
Destination	Hôpital Cochin

	One carrier
Layer thickness (mm)	0.33
Filling density	100%
Wall thickness	1.98
Print duration	3 h 01 min
ABS quantity (cm3)	50.921
Support quantity (cm3)	37.453
Raw material costs (€)	14.36 €

7.3.29 Table hold

General equipment GE29

This is to prevent tables from moving.

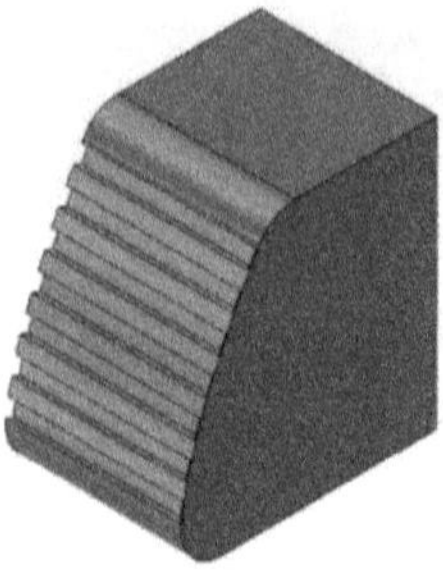

Date of first request	July 2020
Origin of the request	Reproduction medicine (Hôpital Cochin)
People involved in design	BONE 3D engineer
Quantity produced	5
Destination	Hôpital Cochin

	One holder
Layer thickness (mm)	0.33
Filling density	100%
Wall thickness	0.81
Print duration	1 h 51 min
ABS quantity (cm3)	7.622
Support quantity (cm3)	6.607
Raw material costs (€)	3.38 €

7.3.30 Maintenance nut

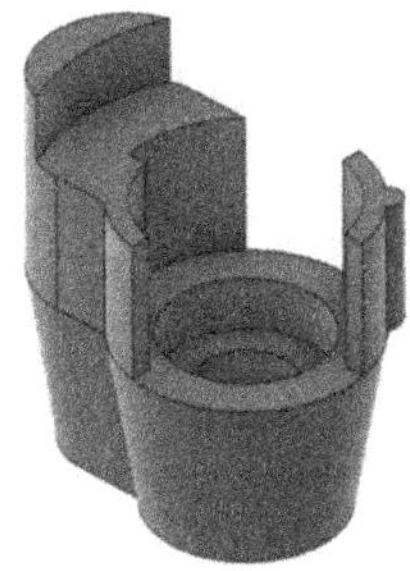

General equipment GE30

This piece is a specific maintenance nut that was broken and needed to be fixed, without any equivalent available on the market.

Date of first request	July 2020
Origin of the request	Maintenance (Hôpital Cochin)
People involved in design	BONE 3D engineer
Quantity produced	1
Destination	Hôpital Cochin

	One nut
Layer thickness (mm)	0.33
Filling density	100%
Wall thickness	1.98
Print duration	41 min
ABS quantity (cm3)	9.926
Support quantity (cm3)	3.027
Raw material costs (€)	1.98 €

7.3.31 Fenwick handle

General equipment GE31

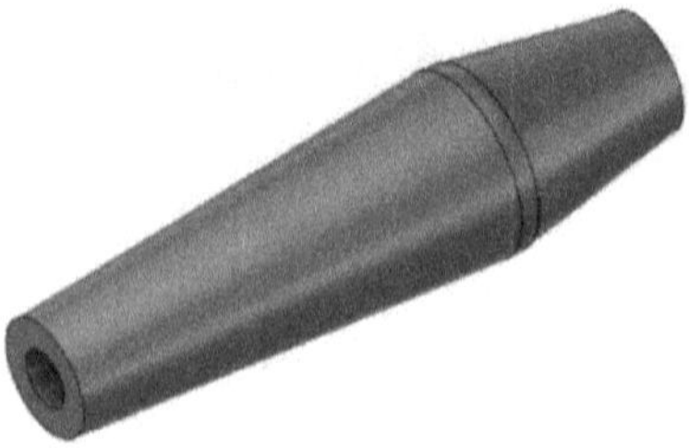

This piece is a Fenwick handle.

Date of first request	June 2020
Origin of the request	Maintenance (Hôpital Cochin)
People involved in design	BONE 3D engineer
Quantity produced	11
Destination	Hôpital Cochin

	One fenwick handle
Layer thickness (mm)	0.33
Filling density	100%
Wall thickness	1.98
Print duration	2 h 06 min
ABS quantity (cm3)	45.528
Support quantity (cm3)	2.212
Raw material costs (€)	7.88 €

7.3.32 Wardrobe handle

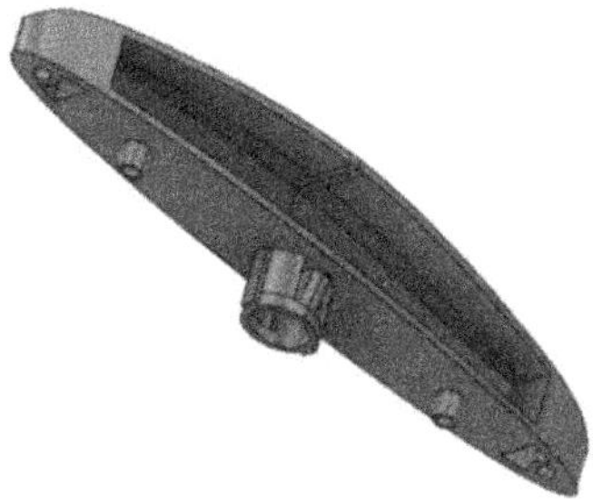

General equipment GE32

This piece is wardrobe handle.

Date of first request	July 2020
Origin of the request	Maintenance (Hôpital Cochin)
People involved in design	BONE 3D engineer
Quantity produced	10
Destination	Hôpital Cochin

	One wardrobe handle
Layer thickness (mm)	0.33
Filling density	100%
Wall thickness	1.98
Print duration	1 h 54 min
ABS quantity (cm3)	31.572
Support quantity (cm3)	21.36
Raw material costs (€)	8.58 €

7.3.33 Drawer spare part №1

General equipment GE33

This piece was designed for specific drawers from the Hôpital Necker - Enfants Malades operating room. Spare parts were not available for sale.

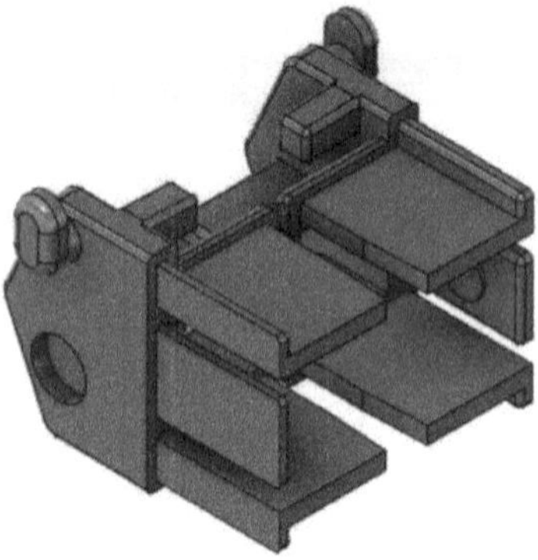

Date of first request	June 2020
Origin of the request	Maintenance (Hôpital Necker - Enfants Malades)
People involved in design	BONE 3D engineer
Quantity produced	4
Destination	Hôpital Necker - Enfants Malades

	One drawer spare part
Layer thickness (mm)	0.33
Filling density	100%
Wall thickness	1.98
Print duration	1 h 07 min
ABS quantity (cm3)	15.646
Support quantity (cm3)	12.338
Raw material costs (€)	4.46 €

7.3.34 Drawer spare part №2

General equipment GE34

This piece was designed for specific drawers from the Hôpital Necker - Enfants Malades operating room. Spare parts were not available for sale.

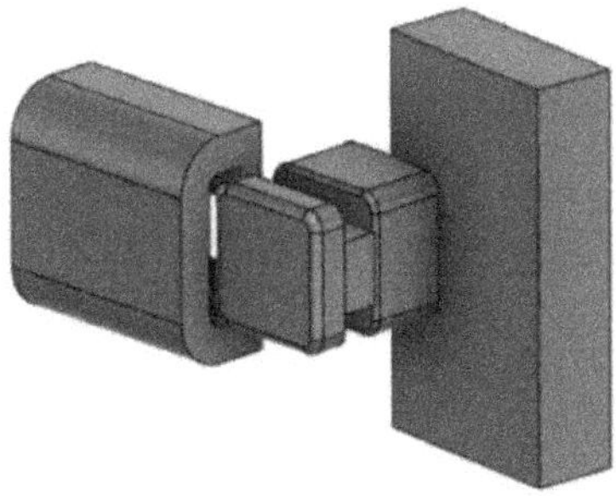

Date of first request	June 2020
Origin of the request	Maintenance (Hôpital Necker - Enfants Malades)
People involved in design	BONE 3D engineer
Quantity produced	1
Destination	Hôpital Necker - Enfants Malades

	One drawer spare part
Layer thickness (mm)	0.33
Filling density	100%
Wall thickness	1.98
Print duration	20 min
ABS quantity (cm3)	3.452
Support quantity (cm3)	2.529
Raw material costs (€)	0.83 €

7.3.35 Door hold

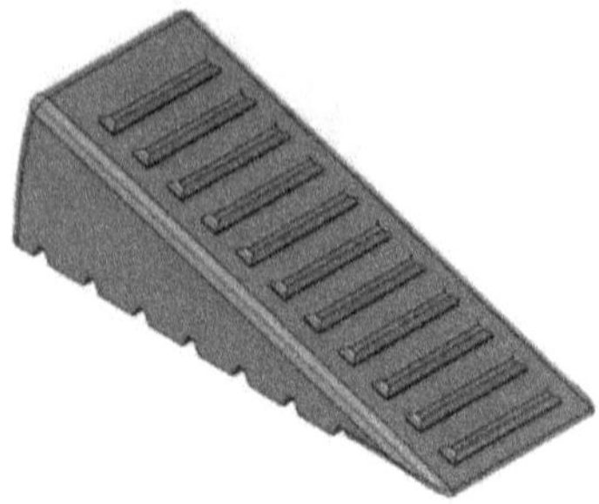

General equipment GE35

This piece is a door holder.

Date of first request	July 2020
Origin of the request	Maintenance (Hôpital Cochin)
People involved in design	BONE 3D engineer
Quantity produced	25
Destination	Hôpital Cochin

	One door holder
Layer thickness (mm)	0.25
Filling density	100%
Wall thickness	0.81
Print duration	4 h 40 min
ABS quantity (cm3)	33.192
Support quantity (cm3)	4.342
Raw material costs (€)	9.60 €

7.3.36 Corner-shaped maintenance piece

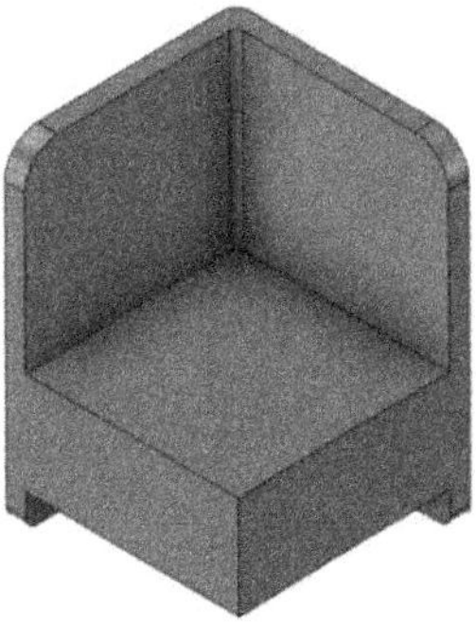

General equipment GE36

This piece is a specific support that the occupational therapy unit required.

Date of first request	June 2020
Origin of the request	Occupational therapy (Hôpital Cochin)
People involved in design	BONE 3D engineer
Quantity produced	8
Destination	Hôpital Cochin

	One support
Layer thickness (mm)	0.33
Filling density	100%
Wall thickness	1.98
Print duration	42 min
ABS quantity (cm3)	20.661
Support quantity (cm3)	2.976
Raw material costs (€)	3.80 €

8. Academic projects developed within the platform: approaches and perspectives

Besides projects specifically related to the management of the pandemic, the availability of 3D printers within a trust of academic hospitals gave rise to a vast number of academic and artistic projects that contributed to the adoption of the platform by a large community of health professionals.

The 3D printers located within Hôpital Cochin, with engineers available for designing new projects, were quickly spotted by academics from the various AP-HP university hospitals. Our team started working on a series of projects that provided a good prequel of the integration of a 3D platform within an academic environment, with a focus on the different possible approaches for such a collaboration.

8.1 Craniofacial simulators for medical students: top-down approach

In 2019, 72.000 euros were awarded to the maxillofacial surgery department of Hôpital Necker - Enfants Malades from the Agence Régionale de Santé (ARS) Île-de-France together with iLumens and Université de Paris[1], in order to develop 4 3D-printed simulators dedicated to the teaching of disorders of the craniofacial region. The design of the simulators was performed with BONE 3D and the following projects were chosen, with a medical project manager for each simulator

→ Fronto-facial monobloc advancement simulator (maxillofacial surgery) (Figures 42 & 43),

→ Middle ear examination (ENT) (Figure 44)

→ Dental implant placement simulator (oral surgery) (Figure 45),

→ Oculomotricity simulator (ophthalmology).

1 HEADSOFF : simulation pour enseigner les pathologies de la tête et du cou', C2019DOSRH035.

All projects were co-supervised by surgeons and by engineers from BONE 3D based on exchanges between each project manager and developers.

This project was not related to the 3D COVID project but the availability of the engineers and the printers during this period led to very fast development of the simulators. The platform itself became a natural meeting point between the 4 surgeons managing the projects and involved in the design of the models (Figures 43 & 44). This process was a good illustration of the fruitful interactions between health professionals and 3D designers in educational projects in a dedicated convenient place located within an academic hospital.

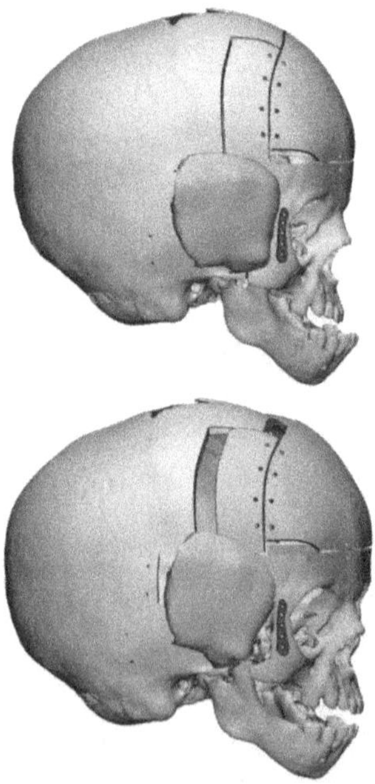

43.

Fig. 43. Simulation of the temporal muscle in the monobloc advancement model. Intermediate 3D design from one out of many interations between developers and surgeons.

The 4 simulators have been used for teaching at the Université de Paris from March 2021. Their whole development process took less than a year. They will be manufactured for the Université de Paris but also become a commercial product for BONE 3D, with royalties for AP-HP and the Université de Paris.

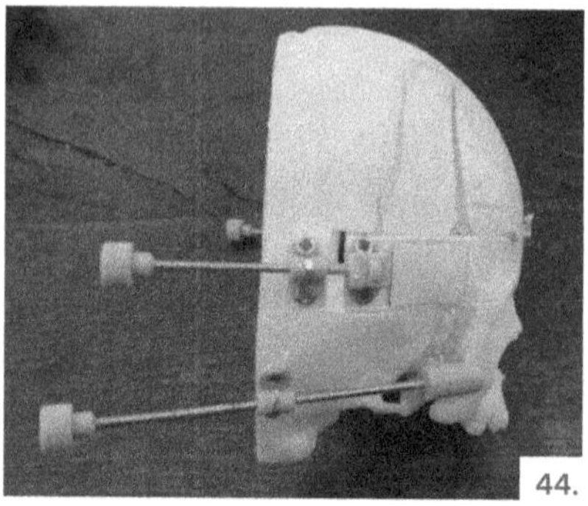

44.

Fig. 44. Intermediate design of the monobloc model with indications by surgeons drawn on the model to direct modifications by engineers.

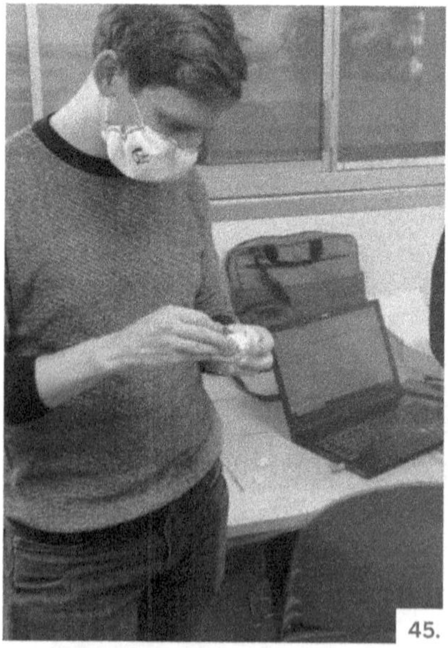

45.

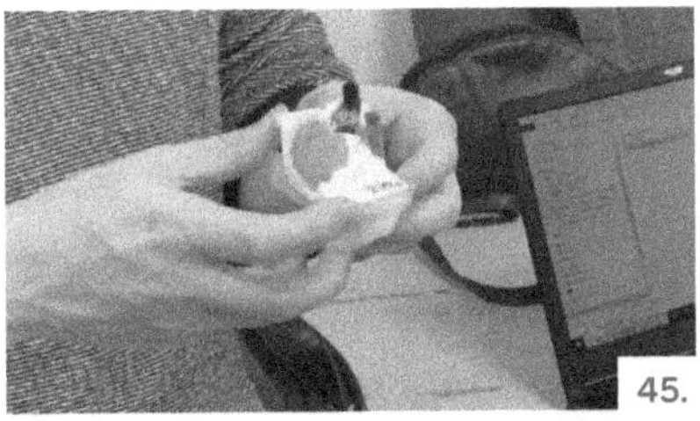

Fig. 45. Discussions on the design of the ear model between an ENT surgeon (AP-HP) and a designer (BONE 3D).

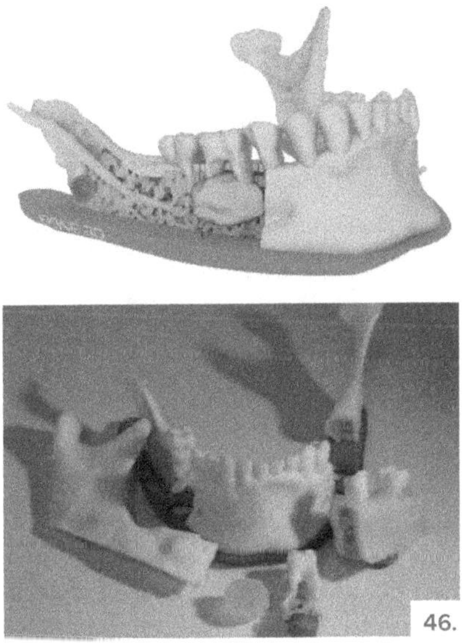

Fig. 46. Final rendering and prototype of the oral surgery model.

8.2 Modeling orthopaedic tumours for a large reference center: bottom-up approach

The orthopaedic surgery department at Hôpital Cochin, where the printers were settled, is notorious nationwide for tumour surgery and acts as a reference center for these conditions. This field of orthopaedics is particularly in need for anatomical models. A trainee from this department, who was personally involved in 3D printing, reached our team in October 2020 and started a very fruitful collaboration with our engineers, both for developing specific models for his patients (Figure 46), but also by launching larger scale projects for specific simulators dedicated to complex hip resections in sarcoma surgery (Figure 48).

As opposed to the project detailed in paragraph 8.1, which was a top-down approach with a strong institutional background, the collaboration with this trainee showed that 3D platforms within hospitals were also suited for bottom-up academic projects relying on strong and motivated individuals. From October 2020 to May 2021, more than 50 models were produced under the initiative of this trainee and the orthopaedic surgery department of Hôpital Cochin (Figure 49).

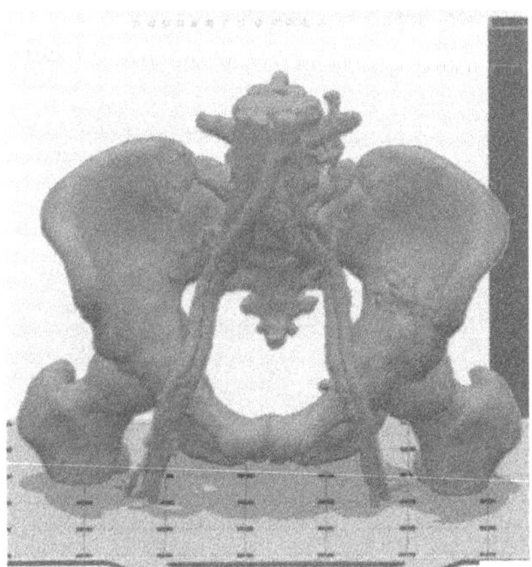

Fig. 47. Patient-specific model for a pelvic sarcoma.

Date of first request	04/12/2020
Origin of the request	Orthopedic surgery trainee
People involved in design	Orthopedic surgery trainee
Quantity produced	2
Destination	Orthopedic surgery (Hôpital Cochin)

	One model
Layer thickness (mm)	0.25
Filling density	100%
Wall thickness	1.54
Print duration	2 d 23 h 01 min
ABS quantity (cm3)	1090.546
Support quantity (cm3)	395.656
Raw material costs (€)	245 €

Printing characteristics of the pelvic sarcoma individual model, as an example of an elaborate anatomical model for clinical use.

Printing characteristics of the bladder model, as an example of a subpart of an anatomical teaching model in the process of being designed by an orthopaedic surgery trainee.

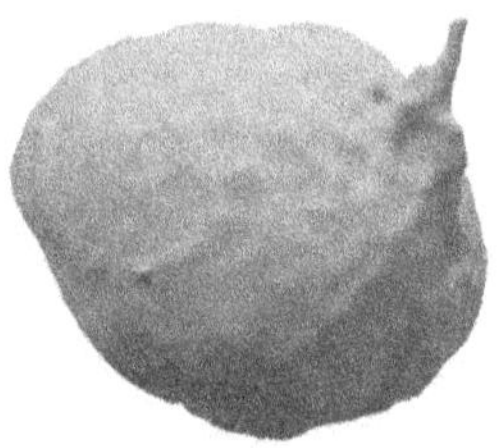

48.

Fig. 48. Prototype for a bladder printed in TPU to be included in a model for pelvic sarcoma resection surgery.

Date of first request	04/12/2020
Origin of the request	Orthopedic surgery trainee
People involved in design	Orthopedic surgery trainee
Quantity produced	1
Destination	Orthopedic surgery (Hôpital Cochin)

	One model
Layer thickness (mm)	0.25
Filling density	100%
Wall thickness	0.81
Print duration	12 h 54 min
ABS quantity (cm3)	87.21
Support quantity (cm3)	19.529
Raw material costs (€)	27.75 €

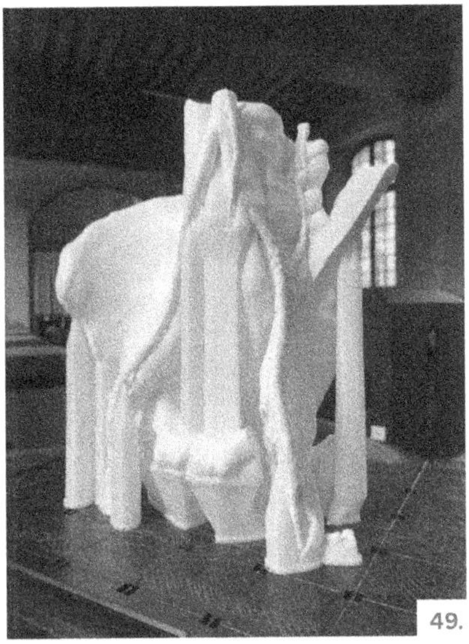

49.

Fig. 49. Hip tumour model designed with an orthopaedic surgery trainee fresh out of the Stratasys F370 FMD printer before post-treatment.

8.3 A model for training anaesthesiologists for a difficult facial block: importance of raw data

This project is another illustration of the academic use an integrated 3D platform. An anaesthesiologist from Hôpital Necker - Enfants Malades was writing a paper on the specific issues raised by pterygo-palatine blocks in patients with bleeding disorders. The paper was based on a case series and the main author wished to include a 3D-printed model into her paper. This main author heard about our initiative and reached our team. We designed a skull model with the pterygo-palatine ganglion and the maxillary artery (Figure 49). The model was printed and photographed with the needle of the block in its proper clinical position. The model will also be secondarily used to teach pterygo-palatine blocks to anaesthesiology trainees.

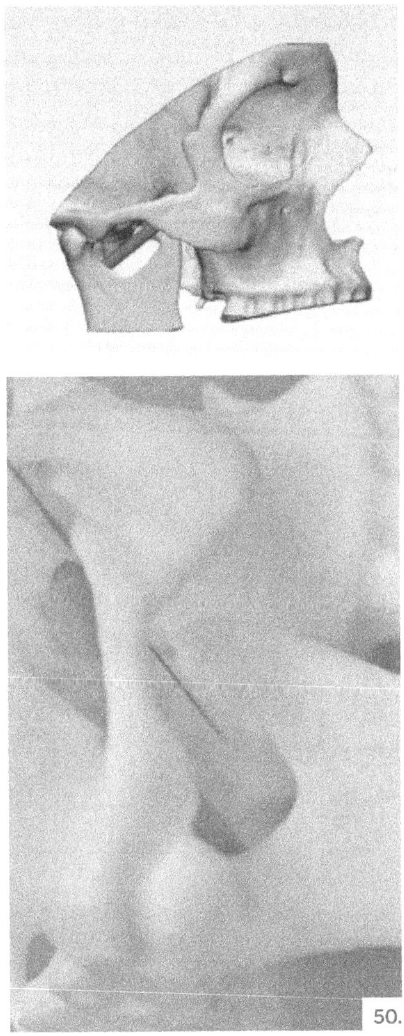

50.

Fig. 50. 3D rendering and 3D-printed model of the pterygo-palatine block showing the position of the needle relative to the ganglion and the maxillary artery.

This project is an illustration of another crucial point of locating a 3D printing platform within an academic hospital: the availability of clinical data. The computers managing the printers were also connected to the central imaging database of AP-HP (PACS) and thus to an immense number of images that could be used to design models. According to the EU ethical laws, such projects require a registration with the local Data Protection Officer and the information of the patients when their data is used. Despite these moderate constraints, managed in a straightforward way by academics who are used to the process, the on-site availability of clinical data within a 3D platform is an invaluable advantage for the promotion of scientific and educational projects.

8.4 A clitoris model for demonstration in a shelter for women with genital mutilations: social 3D-printing

A gynaecologist at the Maison des Femmes of Saint-Denis, in the North of Paris, reached our team to ask if we could produce educational models for women who have been victims of genital mutilations. Her center already had access to several commercial models, but she needed several modifications and eventually production at cheaper prices (Figure 50).

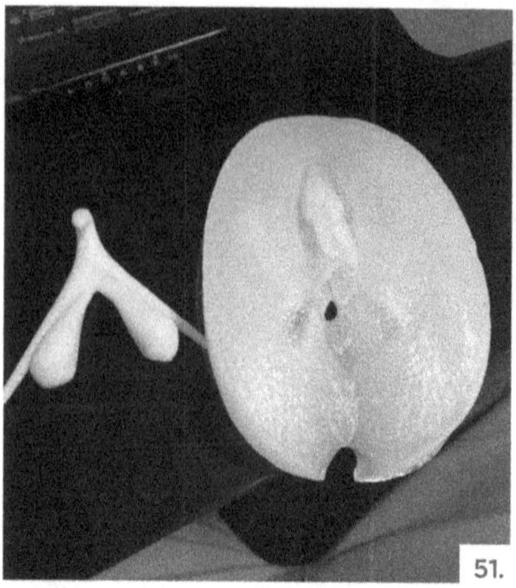

51.

Fig. 51. Clitoris models produced for the 'Maison des Femmes' (Saint-Denis).

The technical aspects of this project were standard for the remarkable characteristics of polyjet 3D-printers. This project was nevertheless in the sense that it highlighted the potential role of 3D-printing in supporting specific social causes: the specificity of 3D-printing lies in the fact that it can produce visually striking objects that reinforce sanitary messages, especially for targets that would be little receptive to verbal communication due to language or cultural issues for instance.

8.5 Simplified anatomical model for a medical refuge for migrants: another example of social 3D-printing

Hôtel-Dieu, a central hospital in Paris, is the home of a Permanence d'Accès aux Soins de Santé (PASS), a specific department dedicated to basic care for socially deprived patients including many migrants who do not speak French. The head nurse at PASS reached us because he needed a simple anatomical model to explain the basics of anatomy to the patients managed in PASS – for instance to explain where and what the liver is to a patient who is diagnosed with hepatitis. He showed us a famous cartoon by Fritz Kahn, a major German illustrator, as a potential model (Figure 52). This project illustrates the fact that academic 3D printing can tackle many unexpected aspects of patient education. This example and the model from section 8.4 highlight the relevance of a specific social use of 3D-printing with many perspectives, especially if a freely available academic platform is settled within a large hospital trust.

8.6 Producing 3D skull models for a reference centre for craniofacial malformations: increased efficiency and security

Hôpital Necker - Enfants Malades is a reference centre for craniofacial malformations. Anatomical models are commonly ordered to private companies for preparing complex facial reconstructions. To order these models, patient files are currently transferred using non-secure methods such as emails or free transfer applications. The 3D COVID platform has offered an alternative to external providers and has produced a large series of models using FDM technology (Figure 53) and polyjet technology (Figure 54). This process is more fluid and secure than the previous workflow used to obtain anatomical models. It also allows to keep data within an academic environment, envision further development and prevent private partners to build databases that then can secondarily exploit without any benefit for the ublic structures that provided the raw images.

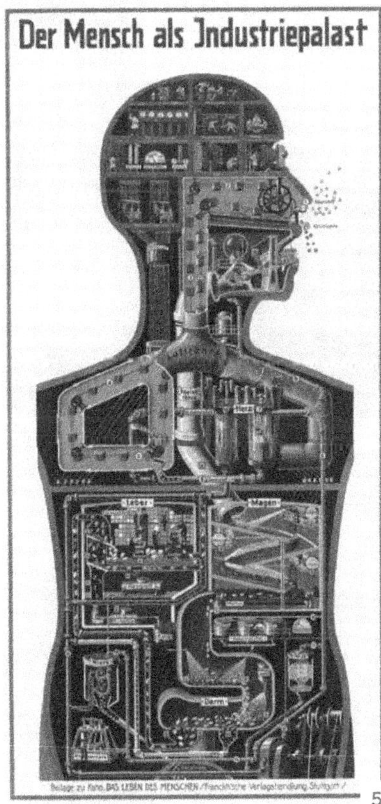

52.

Fig. 52. Cartoon by Fritz Kahn to be used as a template for an educational model for refugees managed at Hôtel-Dieu in central Paris.

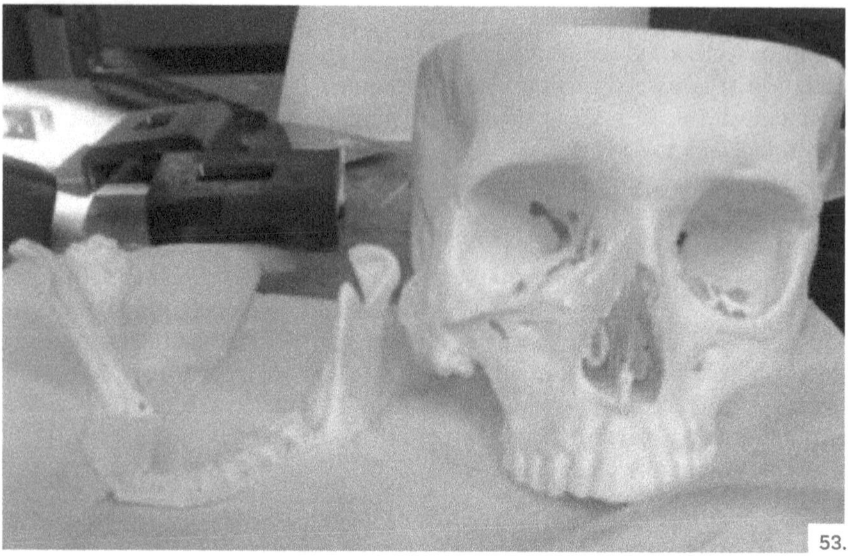

53.

Fig. 53. Anatomical model for left coronoid hypertrophy used to assess the anatomical conflict before planning resection surgery. Request of the maxillofacial surgery department, Hôpital Necker - Enfants Malades

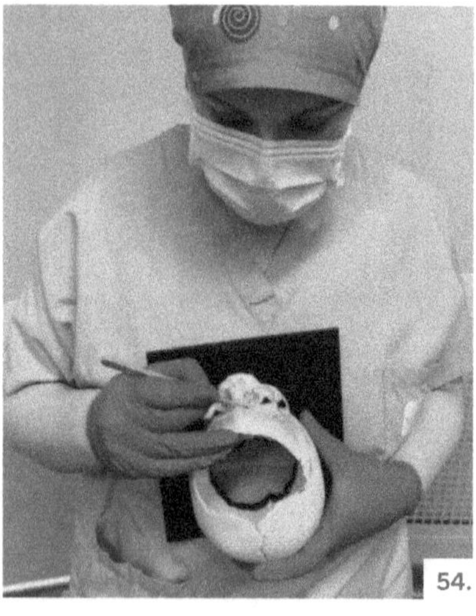

54.

Fig. 54. Surgical model for trigonocephaly being used by the Craniofacial Surgery Unit, Hôpital Necker - Enfants Malades.

8.7 Developing 10 models for benign jaw tumours: a medical thesis project - 3D printing, formal academic life, and valorisation

Benign jaw tumours are a tricky chapter in the training of maxillofacial and oral surgeons. These lesions have complex 3D structures and various anatomical relationships with teeth and nerves for instance, that can be clearly highlighted using anatomical models.

An oral surgery trainee dedicated her medical thesis the design of 10 anatomical models of the most relevant benign jaw tumours. These models were printed using the Stratasys J735 at Hôpital Necker - Enfants Malades and will be secondarily

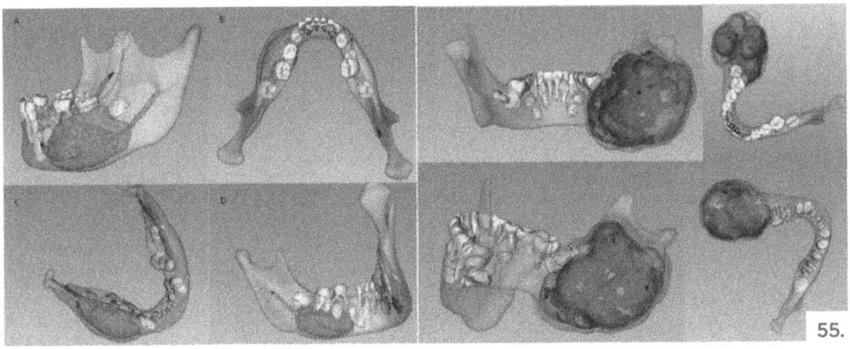

55.

adapted to become commercial products co-marketed by Université de Paris and BONE 3D. Here 3D-printing was used to contribute to the standard academic life of a large university hospital, with valorisation perspective arising from an MD project, which an interesting characteristic of the use of 3D printing.

Fig. 55. 3D models of benign jaw tumors: left = juvenile ossifying fibroma; right = anyvrysmal cyst.

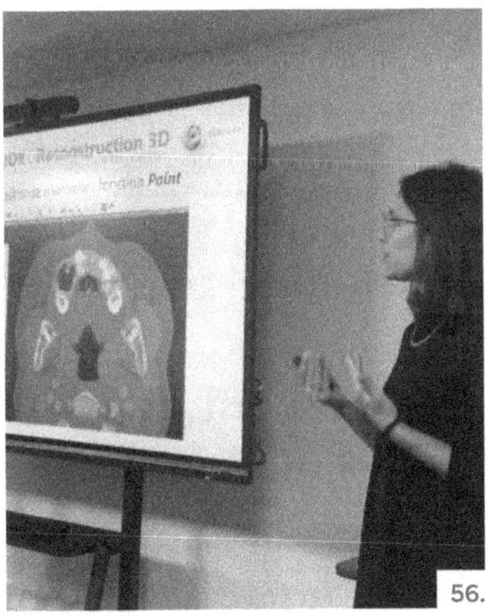

56.

Fig. 56. The trainee during her MD vivo (December 2020) at the Université de Paris, on 3D models of benign jaw tumors designed in collaboration with the AP-HP 3D platform.

8.8 Awarding students at Université de Paris: personalized trophees – positive reinforcement during the pandemic

Université de Paris is the home of the largest medical school in Europe. This university offers medical students several courses dedicated to 3D design and 3D printing:

→ An undergraduate 20h course 'Introduction to computer-aided surgery', for medical student, where the basics of segmentation and 3D design, as well as some general notions of 3D printing are offered to students

→ A post-graduate 70h course offering more advanced notions on the same topics, with clear clinical examples, intended for surgery trainees (Diplôme d'Université 'Planification chirurgicale et Médecine Personnalisée').

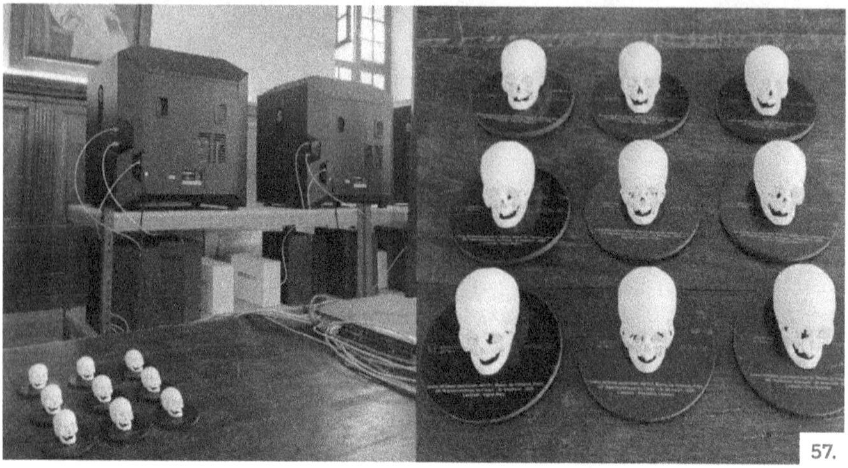

57.

Fig. 57. 3D-printed awards for medical students at the Université de Paris after passing exams of undergraduate computer design courses.

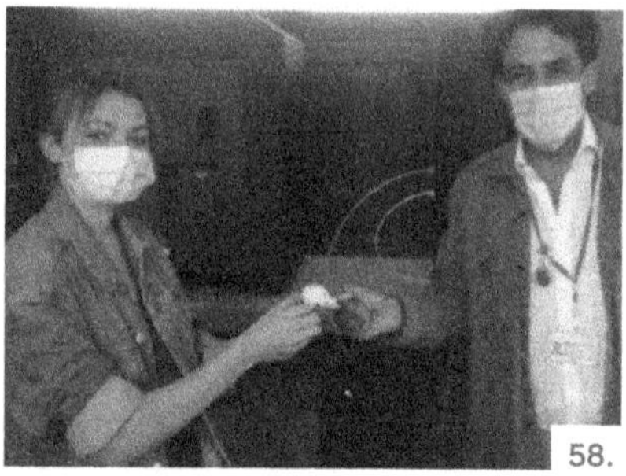

58.

Fig. 58. Medical student at the Université de Paris receiving a 3D-printed award after passing her exams.

The students attending the undergraduate 20h course in 2020 were awarded personalized trophies printed using polyjet printers (Figure 57), representing a skull with an intentional deformation for the Toulouse region in South-West France. In a context of severe disturbance in academic life, it appeared as a symbolic gesture to provide some level of positive reinforcement to medical students. The awards were given to students within the premises of the AP-HP 3D platform, in accordance with the distanciation rules imposed by the pandemic (Figure 58). As student life was deeply disturbed and impoverished during the pandemic, simple events such as award ceremonies, with the delivery of personalised gimmicks produced thanks to 3D-printing, contributed to keep the links between students and the university alive.

8.9 Medical thesis viva voce during confinement: printing Hippocrates in 3D - a case of academic emergency

Traditionally, medical theses viva voce end with the Hippocratic Oath, the student standing in front of a Hippocrates bust. For all viva occurring during Winter 2021, the Université de Paris was closed to students due to the virus so that there was no access to a Hippocrates bust. One of such busts was thus printed[2] in small size using polyjet printers and the Oath took place according to traditions (Figure 59), which may seem anecdotical but has a major symbolic value for graduating medical students and their families.

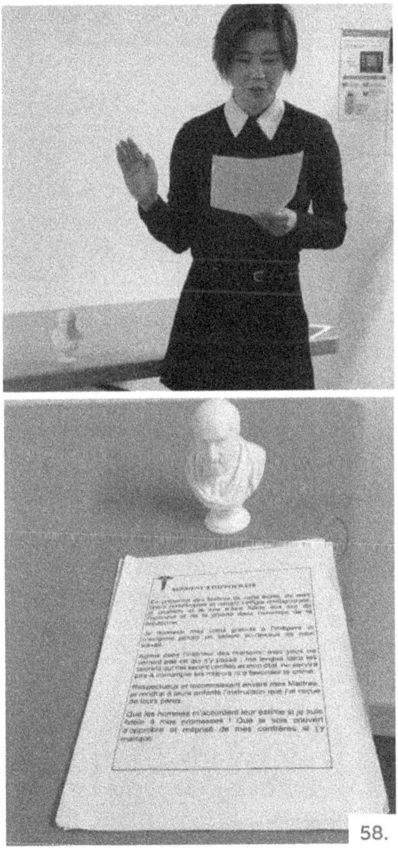

58.

Fig. 59. 3D-printed Hippocrates bust provided for an MD viva passed when Université de Paris was closed due to the pandemic.

2 Based on free online STL files: https://www.myminifactory.com/object/3d-print-hippocrates-80484

8.10 Fracture device for a biomaterial laboratory at Université de Paris – interactions with research institutions

Most of the interactions of the 3D COVID core team were with clinical departments. Nevertheless, several projects with fundamental research laboratories were also conducted. An orthopaedic surgeon at Lariboisière hospital put the team in touch with a biologist working at the Inserm laboratory UMR1132 dedicated to bone and cartilage biology. This researcher was working on fracture consolidation in rodents and for this, needed a specific fracture device for which he only had designs published in the literature [3] (Figure 60).

Based on the published designed, the fracture device was reproduced by the team using a combination of 3D printing and usual manufacture, and successfully used by researchers.

3 Zondervan, R.L., Vorce, M., Servadio, N., Hankenson, K.D. Fracture apparatus design and protocol optimization for closed-stabilized fractures in rodents. J Vis Exp 2018;138:e58186.

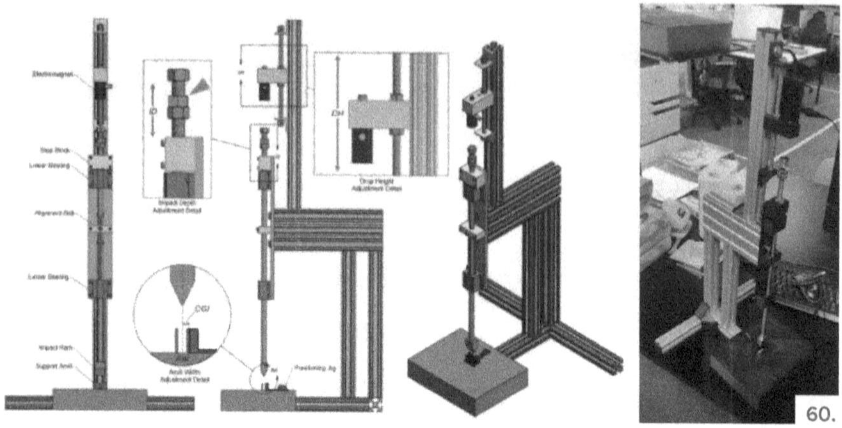

60.

Fig. 60. Design of the fracture device from the literature and device produced by 3D COVID for INSERM1132.

These examples – from anecdotical applications to promising innovations – demonstrate that a 3D printing platform located centrally in a large academic hospital is promptly adopted by academics from diverse backgrounds and serves missions such as education, training, fundamental research, social projects, and links with students. The social role of 3D printing is particularly relevant in a context of sanitary crisis.

9. Artistic and collaborative projects

3D printing is a major source of inspiration for artists. As a preliminary approach, a set of artistic projects were conducted using the production capabilities of the printers of the 3D COVID platform and the design skills of BONE 3D engineers. These initial actions pave the way for an integration of artistic projects within the long-term AP-HP 3D printing platform project.

Artistic projects are also a wonderful occasions for health professionals from different backgrounds to interact, and for patients to establish new types of exchanges with their care providers.

9.1 Jean-Denis Cochin, Saint-Roch and COVID-19

Visual artist Olga Kisseleva is a renowned specialist in the connections between art and science, also working as an associate professor at Sorbonne Université. After visiting the premises of the AP-HP 3D printing facility, Kisseleva proposed a project based on the 3D scan of a bust of Jean-Denis Cochin, the founder of Hôpital Cochin, located in the church of the Port-Royal abbey, right next to the place where the printers have been positioned (Figure 61). The Cochin bust was optically 3D scanned by the BONE 3D team using an ARTEC Spider 3D scanner.

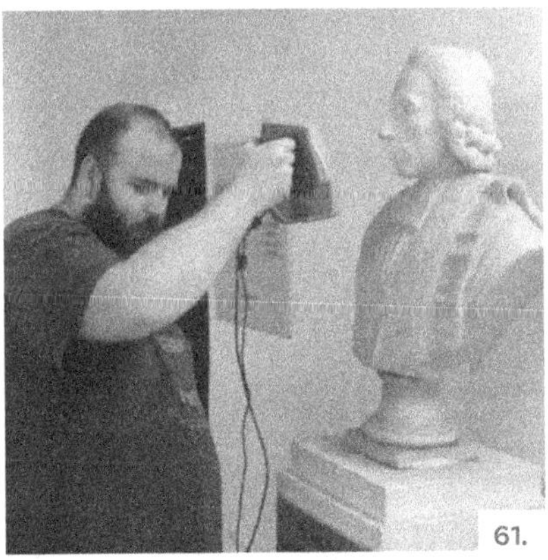

61.

Fig. 61. BONE 3D technician scanning Cochin using an Artec Spider 3D camera.

Kisseleva's project consisted in submitting the 3D image of the Cochin scan to various virtual viral attacks simulating the mechanisms of COVID injuries (Figure 62). The damaged Cochin face would then be treated using an anti-virus. The whole range of decaying and recovering Cochins was finally 3D printed An exhibition of the whole series of busts was organised within Port-Royal Abbey in November 2021 (Figure 63).

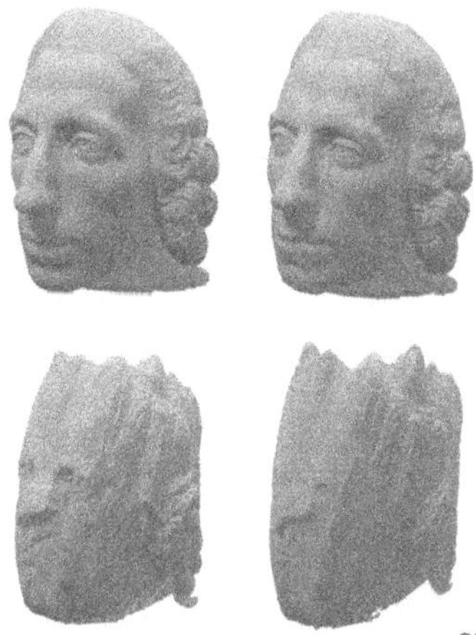

62.

Fig. 62. Three stages of progressive deconstruction of Cochin's bust, starting from the initial scan (upper left).

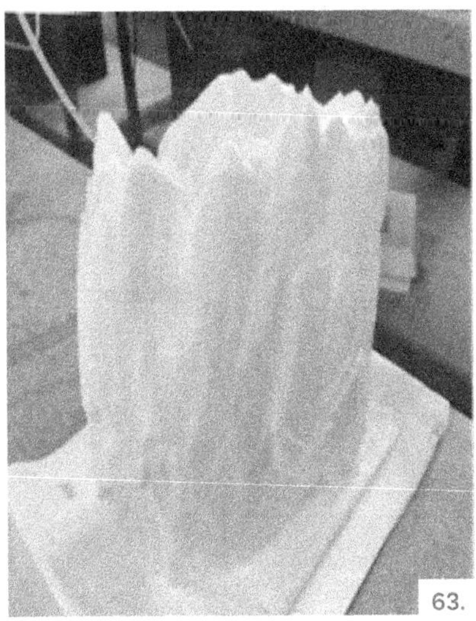

63.

Fig. 63. Later stage deconstruction Cochin heads before post-treatment.

The data on the four busts of Figure 61 are the following, with a layer thickness of 0.25, a filling density of 100 % and a wall thickness of 1.52 for all prints:

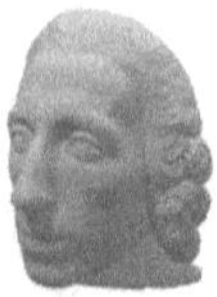	**Print duration**	3 days 8 hours 24 min
	ABS quantity	11110.02 cm^3
	Support quantity	422.29 cm^3
	Raw material cost	252€
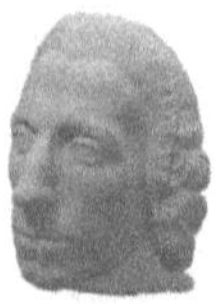	**Print duration**	2 days 7 hours 52 min
	ABS quantity	354.678 cm3
	Support quantity	455.427 cm3
	Raw material cost	133€
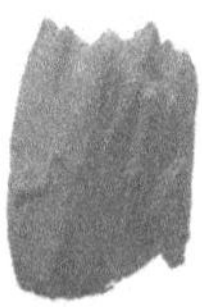	**Print duration**	1 days 19 hours 19 min
	ABS quantity	318.87 cm^3
	Support quantity	338.249 cm^3
	Raw material cost	108€
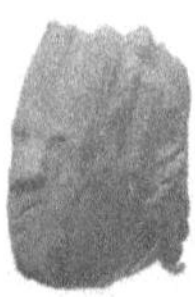	**Print duration**	2 days 7 hours 28 min
	ABS quantity	644.484 cm^3
	Support quantity	332.087 cm^3
	Raw material cost	161€

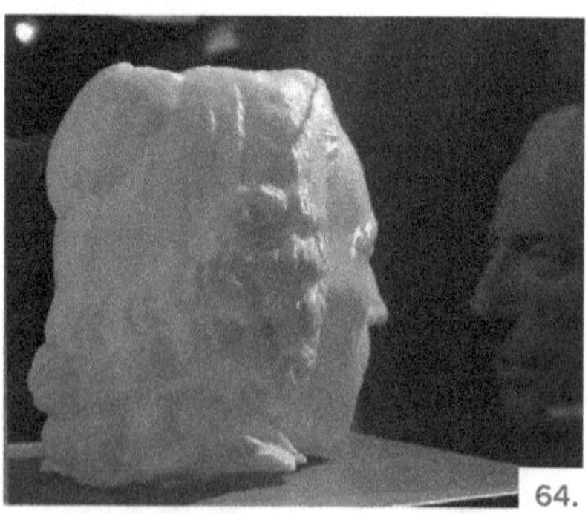

64.

Fig. 64. The Kisseleva 'Anticorps' exhibition within Port-Royal Abbey, next to the location of the 3D printing platform.

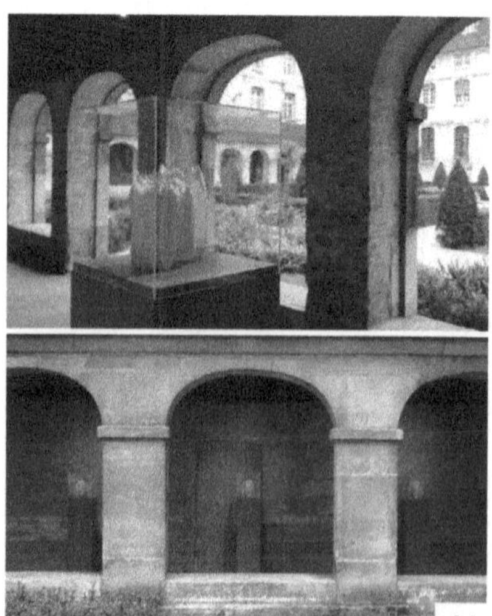

64.

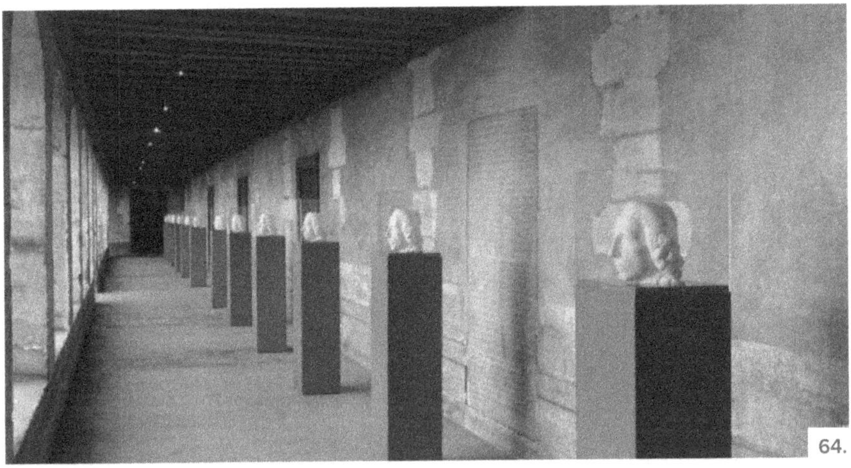

64.

9.2 Interactive tunnels for healthcare professionals

By collaborating with Kisseleva it became clear that the platform, by its technical facilities and its exceptional premises, had a high potential for building art-science collaborative projects.

To investigate this perspective further, the 3D COVID core team contacted a prominent curator, former head of the Espace Culturel Louis Vuitton, who introduced two artists to the 3D COVID team: Laurent Saksik and Alain Blondel, both with strong backgrounds in various collaborations with scientist and engineers.

The initial project Saksik and Blondel proposed was the design of a small series of 15 cm building blocks that could be assembled by health professionals and patients to form large tunnels through which they could walk, thus symbolising various personal journeys in this pandemic period (Figure 64). After a prototyping phase with the engineers of the team, it became clear that FDM printing and ABS were not adapted to producing these blocks. Initial prototypes would eventually disintegrate under the mechanical constraints of the arches of the tunnels (Figure 65). The project was terminated without reaching the state of a convincing prototype.

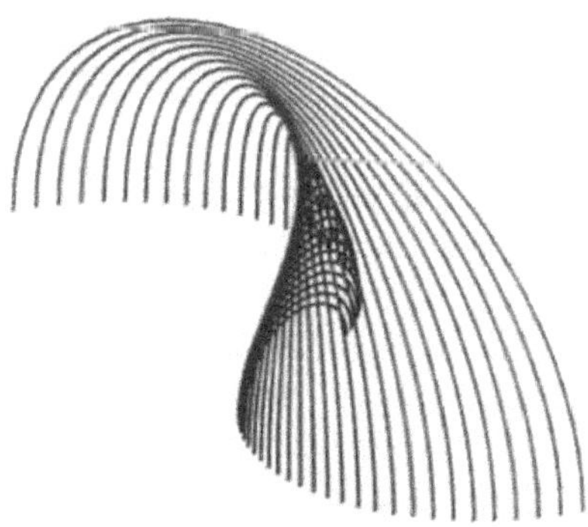

65.

Fig. 65. 3D rendering of a tunnel designed by Saksik and Blondel, to be assembled by health professionals and patients using individual 3D-printed modules.

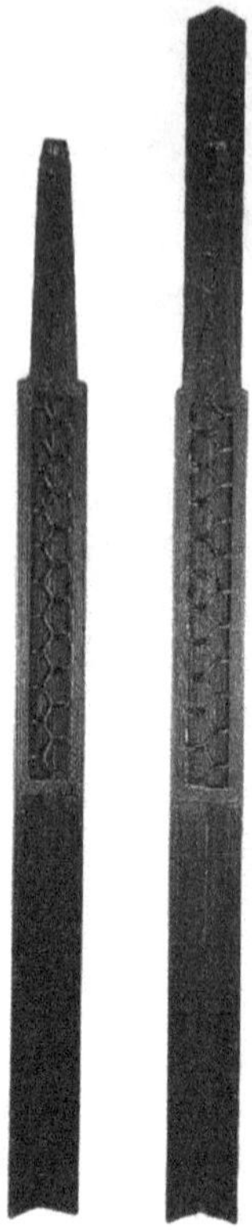

66.

Fig. 66. A broken module printed in ABS designed for building 3D tunnels.

9.3 Building clouds

Saksik and Blondel proposed a second interactive project after the technical failure of their initial idea. This project also involved health professionals and patients and consists in building clouds based in 3D-printed puzzle pieces. Four basic shapes were designed by Saksik and Blondel (Figure 66), which could be variously combined to form larger scale clouds (Figure 67). As in the first project, the creative project was integrated into the life of the hospital and the objects that would arise from this project had a symbolic link with the journey and hopes of both health professionals and patients. The design of this project is ongoing. The building blocks of the clouds are being designed to be polyjet-printed.

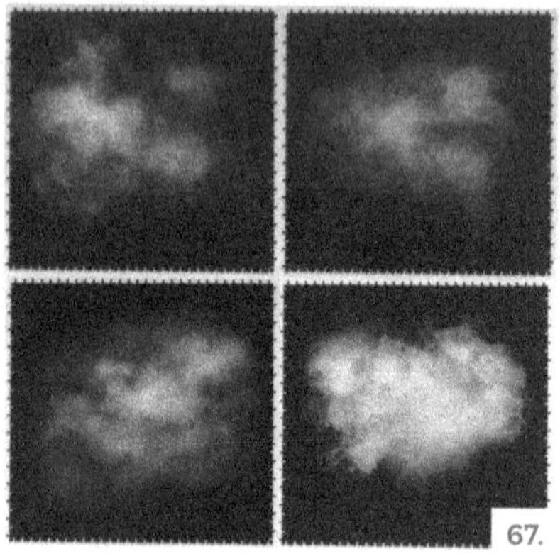

67.

Fig. 67. Mobiles Immobiles project – Laurent Saksik & Alain Blondel – 4 elementary clouds.

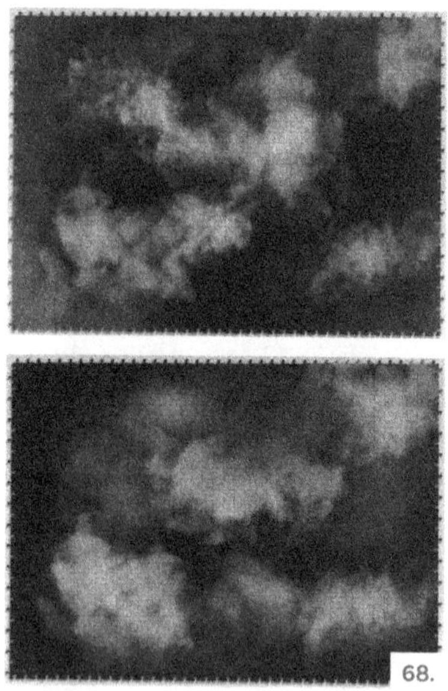

68.

Fig. 68. Two examples of combinaisons based on the 4 elementary cloud elements.

9.4 Reconstructing the face of war victims on sculptures

A young Parisian sculptor, Thomas Waroquier , has recently designed a series of busts of war victims from several XXth century conflicts (WWI, Irak-Iran war). Waroquier reached our platform with the project to 3D scan his sculptures, perform virtual surgery on them and then print the results of the virtual reconstructions. A first work reprensenting an Iranian soldier wounded in the 1980s has been scanned and is currently undergoing virtual reconstruction (Figure 69).

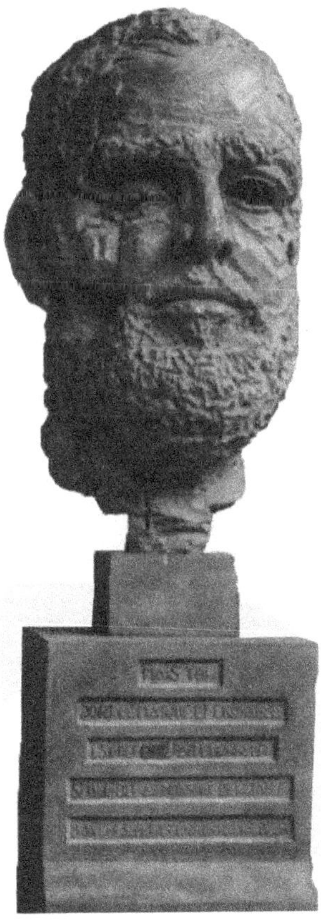

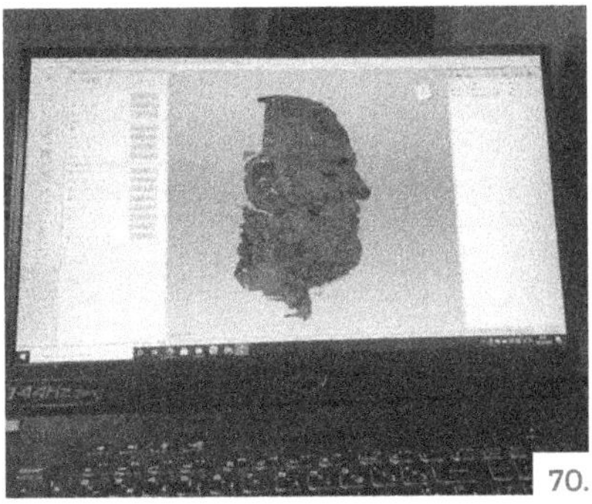

70.

Fig. 70. Bust of an Irak-Iran war victim by Waroquier scanned in 3D and ready for virtual facial reconstruction.

A 3D printing facility within a hospital offers infinite creative perspective to artists. Furthermore, when creative processes implicate health professionals and patients, they can constitute links within and between their communities. Art is one of the only tools that can put patients and health pracitioners in contact outside professional interactions.

10. Press and media: extensive list

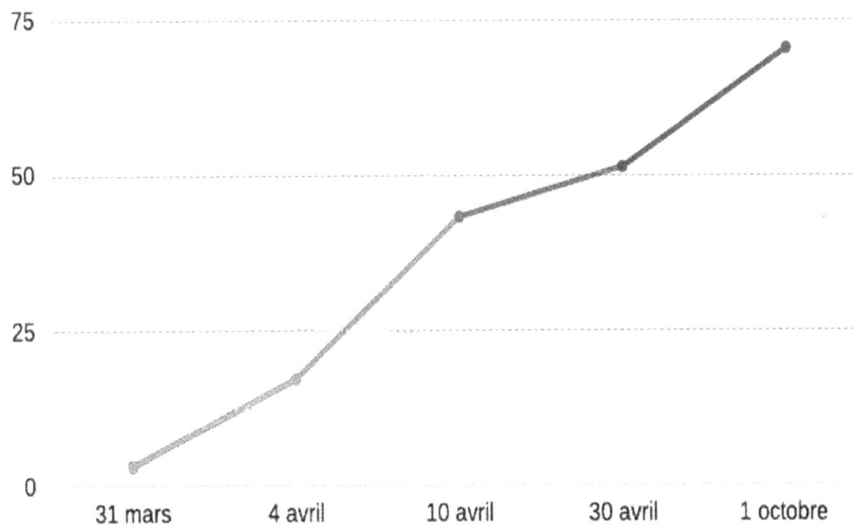

71.

Fig. 71. Press coverage of 3D COVID, in number of occurrences over time.

Media coverage for 3D COVID was impressively extensive, thanks to the support of Image7 and of the communication team of AP-HP. Most major French TV, radio and press covered the work performed at 3D COVID (Figure 70). A press day was organised by AP-HP the 3rd of April with high media attendance (Figures 71 & 73).

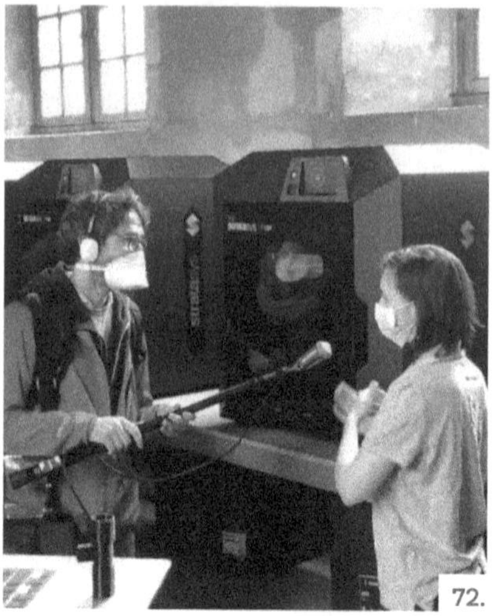

72.

Fig. 72. BONE 3D engineer being in-terviewed at the press day April 3rd 2020.

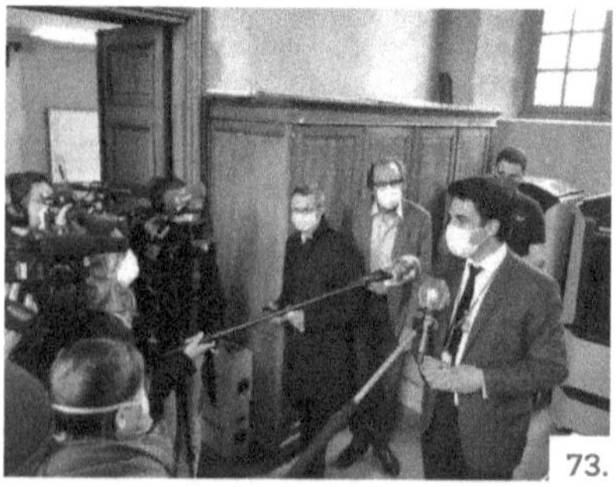

73.

Fig. 73. BONE 3D core team being interviewed at the press day on April 3rd 2020, with Université de Paris and AP-HP officials in the back-ground.

Furthermore, during the active phases of the pandemic, two events led to spe-cific interactions with media. When delivering contact-free door handle to the public schools of the 5th district of Paris (Figure 74), our team interacted with the Mayer of this district (Figure 75). The Mayer was a strong support of our project. We also took part in delivering and mounting face shields for the inhabitants of the district wit-hin the premices of the 5th district city hall (Figure 76).

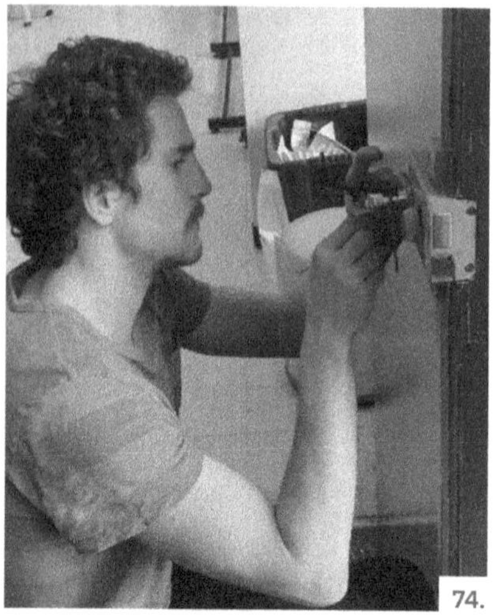

74.

Fig. 74. BONE 3D engineer fixing contact-free door handles in a pri-mary school of the 5th district in Paris on May 6th 2020.

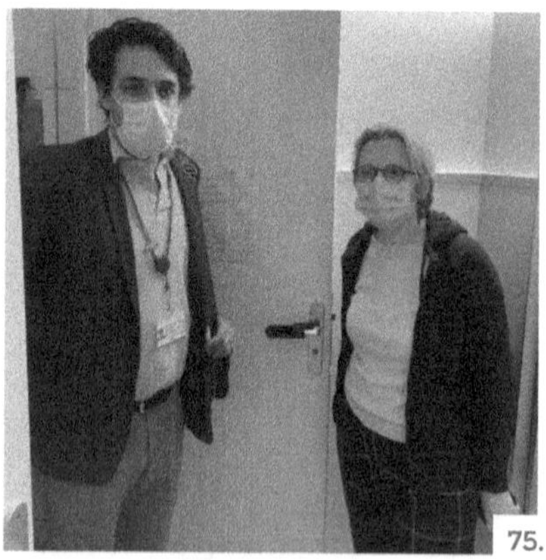

75.

Fig. 75. Medical coordinator with the Mayer of the 5th district instal-ling contact-free door handles in a primary school of the 5th district in Paris on April 16th 2020.

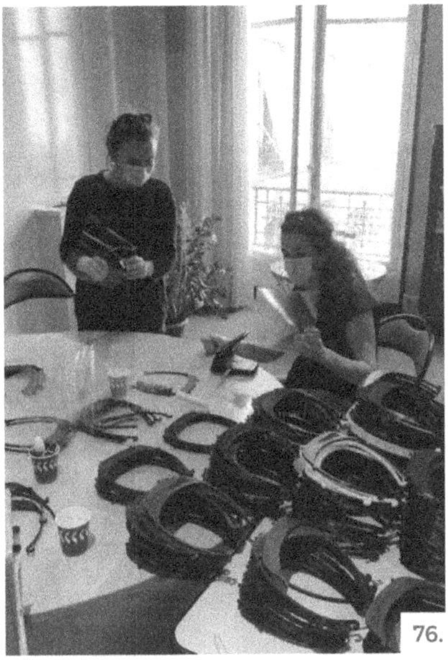

76.

Fig. 76. Delivering face shields to the city hall of the 5th district of Paris on April 20th 2020.

Furthermore, on the 3rd of June, the First Lady unexpectedly visited the 3D platform together with AP-HP and Hopital Cochin heads (Figure 77). The First Lady was very interested in the maintenance solutions provided by our platform and invited the team to visit the presidential palace in order to evaluate potential needs. The visit took place on the 29th of September and was coordinated by the head of resource and modernisation of the Élysée palace (Figure 78). We determined that one department could have potential 3D printing needs, namely the mechanical engineering unit managing the presidential cars, but they already had acquired an FDM machine and one of the mechanics working there had advanced skills in 3D design.

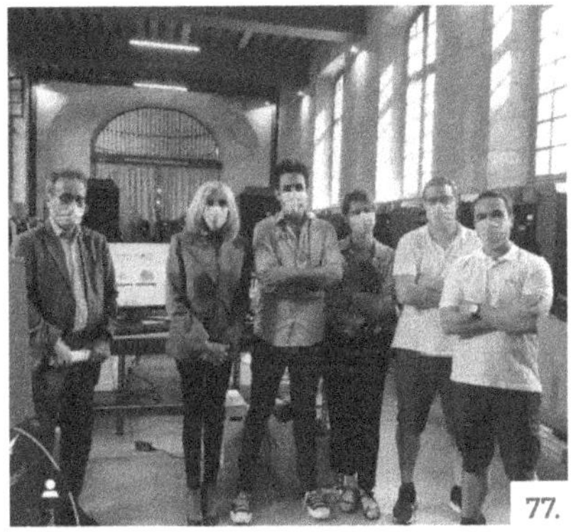

77.

Fig. 77. First lady visit at the AP-HP 3D platform. From left to right: AP-HP head, First Lady, 3D COVID core team, Hôpital Cochin head, 3D COVID core team.

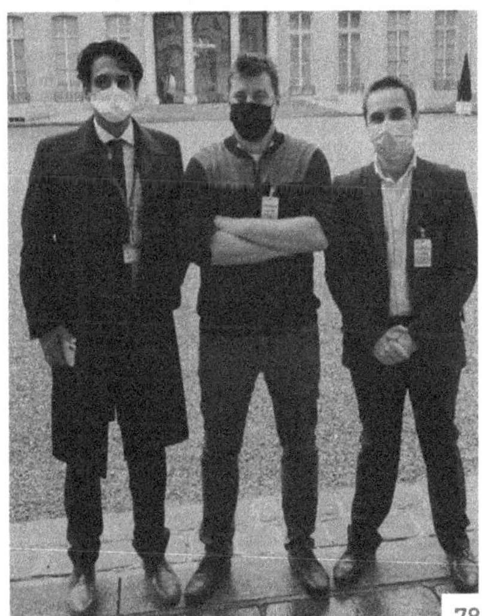

78.

Fig. 78. The COVID 3D team at the presidential palace.

10.1 Selection of most relevant citations

be judged from the peer-reviewed scientific output in the near future.

The response to the crisis was data-driven, thanks to a single institutional data platform fed by a single information system, providing important decision making parameters (eg, length of stay, treatment, clinical pathway) in real time.

Large-scale initiatives were rapidly developed. Each day, a farm of 63 3D printers manufactured 1000 parts of various medical devices, bypassing a slow supply chain and avoiding disabled equipment. The Covidom telemedicine platform monitored more than 50 000 patients at home (appendix).[3]

A region-wide patient-tracing programme, COVISAN, was set up.[4] Devised by AP-HP under the umbrella of the regional health authority, the COVISAN programme brought together local authorities, general practitioners, non-governmental organisations, and private companies,

2 European University Hospital Alliance. University hospitals urgently call for more European collaboration to prevent drug shortages. March 31, 2020. http://www.euhalliance.eu/2020/03/31/university-hospitals-urgently-call-for-more-european-collaboration-to-prevent-drug-shortages/ (accessed May 1, 2020).

3 Assistance Publique-Hôpitaux de Paris. COVIDOM: une solution de télésuivi à domicile pour les patients porteurs ou suspectés Covid-19 co-construite par l'AP-HP et Nouveal e-santé. March 12, 2020. https://www.aphp.fr/contenu/covidom-une-solution-de-telesuivi-domicile-pour-les-patients-porteurs-ou-suspectes-covid-19 (accessed May 1, 2020).

4 Piarroux R, Riou B. Coronavirus: pour déconfiner sans provoquer une deuxième vague, une approche centrée sur le patient. April 27, 2020. https://www.lemonde.fr/idees/article/2020/04/27/coronavirus-pour-deconfiner-sans-provoquer-une-deuxieme-vague-une-approche-centree-sur-le-patient_6037850_3232.html (accessed May 1, 2020).

The COVID-19 MS Coalition—accelerating diagnostics, prognostics, and treatment

Mass spectrometry-based analysis can answer questions broadly falling into two categories. The first concerns multi-omic profiling of the host response, correlating prognosis with disease severity. Robust biomarkers will further our understanding of disease mechanisms and the susceptibility of certain clinical groups. The most valuable of these prognostic markers will be those indicating the transition from a beneficial immune response to one that is harmful, ultimately resulting in respiratory distress. Such data will facilitate public health efforts for population screening, defining high-risk patients, tracking disease progression, and identifying sources of vulnerability that will permit treatment stratification and minimise or prevent future coronavirus pandemics.

The second category concerns the SARS-CoV-2 viral spike glycoprotein, which is not only key for host-cell attachment but is also a major target for neutralising antibodies elicit-

For the **Covidom application** see https://www.nouveal.com/covidom-le-suivi-des-patients-porteurs-du-covid-19/

For the **COVISAN programme** see https://www.aphp.fr/actualite/lancement-de-covisan-un-dispositif-de-suivi-renforce-des-personnes-covid

Published Online May 27, 2020 https://doi.org/10.1016/S0140-6736(20)31211-3

The Lancet. Assistance Publique - Hôpitaux de Paris' response to the COVID-19 pandemic - 26/05/20

La nouvelle vie des imprimantes 3D de l'AP-HP

Installée en plein confinement, la batterie d'imprimantes 3D des Hôpitaux de Paris tourne à plein régime. Une initiative qui pourrait faire école et même s'exporter.

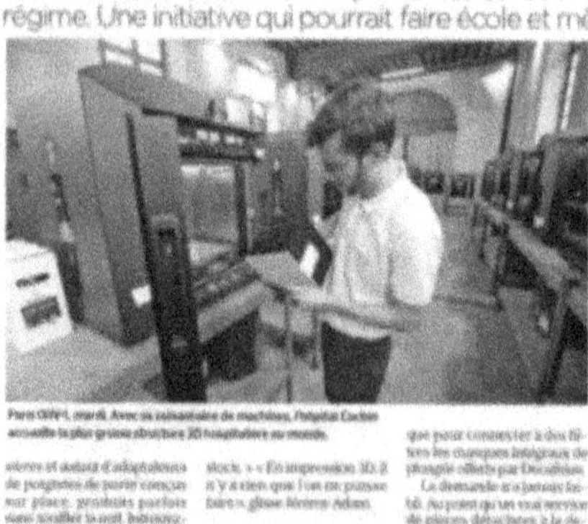

Une centaine de références déjà sorties

Le Parisien. La nouvelle vie des imprimantes 3D de l'AP-HP – 01/10/20

Capital. Petits et grands patrons,

Sans prétendre décerner des médailles, Capital a voulu d'ores et déjà saluer tous ces combattants d'une guerre économique pas ordinaire. Elle révèle l'incroyable capacité d'adap tation de nos industries, la place centrale du numérique, et surtout l'esprit de solidarité qui habite bien plus souvent qu'on ne le croit nos entrepreneurs. Il y a ceux qui ont fait des dons financiers (20 millions d'euros d'Hermès pour l'Assistance publique-Hôpitaux de Paris, l'AP-HP, tandis que Kering, lui, paie des imprimantes 3D) ou de matériel, combinaisons, défibrillateurs (Renault, PSA) ; ceux qui ont choisi de ne pas alourdir les finances publiques en prenant totalement à leur charge le chômage partiel de leurs collaborateurs (Chanel, Hermès) ; ceux qui

on ne les croyait pas si généreux - 18/05/20
Süddeutsche Zeitung. Dem Virus

Teile. Dringend benötigt wurden Dinge wie Ventile, Intubationsmaterial, Spritzenpumpen, Masken und medizinische Steckverbinder. Die größte Hürde, so der Kopf hinter der Initiative, der Chirurg Roman Khonsari, seien nicht die technischen, sondern die rechtlichen Fragen gewesen, um die Genehmigung der Behörden zu erhalten. Auch Khonsari sieht in der 3-D-Technologie nicht bloß eine Hilfe für die akute Notsituation, sondern auch eine Möglichkeit, zum Beispiel in Katastrophensituationen schnell an Ort und Stelle benötigtes Material herzustellen.

Druck machen - 13/05/20
Le Monde. La mode se paie le luxe de

Grands communicants et combattants de l'ombre

Dans un registre plus insolite, François-Henri Pinault s'est aussi retrouvé à financer l'achat de soixante imprimantes 3D pour l'AP-HP. L'idée émane du Dr Roman Khonsari, chirurgien et maître de conférences à l'université de médecine. Il n'est pas le seul à l'avoir eue, mais ce médecin utilise dans son petit labo de Necker l'une de ces machines pour imprimer des « guides de coupes » avant les interventions sur des enfants souffrant de malformations crâniennes. Martin Hirsch valide son projet illico.

Et ça marche : elles reproduisent vingt-quatre heures sur vingt-quatre des valves pour les respirateurs ou des dispositifs de protection et de confort pour les soignants (équipements pour ouvrir les portes sans les toucher, limiter le frottement des masques sur le visage ou des élastiques derrière les oreilles...). « François-Henri Pinault a dit O.K. sans mégoter ni savoir quel serait précisément le coût de l'opération, précise Roman Khonsari. Personne n'a rien demandé en retour, sauf quelqu'un qui m'a suggéré de mettre #kering sur mes posts. Mais, comme j'ai 300 followers, ça ne sert à rien... »

la solidarité - 20/04/20

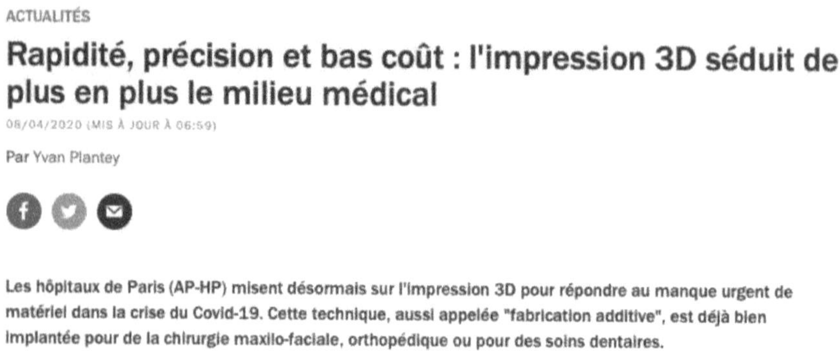

ACTUALITÉS

Rapidité, précision et bas coût : l'impression 3D séduit de plus en plus le milieu médical

08/04/2020 (MIS À JOUR À 06:59)

Par Yvan Plantey

Les hôpitaux de Paris (AP-HP) misent désormais sur l'impression 3D pour répondre au manque urgent de matériel dans la crise du Covid-19. Cette technique, aussi appelée "fabrication additive", est déjà bien implantée pour de la chirurgie maxilo-faciale, orthopédique ou pour des soins dentaires.

France Culture. Rapidité, précision et bas coût : l'impression 3D séduit de plus en plus le milieu médical - 08/04/20

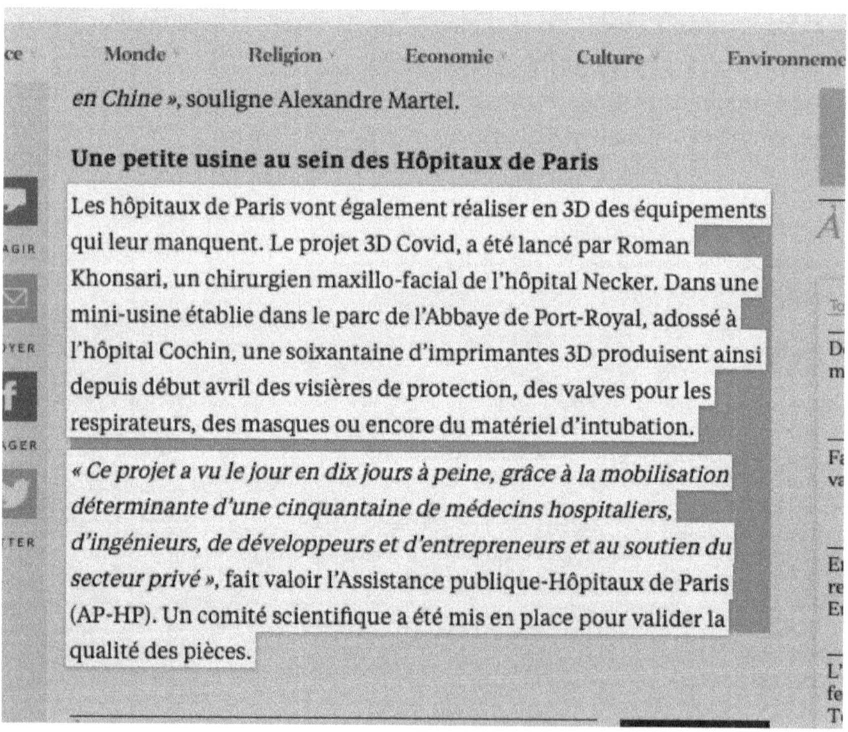

Monde Religion Economie Culture Environneme

en Chine », souligne Alexandre Martel.

Une petite usine au sein des Hôpitaux de Paris

Les hôpitaux de Paris vont également réaliser en 3D des équipements qui leur manquent. Le projet 3D Covid, a été lancé par Roman Khonsari, un chirurgien maxillo-facial de l'hôpital Necker. Dans une mini-usine établie dans le parc de l'Abbaye de Port-Royal, adossé à l'hôpital Cochin, une soixantaine d'imprimantes 3D produisent ainsi depuis début avril des visières de protection, des valves pour les respirateurs, des masques ou encore du matériel d'intubation.

« Ce projet a vu le jour en dix jours à peine, grâce à la mobilisation déterminante d'une cinquantaine de médecins hospitaliers, d'ingénieurs, de développeurs et d'entrepreneurs et au soutien du secteur privé », fait valoir l'Assistance publique-Hôpitaux de Paris (AP-HP). Un comité scientifique a été mis en place pour valider la qualité des pièces.

La Croix. Coronavirus : Des imprimantes 3D pour les 'visières de l'espoir' - 07/04/20

FOCUS

Coronavirus : premières livraisons en 3D à l'AP-HP

L'Assistance Publique - Hôpitaux de Paris (AP-HP) a acquis un parc de 60 imprimantes 3D auprès de Stratasys, le leader américano-israélien du secteur. Installées dans une salle de l'hôpital Cochin de Paris, elles doivent permettre de fabriquer en urgence plusieurs milliers de dispositifs médicaux par semaine.

Les Echos. Coronavirus : premières livraisons en 3D à l'AP-HP - 07/04/20

LE FIGARO

Lire le journal

fabriquer en urgence les milliers de pièces de matériel médical dont les hôpitaux parisiens ont cruellement besoin.

À voir aussi - Coronavirus: l'hôpital Cochin va produire en 3D des équipements médicaux

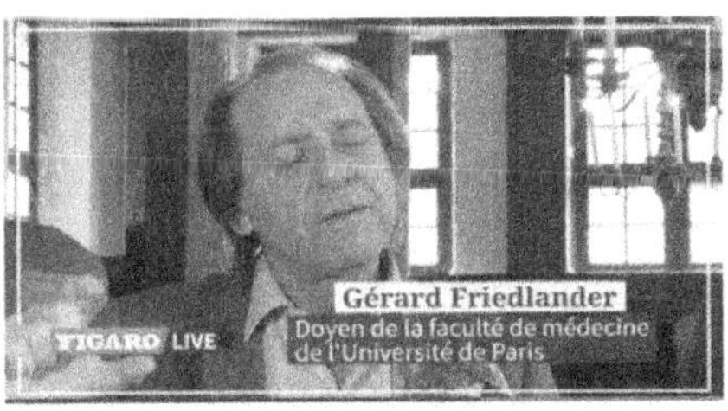

À lire aussi : Une appli de «tracking» contre le Covid-19: le numérique entre fantasme et acceptation

Il n'aura fallu que cinq jours pour que l'idée se concrétise. *«C'est l'université de Paris qui est à l'initiative de ce projet en partenariat avec l'AP-HP, et avec le soutien du groupe Kering»*, affirme Gérard Friedlander, doyen de la faculté de médecine de l'université Paris-

Le Figaro. À Paris, une batterie d'imprimantes 3D pour endiguer le coronavirus - 03/04/20

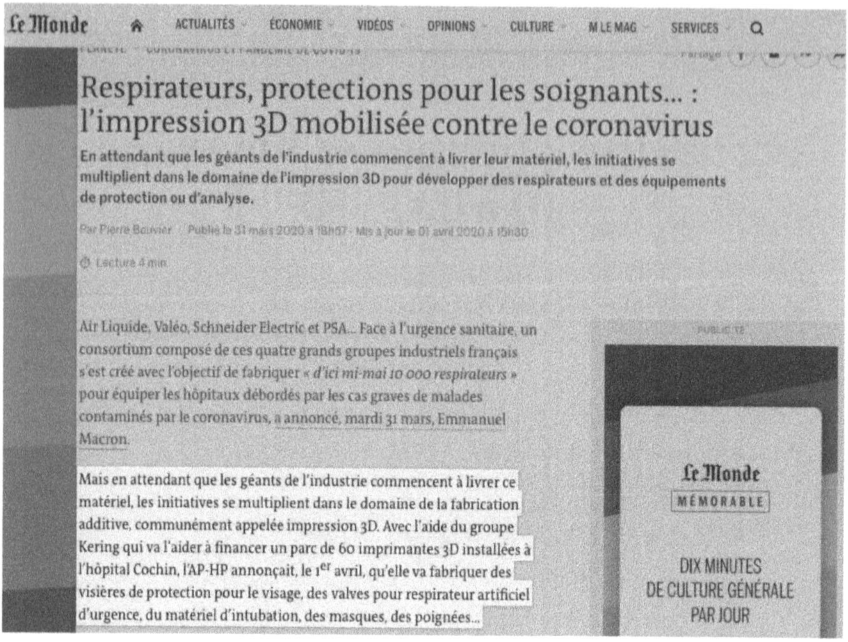

Le Monde — ACTUALITÉS — ÉCONOMIE — VIDÉOS — OPINIONS — CULTURE — M LE MAG — SERVICES

Respirateurs, protections pour les soignants... : l'impression 3D mobilisée contre le coronavirus

En attendant que les géants de l'industrie commencent à livrer leur matériel, les initiatives se multiplient dans le domaine de l'impression 3D pour développer des respirateurs et des équipements de protection ou d'analyse.

Par Pierre Bouvier · Publié le 31 mars 2020 à 18h07 · Mis à jour le 01 avril 2020 à 15h30

Lecture 4 min.

Air Liquide, Valéo, Schneider Electric et PSA... Face à l'urgence sanitaire, un consortium composé de ces quatre grands groupes industriels français s'est créé avec l'objectif de fabriquer *« d'ici mi-mai 10 000 respirateurs »* pour équiper les hôpitaux débordés par les cas graves de malades contaminés par le coronavirus, a annoncé, mardi 31 mars, Emmanuel Macron.

Mais en attendant que les géants de l'industrie commencent à livrer ce matériel, les initiatives se multiplient dans le domaine de la fabrication additive, communément appelée impression 3D. Avec l'aide du groupe Kering qui va l'aider à financer un parc de 60 imprimantes 3D installées à l'hôpital Cochin, l'AP-HP annonçait, le 1er avril, qu'elle va fabriquer des visières de protection pour le visage, des valves pour respirateur artificiel d'urgence, du matériel d'intubation, des masques, des poignées...

Le Monde. Respirateurs, protections pour les soignants : l'impression 3D mobilisée contre le coronavirus - 31/03/20

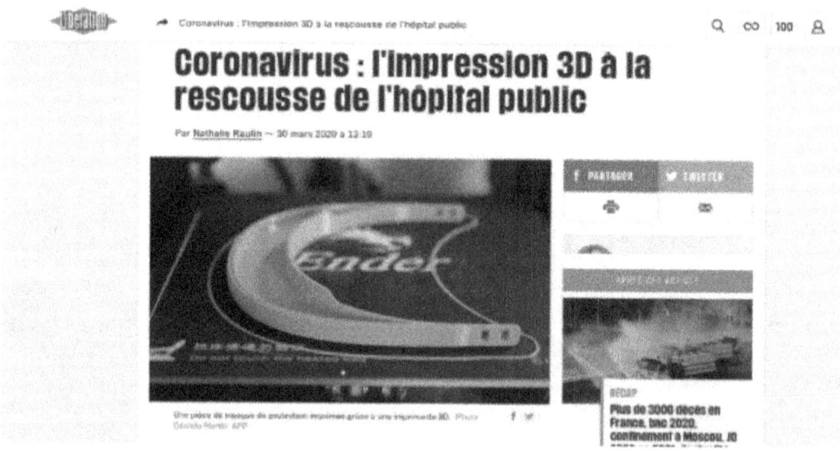

Coronavirus : l'impression 3D à la rescousse de l'hôpital public

Par Nathalie Raulin — 30 mars 2020 à 13:10

Plus de 3000 décès en France, bac 2020, confinement à Moscou, JO

Libération. Coronavirus : l'impression 3D à la rescousse de l'hôpital public - 30/03/20

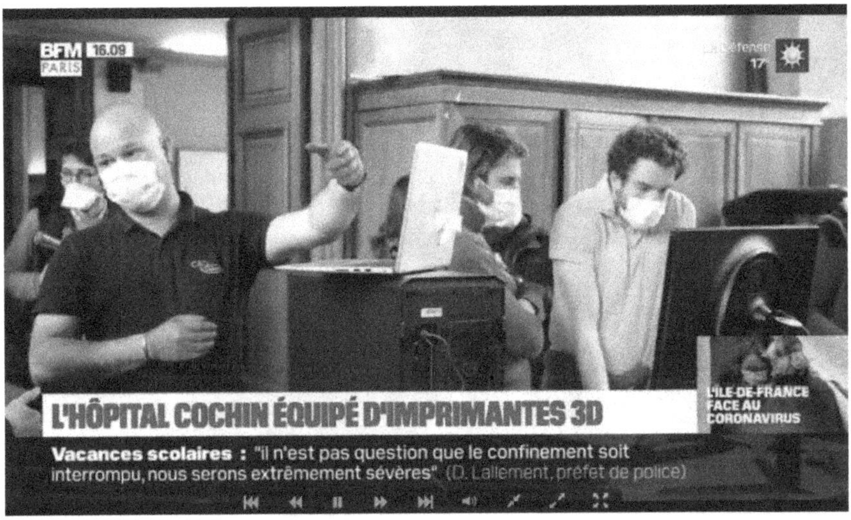
BFM 16.09
PARIS
L'HÔPITAL COCHIN ÉQUIPÉ D'IMPRIMANTES 3D
L'ILE-DE-FRANCE FACE AU CORONAVIRUS
Vacances scolaires : "il n'est pas question que le confinement soit interrompu, nous serons extrêmement sévères" (D. Lallement, préfet de police)

| Emission - BFMTV. 09/04/20

Coronavirus en France : 3D-Covid, un projet d'impression de matériel en 3D à l'AP-HP

Publié le : 06/04/2020 - 17:02 Modifié le : 06/04/2020 - 17:02

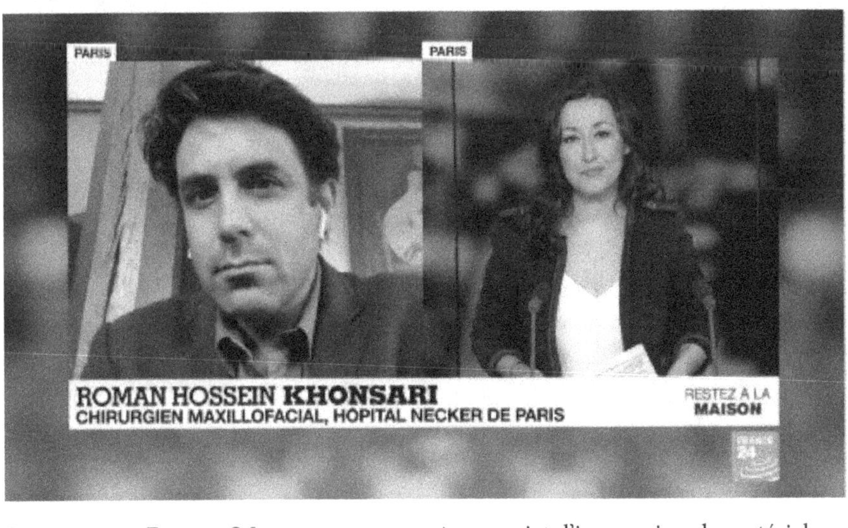
PARIS
PARIS
ROMAN HOSSEIN KHONSARI
CHIRURGIEN MAXILLOFACIAL, HÔPITAL NECKER DE PARIS
RESTEZ À LA MAISON

| Reportage - France 24.
Coronavirus en France : 3D-Covid, un projet d'impression de matériel en 3D à l'AP-HP - 08/04/20

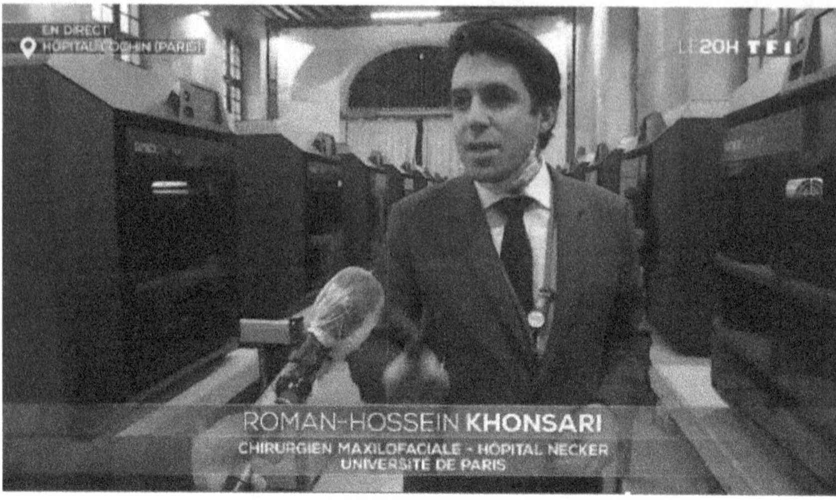

Journal de 20h - TF1. Coronavirus : à Paris, une mini-usine d'impression 3D fournit aux soignants le matériel qui leur manque- 06/04/20

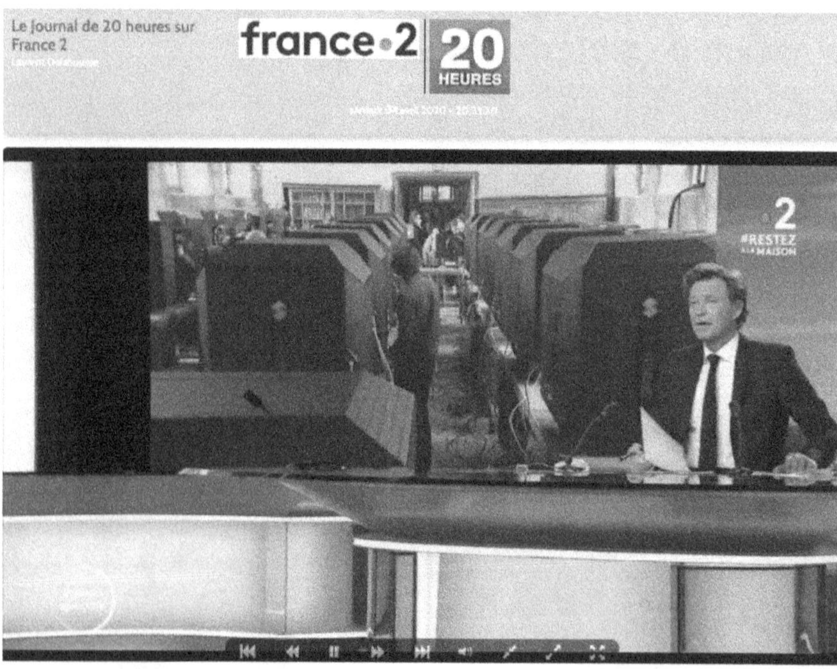

Journal de 20h - France 2. Coronavirus : les hôpitaux de Paris innovent pour fabriquer du matériel médical - 04/04/20

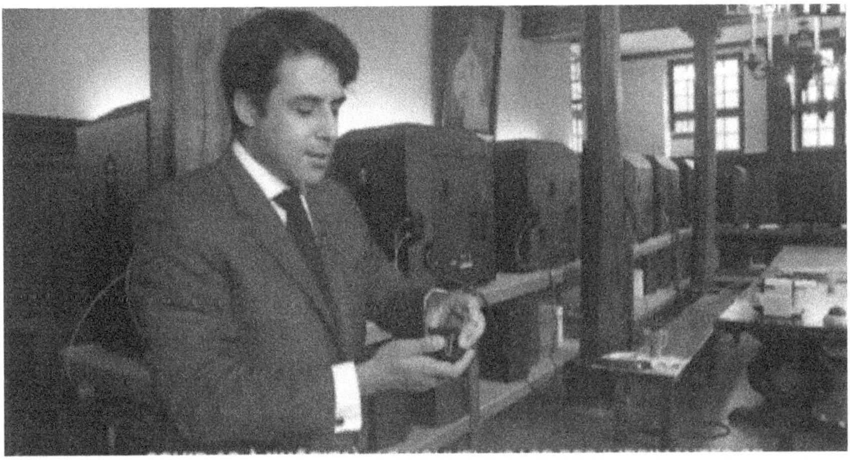

Journal de 20h - TF1.
Coronavirus : le nouvel usage des imprimantes 3D à l'hôpital Cochin - 13/10/20

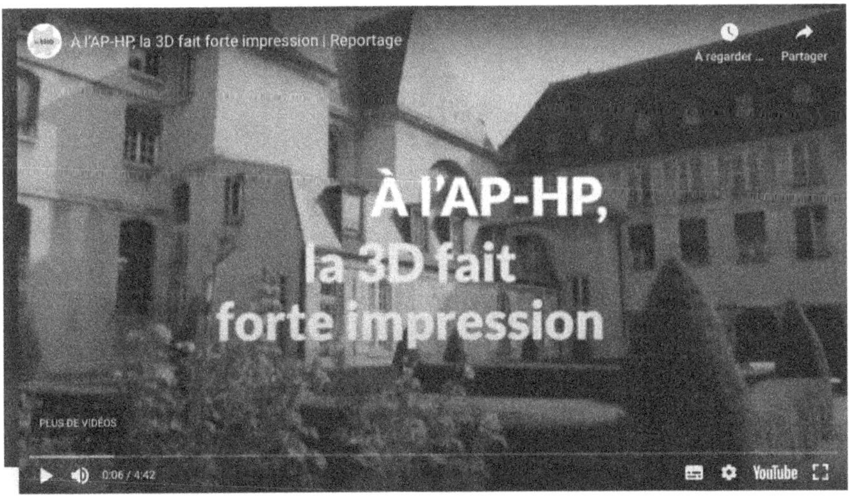

Le Blob - Universsciences.
Coronavirus : À l'AP-HP, la 3D fait forte impression - 13/10/20

10.2 Extensive list of early media citations

Media	Title	Date
Libération	À Paris, l'impression 3D à la rescousse de l'hôpital public	30/03/20
Le Monde	Respirateurs, protections pour les soignants…: l'impression 3D mobilisée contre le coronavirus	31/03/20
AP-HP	Fabrication de matériel critique en 3D pour les soignants et les patients rendue possible par le soutien de Kering	01/04/20
Le voix du Nord	Coronavirus : les hôpitaux de Paris vont produire en 3D les équipements manquants	01/04/20
Maddyness	L'impression 3D peut-elle pallier le manque de matériel des hôpitaux ?	01/04/20
Hospimedia	60 imprimantes 3D s'installent à Cochin pour fabriquer du matériel critique	01/04/20
Doctissimo	Les hôpitaux de Paris vont produire en 3D les équipements qui leur manquent	01/04/20
CNEWS	CORONAVIRUS : quand l'impression 3D vient au secours des hôpitaux	02/04/20
Le Parisien	L'AP-HP va imprimer en 3D les équipements qui manquent dans ses hôpitaux	03/04/20
Le Figaro	À Paris, une batterie d'imprimantes 3D pour endiguer le coronavirus	03/04/20
TechHospital	3D Covid, un projet d'impression de matériel en 3D à l'AP-HP	03/04/20

Journal international de médecine	La 3D contre la pénurie d'équipements médicaux	04/04/20
Science & Vie	L'impression 3D s'attaque au coronavirus	04/04/20
RF1	Coronavirus : l'hôpital Cochin va produire en 3D le matériel médical qui fait défaut	04/04/20
L'Usine Digitale	Covid-19 : L'AP-HP se dote de 60 imprimantes 3D pour pallier la pénurie de matériel médical	06/04/20
Pressecitron	Les Hôpitaux de Paris investissent 2 millions d'euros dans l'impression 3D	06/04/20
L'Usine Nouvelle	L'AP-HP s'arme de 60 imprimantes 3D à Paris pour lutter contre le Covid-19	06/04/20
ZDNET	L'AP-HP met en place un parc d'impression 3D pour lutter contre le Covid-19	06/04/20
3Dnatives	L'AP-HP se dote de 60 imprimantes 3D pour concevoir des dispositifs médicaux en urgence	06/04/20
Génération Nouvelles Technologies	Coronavirus : un parc de 60 imprimantes 3D dans un hôpital pour aider les soignants et patients	06/04/20
AQUAE	COVID-19 : des imprimantes 3D pour combler les besoins de l'AP-HP	06/04/20
Campus Matin	Covid-19 : les membres d'Université de Paris fabriquent du matériel pour les soignants	06/04/20
La revue du Digital	Les hôpitaux de Paris se dotent d'imprimantes 3D en grande quantité pour lutter contre le Covid-19	06/04/20
A3DM	Rencontre avec Roman Hossein Khonsari, chirurgien responsable de l'impression 3D de crise pour l'AP-HP	06/04/20

Journal du Geek	Pour pallier le manque de matériel, les hôpitaux de Paris se lancent dans l'impression 3D	07/04/20
Les Echos	Coronavirus : premières livraisons en 3D à l'AP-HP	07/04/20
SiecleDigital	Paris : l'impression 3D devient une arme pour lutter contre le Covid-19	07/04/20
La Croix	Coronavirus : Des imprimantes 3D pour les « visières de l'espoir »	07/04/20
Clubic	Coronavirus : à l'hopital Cochin, des dizaines d'imprimantes 3D pour imprimer protections et valves	07/04/20
La Tribune	Covid-19 : le monde d'après sera innovant ou ne sera pas	07/04/20
3D printing media network	Parisian hospital system installs 60 Stratasys 3D printers to fight COVID-19	07/04/20
France Culture	Rapidité, précision et bas coût : l'impression 3D séduit de plus en plus le milieu médical	08/04/20
Patients numériques	L'Assistance Publique – Hôpitaux de Paris innove à l'heure du COVID-19	08/04/20
TechHopital	3D-Covid, plateforme d'impression de l'AP-HP, a commencé à livrer le matériel manquant	08/04/20
Industrie Mag	Stratasys : AP-HP installe 60 imprimantes 3D FDM	08/04/20
Industrie&Technologie	[Covid-19] A l'hôpital Cochin, 60 imprimantes 3D produisent des pièces pour dispositifs médicaux et consommables	09/04/20

Carenews	[SOCIAL TECH] Coronavirus : des imprimantes 3D à l'hôpital Cochin	14/04/20
Innovation mutuelle	Covid-19 : des imprimantes 3D pour fabriquer en urgence du matériel hospitalier	16/04/20
Le quotidien du médecin	Covid-19 : les imprimantes 3D, petites mains de l'AP-HP	17/04/20
L'Humanité	COVID 19 : la mobilisation des FABLAB est sans précédent	20/04/20
Usbek & rica	Covid 19 : la mobilisation des makers est sans précédent, l'État et les pouvoirs publics doivent s'en rendre compte	22/04/20
APIVIA	Solidarité en 3D, l'exemple de l'AP-HP	29/04/20
DOCaufutur	Les hôpitaux de l'AP-HP impriment en 3D du matériel médical avec un contrôle qualité garanti par scanner 3D	30/04/20
Süddeutsche Zeitung	Dem Virus Druck machen	13/05/20
DH Magasine	Les hôpitaux de l'AP-HP impriment en 3D du matériel médical avec un contrôle qualité garanti par scanner 3D	13/05/20
L'usine nouvelle	L'impression 3D à la rescousse	14/05/20
Capital	Petits et grands patrons, on ne les croyait pas si généreux	05/20
The Lancet	Assistance Publique– Hôpitaux de Paris' response to the COVID-19 pandemic	26/05/20
Les Échos entrepreneurs	Bone 3D, Feelobject, Dulse : l'impression 3D sort renforcée de la crise sanitaire	25/06/20
Le Parisien	Explications sur la 'phase 2' du projet et le modèle médico-économique mis place au sein de l'AP-HP	01/10/20

France Info	Radio France - L'impression 3D au service de la lutte contre le Covid-19	31/03/20
RMC	RMC Football Show sur RMC Louis Amar	02/04/20
France 2	Le Journal de 20 heures sur France 2	04/04/20
RF1	Informations internationales sur RFI Jeanne Bartoli	05/04/20
France Info	Le Journal de 20 heures sur France 2 -Coronavirus : les hôpitaux de Paris innovent pour fabriquer du matériel médical	05/04/20
France 24	Coronavirus en France : 3D-Covid, un projet d'impression de matériel en 3D à l'AP-HP	06/04/20
LCI	Le Journal de 20 heures sur TF1 - Coronavirus : à Paris, une mini-usine d'impression 3D fournit aux soignants le matériel qui leur manque	06/04/20
PuMS - L'Émission Santé	Coronavirus : l'impression 3D dans les hôpitaux - Dr R. Khonsari #Pour une meilleure santé émission grand public universitaire	13/04/20
France Info	L'impression 3D au service des soignants	10/08/20
Universsiences	A l'AP-HP la 3D fait forte impression	18/09/20
RT France	Impression de crise à l'AP-HP	10/10/20
TF1	COVID19 - Le nouvel usage des imprimantes 3D à l'hôpital Cochin.	13/10/20
France Inter	Emission grand angle	13/10/20
France 3	Phase 2 projet 3Dcovid – 20h	15/10/20
Loopsider	Impression de crise à l'AP-HP	29/10/20

11. Genesis of this report

Early April 2020, the head of the Innovation & Technology Transfer Department at Imagine Institute[1], a prominent research institute located within Hôpital Necker - Enfants Malades, got in touch with Khonsari and introduced him to two consultants working at Alcimed[2], a brand specialised in tech with specific expertise in health. Both consultants were eager to contribute pro bono to 3D COVID, independently of Alcimed, during the sanitary crisis period.

After discussions with Khonsari, the Alcimed team agreed to work on the structure of a report that would provide a comprehensive account of our experience at 3D COVID. Within a few days, a group formed to start collecting data for this report. Two initial members of the 3D COVID team offered their support to the consultants, and included two friends to assist them in data collection: the chief technology officer at LegalPlace[3] and an engineer in charge of internal affairs at IRSN[4].

Key people involved in the 3D COVID project were interviewed by the report team and a first version of this document was released the 13th of May 2020. This initial version corresponded to chapter 1 of the current version. The report was considerably augmented by Khonsari and several interns (including Laura Laliève) to reach the current version, (BONE 3D staff members) also worked, mostly regarding the production metrics and the information on devices. Benjamin Demoury, MD student, contributed to the last stages of page setting. Final design and editing was perfomed by medical illustrator Emma Blanc-Tailleur.

1 Imagine Institute, Institut des Maladies Génétiques : https://www.institutimagine.org
2 Alcimed, a consulting brand with specific expertise in health : https://www.alcimed.com
3 LegalPlace, online legal services for French companies : https://www.legalplace.fr
4 Institut de Radioprotection et de Sûreté Nucléaire, the national body in charge of nuclear safety : https://www.irsn.fr

12. Supplementary materials

12.1 Initial business plan

TRESORERIE PREVISIONNELLE	2020									2021			
	Avril	Mai	Juin	Juillet	Aout	Septembre	Octobre	Novembre	Décembre	Janvier	Février	Mars	Avril
Dons Particuliers													
Dons Entreprises													
Financement AP-HP													
RECETTES	0	0	0	0	0	0	0	0	0	0	0	0	0
DEPENSES													
Achats matériels	893 950 €												
Achats matières consommables	82 667 €	38 640 €	19 320 €	0									
Fournitures - divers	2 000 €	2 500 €	2 500 €	2 500 €									
SALAIRES NETS (75 %)													
Coordinateur	3 000 €	2 250 €	2 250 €	2 250 €									
Prestation BONE 3D	80 000 €	80 000 €	80 000 €	80 000 €									
Livreur	2 000 €	2 000 €	2 000 €	2 000 €									
CHARGES SOCIALES													
Part salariale (25 %)	1 667	28 333	28 083	28 083									
Part patronale (45 %)	3 000	50 550	50 550	50 550									
TOTAL DES DÉPENSES	1 068 284	204 273	184 703	165 383	0	0	[illegible]	0	0	0	0	0	0
RECETTES - DÉPENSES	-1 068 284	-204 273	-184 703	-165 383	0	0	[illegible]	0	0	0	0	0	[illegible]
CUMUL	-1 068 284	-1 272 557	-1 457 260	-1 622 644	-1 622 644	-1 522 644	-1 622 644	-1 622 644	-1 622 644	-1 622 644	-1 622 644	-1 622 644	-1 622 644

INVESTISSEMENTS 2020		Durée d'amortissements (ans)	Amortissements			
	Montant		2020	2021	2022	2023
Achats machines						
Fortus F120	595 100 €	3	148 775	198 367	198 367	49 592
Fortus F170	278 000 €	3	69 500	92 667	92 667	23 167
Cuve SCA 3600	20 850 €					
Total	893 950 €		218 275 €	291 033 €	291 033 €	72 758 €

SALAIRES 2020	Brut	Mois	Total
PERMANENTS			
Coordinateur	3 000 €	4	12 000 €
Prestation BONE 3D	80 000 €	4	320 000 €
Bénévoles	278 000 €		69 500
Opérateur production		4	0 €
Livreur	2 000 €	4	8 000 €
SALAIRES BRUTS			340 000 €
CHARGES SOCIALES		45 %	153 000 €
SALAIRES ET CHARGES			493 000 €

PRODUCTION							
MOIS	Avril	Mai	Juin	Juillet	Août	Septembre	Total
NOMBRE MACHINES TOTAL	62	60	30	0	0	0	
Produits							
Visières	4 830	4 830					9 660
Masques	6 827	6 827	6 827				20 481
Dispositif 3	560	560	560	560			2 240
Dispositif 1	560	560	560	560			2 240
Dispositif 2	560	560	560	560			2 240
Valves	493						493
TOTAL	13 829	13 337	8 507	1 680	0	0	37 353

PRODUCTION

SEMAINE	01	02	03	04	Total
NOMBRE MACHINES TOTAL	62	62	62	62	
Produits					
Visières	1 208	1 208	1 208	1 208	4 830
Masques	1 707	1 707	1 707	1 707	6 827
Dispositif 3	140	140	140	140	560
Dispositif 1	140	140	140	140	560
Dispositif 2	140	140	140	140	560
Valves	493				493
TOTAL	3 827	3 334	3 334	3 334	13 829

PRODUCTION

JOUR	01	02	03	04	05	06	07	Total
NOMBRE MACHINES TOTAL	62	62	62	62	62	62	62	
Produits								
Visières	173	173	173	173	173	173	173	1 208
Masques	244	244	244	244	244	244	244	1 707
Dispositif 3	20	20	20	20	20	20	20	140
Dispositif 1	20	20	20	20	20	20	20	140
Dispositif 2	20	20	20	20	20	20	20	140
Valves	70	70	70	70	70	70	70	493
TOTAL	547	547	547	547	547	547	547	3 827

J	Fortus F170	Stratasys J750	Nombre unités total
NOMBRE MACHINES TOTAL	60	2	60
Produits			
Visières	173		173
Masques	244		244
Dispositif 3			5
Dispositif 1			5
Dispositif 2			20
Valves		70	70
TOTAL	416	70	517

COÛT/UNITÉ CONSOMMABLES	Total Coûts Avril	Total Coûts Mai	Total Coûts Juin	Total Coûts Juillet	Total Coûts Août	Total Coûts Septembre	Total Coûts
4	19 320	19 320	0	0	0	0	38 640
2,83	19 320	19 320	19 320	0	0	0	57 960
0	0	0	0	0	0	0	0
0	0	0	0	0	0	0	0
0	0	0	0	0	0	0	0
89,38	0	0	0	0	0	0	44 027
	82 667	**38 640**	**19 320**	**0**	**0**	**0**	**140 627**

TOTAL BESOINS AP-HP

PRODUITS	Total
Visières	10 000 €
Masques	20 000 €
Dispositif 3	2 000 €
Dispositif 1	2 000 €
Dispositif 2	2 000 €
Valves	500
TOTAL	**36 500**

CAPACITÉS DE PRODUCTION TOTALES

	Nombre machines	Fortus F170	Stratasys J750	Nombre unités total/jour
PRODUITS				
Visières	30	173		173
Masques	30	244		244
Sous-total	60	416		416
Valves	2		**70**	**70**
TOTAL	**62**	**416**	**70**	**487**

FORTUS F170	60	Durée fonctionnement (heures/jour)	Temps production (heures)	Total nombre unités porduites/ jour
PRODUITS				
Visières		23	4,00	6
Masques		23	2,83	8
TOTAL				**14**

STRATASYS J750	2	Durée fonctionnement (heures/jour)	Temps production (heures)	Total nombre unités porduites/ jour
PRODUITS				
Valves		23	0,65	35
TOTAL				**35**

Cuve de solubilisation SCA 1200	4	Durée fonctionnement (heures/jour)	Temps production (heures)	Total nombre unités porduites/ jour
PRODUITS				
Visières		23	4,00	6
Masques		23	0,65	35
TOTAL				**41**

COÛT/UNITÉ CONSOMMABLES				
VISIÈRE PRUSA	poids polyjet (g)	Coût unité	Coût matières premières (kg)	Coût/ unite
ÉLÉMENTS				
Headband imprimé 3D	32	0.001	200	6.40000
Visière plastique	1	0.05	1	0.0500
Revêtement silicone	1	0.5	1	0.50000
Adaptateur bande élastique	2	1.5	1	3.0000
Bande élastique	1	2	1	2.0000
Matériau support	1	0.05	1	0.0500
Supplément pertes				
TOTAL				**12.0000**

COÛT/UNITÉ CONSOMMABLES

MASQUE	poids matières premières (g)	Coût unité	Coût matières premières (kg)	Coût/ unité
ÉLÉMENTS				
Masque imprimé 3D	37	0.001	200	7.4000
Textile	5	0.001	1	0.0050
Revêtement silicone	1	1.1	1	1.1000
Matériau support	50	0.001	0	0.0000
TOTAL				**7.4050**

COÛT/UNITÉ CONSOMMABLES

VALVE	poids matières premières (g)	Coût unité	Coût matières premières (kg)	Coût/ unité
ÉLÉMENTS				
Socle imprimé 3D				89.3800
TOTAL				**89.3800**

DISPOSITIF 1	poids matières premières (g)	Coût unité	Coût matières premières (kg)	Coût/ unité
ÉLÉMENTS				
Socle imprimé 3D	25	0.001	250	0.0000
TOTAL				**0.00**

DISPOSITIF 2	poids matières premières (g)	Coût unité	Coût matières premières (kg)	Coût/ unité
ÉLÉMENTS				
Socle imprimé 3D	25	0.001	250	0.0000
TOTAL				**0.00**

DISPOSITIF 3	poids matières premières (g)	Coût unité	Coût matières premières (kg)	Coût/ unité
ÉLÉMENTS				
Socle imprimé 3D	25	0.001	250	0.0000
TOTAL				**0.00**

12.2 Regulations on personal protection equipment 1/2

Ministère de l'économie et des finances

Ministère du travail

NOTE d'INFORMATION du 30 avril 2020

Objet : Equipements de protection individuelle : adaptation de la procédure d'évaluation de la conformité des visières de protection dans le cadre de la lutte contre le COVID-19

Dans le contexte de situation sanitaire sans précédent que connaît la France dans le cadre de la pandémie de COVID-19, la présente note fixe en annexe la procédure d'évaluation de la conformité par des organismes notifiés des visières de protection destinées à la lutte contre le COVID-19 pour lesquelles la procédure de mise sur le marché est adaptée par l'instruction interministérielle n° DGT/DGS/DGCCRF/DGDDI/2020/63 du 23 avril 2020 relative à la mise en œuvre de la recommandation (UE) 2020/403 de la Commission européenne du 13 mars 2020.

Cette procédure d'évaluation de conformité adapte les exigences techniques fixées par la norme harmonisée EN 166 : 2001 « protection individuelle de l'œil_spécifications » afin de garantir la disponibilité des visières de protection sur le marché tout en veillant à assurer un niveau adéquat de protection de la santé et de la sécurité des utilisateurs. Elle a été établie sur le fondement des recommandations techniques formulées par la coordination française des organismes notifiés pilotée par EUROGIP[1].

Les équipements de protection individuelle faisant l'objet de la présente procédure peuvent être mis à disposition sur le marché national jusqu'au 1er septembre 2020.

Le directeur général du travail

Le directeur général des entreprises

[1] EUROGIP : Groupement d'intérêt public entre la CNAMTS et l'INRS œuvrant sur différents aspects liés à la santé et la sécurité au travail au plan européen

Annexe I : Procédure d'évaluation UE de type des visières de protection des yeux selon la fiche d'interprétation des règles EUROGIP « REPI N° R8.01 »

La visière de protection contre le SRAS CoV-2 (COVID-19) est un équipement de protection individuelle de catégorie III au sens de l'annexe I du règlement européen EU 2016/425, compte tenu du fait qu'elle est destinée à protéger l'utilisateur contre un agent biologique nocif.

Les exigences de la norme harmonisée EN 166 : 2001 « protection individuelle de l'œil_spécifications » sont applicables à l'exception des adaptations suivantes :

7.1.2.1 Puissances optiques sphérique, prismatique et astigmatique
La visière doit répondre aux exigences de la classe optique 2 au minimum.

7.1.4.2.2 Solidité renforcée
Une déformation de l'oculaire tel que décrit en b) est tolérée.
Note : l'exigence du point d) s'applique à l'ensemble du protecteur, y compris le serre-tête.

7.1.5 Résistance au vieillissement
Essai non exigé

7.1.6 Résistance à la corrosion
Essai non exigé

7.1.7 Résistance à l'inflammation
Essai non exigé

7.2.4 Protection contre les gouttelettes et projections liquides
L'essai de projections liquides doit être réalisé en prenant en compte la zone étendue EFIJ telle que définie dans la figure 11 de l'EN 168 : 2002 et modifiée telle que ci-dessous.

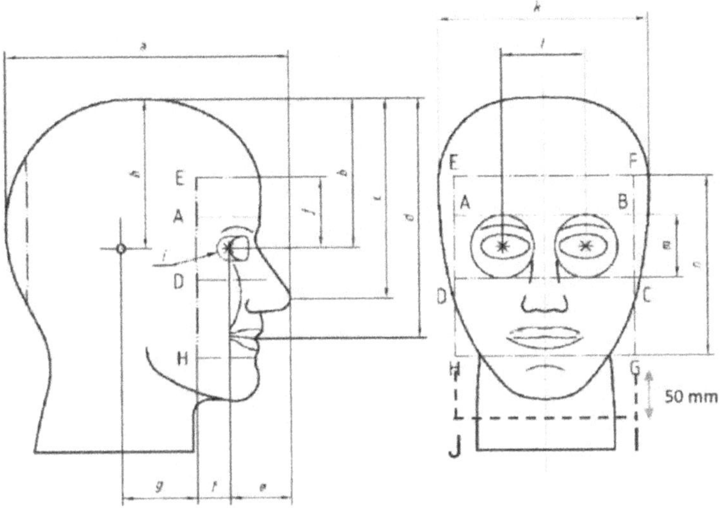

Figure 11 — Tête artificielle de référence

9. Marquage

La référence de la norme EN 166 ne doit pas apparaître sur la monture de la visière, ni sur le packaging.
La référence de la présente fiche doit apparaître sur le produit, à savoir R8.01.
Le champ d'application d'utilisation doit apparaître, à savoir uniquement la mention « COVID 19 ».
Le marquage symbole 3 au titre de l'essai projection liquide doit apparaître.

10. Informations fournies par le fabricant

- Les informations fournies par le fabricant doivent accompagner chaque plus petit emballage commercial disponible. Les informations fournies par le fabricant doivent être au moins dans la ou les langues officielles du pays de destination.
- Les informations fournies par le fabricant doivent contenir toutes les informations nécessaires sur :
  - les limites d'utilisation ;
  - les contrôles avant utilisation ;
  - l'enfilage, l'installation et l'ajustement ;
  - l'utilisation ;
  - le cas échéant, l'entretien (par exemple, nettoyage, désinfection) ;
  - le stockage ;
  - la signification de tout symbole ou pictogramme utilisé pour l'équipement.
- Les informations doivent être claires et compréhensibles. Si elles sont utiles, des illustrations, des numéros de pièces, des marquages doivent être ajoutés.
- L'information doit fournir des recommandations quant au moment où la visière doit être jetée ou remplacée.
- Avec l'absence de l'essai inflammabilité, une alerte spécifique doit être introduite :
  " Matériau inflammable : tenir éloigné d'une flamme ou source de chaleur "
- Les informations à fournir par le fabricant doivent comprendre la phrase " Cette visière est fabriquée uniquement pour la protection COVID-19. Cette visière n'est pas une visière à usage général et ne doit pas être utilisée à des fins autres que la protection contre COVID-19. Elle protège les porteurs des grosses gouttelettes émises immédiatement après une toux par une personne à proximité et face à l'écran, mais ne protège pas des particules restant en suspension. Cette visière vient en complément des protections de voies respiratoires adéquates. L'exigence de protection contre les produits nocifs est couverte par l'essai de projection telle que défini au§ 7.2.4 de l'EN 166 :2001.".

12.3 Supplementary material 3: regulation on personal protection equipment and medical devices 2/2

Bulletin officiel du ministere du travail

Travail, emploi, formation professionnelle

Travail et gestion des ressources humaines

Instruction interministérielle n° DGT/DGS/DGCCRF/DGDDI/2020/63 du 23 avril 2020 relative à la mise en œuvre de la recommandation (UE) 2020/403 de la Commission européenne du 13 mars 2020 relative aux procédures d'évaluation de la conformité et de surveillance du marché dans le contexte de la menace que représente le COVID-19
NOR : *MTRT2010499J*

Date d'application : immédiate.

Catégorie

Interprétation à retenir, sous réserve de l'appréciation souveraine du juge, lorsque l'analyse de la portée juridique des textes législatifs ou réglementaires soulève une difficulté particulière.

Résumé

La présente instruction abroge et remplace les instructions interministérielles n° 2020/55 du 31 mars 2020 et n° 2020/57 du 5 avril 2020 relatives à la mise en œuvre de la recommandation (UE) 2020/403 de la Commission européenne du 13 mars 2020 relative aux procédures d'évaluation de la conformité et de surveillance du marché dans le contexte de la menace que représente le COVID-19. Elle décline les préconisations de la Commission européenne visant à adapter les conditions de mise sur le marché des équipements de protection individuelle de type masques FFP1, FFP2 et FFP3, lunettes et visières de protection et des dispositifs médicaux de type masques chirurgicaux afin de garantir leur disponibilité en veillant à ce que les équipements et dispositifs médicaux ainsi mis sur le marché continuent à assurer un niveau adéquat de protection de la santé et de la sécurité des utilisateurs.

Mots-clés

Équipements de protection individuelle - dispositifs médicaux – masques – lunettes – visières - conformité - mise à disposition sur le marché.

Mention Outre-mer

Le texte s'applique en l'état dans ces territoires, et ne contient pas de dispositions spécifiques.

Références

→ Règlement (UE) 2016/425 du Parlement européen et du Conseil du 9 mars 2016 relatif aux équipements de protection individuelle et abrogeant la directive 89/686/CEE du Conseil;
→ Directive 93/42/CEE du Conseil du 14 juin 1993 relative aux disposi-

tifs médicaux ;
→ Règlement (UE) 2017/745 du Parlement européen et du Conseil du 5 avril 2017 relatif aux dispositifs médicaux, modifiant la directive 2001/83/CE, le règlement (CE) n° 178/2002 et le règlement (CE) n° 1223/2009 et abrogeant les directives du Conseil 90/385/CEE et 93/42/CEE ;
→ Recommandation (UE) 2020/403 relative aux procédures d'évaluation de la conformité et de surveillance du marché dans le contexte de la menace que représente le COVID-19 du 13 mars 2020 ;
→ Code de la santé publique, notamment ses articles L. 3131-12, L. 3131-16, L.5311-1, L. 5211-1, R. 5211-19 ;
→ Code du travail, notamment ses articles L. 4311-1 et suivants ;
→ Code des douanes, notamment son article 38 ;
→ Décret n° 2020-293 du 23 mars 2020 prescrivant les mesures générales nécessaires pour faire face à l'épidémie de COVID-19 dans le cadre de l'état d'urgence sanitaire.

Instructions abrogées

→ Instruction interministérielle n° 2020/55 du 31 mars 2020 relative à la mise en œuvre de la recommandation (UE) 2020/403 de la Commission européenne du 13 mars 2020 relative aux procédures d'évaluation de la conformité et de surveillance du marché dans le contexte de la menace que représente le COVID-19 ;
→ Instruction interministérielle n° 2020/57 du 5 avril 2020 modifiant l'instruction interministérielle n° 2020/55 du 31 mars 2020.

Annexes

→ Annexe I : Equivalence des normes pour les équipements de protection individuelle (masques FFP1, FFP2 et FFP3) ;
→ Annexe II : Equivalence des normes pour les dispositifs médicaux (masques chirurgicaux) ;
→ Annexe III : Equivalence des normes pour les équipements de protection individuelle (lunettes et visières de protection).

Dans le contexte de la menace que représente le COVID-19, les masques, les lunettes et les visières de protection répondant à la définition d'équipements de protection individuelle (EPI) ou de dispositif médical (DM) sont essentiels pour les professionnels de la santé, les équipes de première intervention et les autres personnes participant aux efforts visant à contenir le virus et éviter sa propagation.

I – Mise à disposition des équipements de protection individuelle et des dispositifs médicaux pour les professionnels de santé

Les équipements de protection individuelle, tels que les masques de type FFP1, FFP2 et FFP3, les lunettes et visières de protection, d'une part, et les masques répondant à la définition de dispositifs médicaux dits « masques chirurgicaux », d'autre part, importés par l'Etat ou l'un de ses opérateurs sans apposition du marquage CE, peuvent être mis à disposition uniquement des professionnels de la santé sur le territoire national jusqu'au 1er septembre 2020, sous le contrôle de l'autorité de surveillance du marché, conformément aux normes européennes ou conformément aux équivalences de normes figurant aux annexes I, II et III.

Les équipements de protection individuelle tels que les masques de type FFP1, FFP2 et FFP3, les lunettes et visières de protection et les masques répondant à la définition de dispositifs médicaux dits 'masques chirurgicaux', fabriqués sur le territoire national ou dans un Etat membre de l'Union européenne et faisant l'objet d'un achat et d'une évaluation mis en place par l'Etat ou l'un de ses opérateurs, sans apposition du marquage CE, peuvent être mis à disposition uniquement des professionnels de la santé sur le territoire national jusqu'au 1er septembre 2020.

Ce principe n'est pas applicable à toute autre filière de distribution ou à tout autre utilisateur professionnel ou particulier.

II – Mise à disposition des équipements de protection individuelle et des dispositifs médicaux pour tous les professionnels

1. Équipements de protection individuelle

Les équipements de protection individuelle tels que les masques de type FFP1, FFP2 et FFP3, les lunettes et visières de protection importés sans apposition du marquage CE peuvent être mis à disposition sur le marché national jusqu'au 1er septembre 2020, sous réserve que les procédures d'évaluation de la conformité prévues par les législations d'harmonisation européenne applicables aient été engagées, et dès lors que le niveau adéquat de santé et de sécurité des produits est constaté par l'autorité de surveillance du marché, conformément aux normes européennes ou conformément aux équivalences de normes figurant aux annexes I et III.

Lorsqu'un marquage CE est déjà apposé sur les équipements concernés importés sans que la totalité du processus d'évaluation de leur conformité ait été effectué, ceux-ci peuvent être mis à disposition sur le marché jusqu'au 1er septembre 2020 sous réserve que les procédures d'évaluation de la conformité prévues par les législations d'harmonisation européenne applicables aient été engagées, et dès lors que le niveau adéquat de santé et de sécurité des produits est constaté par une autorité de surveillance du marché, conformément aux normes européennes ou conformément aux équivalences de normes figurant aux annexes I et III.

Les équipements de protection individuelle tels que les masques de type FFP1, FFP2 et FFP3, les lunettes et visières de protection fabriqués en France ou dans un autre Etat membre de l'Union européenne sans apposition du marquage CE peuvent être mis à disposition sur le marché national jusqu'au 1er septembre 2020, sous réserve que les procédures d'évaluation de la conformité prévues par les législations d'harmonisation européenne applicables aient été engagées, et dès lors que le niveau adéquat de santé et de sécurité des produits est constaté par une autorité de surveillance du marché.

Afin de garantir que les équipements concernés font l'objet d'une évaluation de la conformité, la demande d'examen UE de type au titre de la législation d'harmonisation européenne applicable doit être déposée auprès d'un organisme notifié au titre du règlement (UE) 2016/425 au plus tard à la date de la première mise sur le marché des équipements concernés, qu'il s'agisse d'une importation ou d'une fabrication sur le territoire national ou dans un autre Etat membre de l'Union européenne.

Cela implique que le fabricant ou son mandataire se manifeste auprès de l'organisme notifié par tout moyen afin de formuler une demande d'examen UE de type avant la première mise sur le marché, qu'il s'agisse d'une importation ou d'une fabrication sur le territoire national ou dans un autre Etat membre de l'Union européenne, puis lui transmette le dossier complet dans les 15 jours ouvrés. L'importateur peut également être mandaté par le fabricant pour effectuer cette demande auprès de l'organisme notifié, cette tâche restant sous la responsabilité dudit fabricant. L'organisme notifié saisi de cette demande confirme la prise en compte de celle-ci dans les plus brefs délais et par tout moyen.

L'attention des fabricants et des importateurs est appelée sur le strict respect de l'exigence énoncée au point 1.4 de l'annexe II du règlement (UE) 2016/425, relative aux instructions et aux informations fournies, en vue notamment de préciser les conditions d'emploi de l'équipement de protection individuelle concerné, ainsi que le risque pour lequel ledit équipement a été conçu à des fins de protection.

Ces procédures d'urgence définies en application de la recommandation européenne du 13 mars 2020 conduisent ainsi prioritairement à mettre à disposition des équipements de protection individuelle permettant d'assurer une protection contre le COVID-19.

Par ailleurs, les lunettes et visières ne permettent pas de protéger des particules restant en suspension et n'ont pas l'efficacité des masques de protection respiratoire : elles n'ont pour utilité que de protéger les yeux, qui sont effectivement l'un des points d'entrée du virus ; elles ne peuvent donc pas remplacer l'usage des masques filtrants protégeant le nez et la bouche.

Il est rappelé que l'utilisation des équipements de protection individuelle doit s'inscrire dans le cadre des principes et des règles définis au titre II du livre III de la quatrième partie du code du travail.

2. Dispositifs médicaux

Les masques répondant à la définition de dispositifs médicaux dits « masques chirurgicaux » importés sans apposition du marquage CE peuvent être mis à disposition sur le marché national jusqu'au 1er septembre 2020, sous réserve de l'obtention d'une dérogation consentie par le Directeur général de l'Agence nationale de sécurité du médicament et des produits de santé au titre de l'article R. 5211-19 du code de la santé publique et sous son contrôle, dès lors qu'il constate le niveau adéquat de santé et de sécurité des produits conformément aux équivalences de normes figurant à l'annexe II.

Les masques définis comme des dispositifs médicaux fabriqués en France ou dans un autre Etat membre de l'Union européenne sans apposition du marquage CE peuvent être mis à disposition sur le marché national jusqu'au 1er septembre 2020, sous réserve de l'obtention d'une dérogation consentie par le Directeur général de l'Agence nationale de sécurité du médicament et des produits de santé au titre de l'article R. 5211-19 du code de la santé publique et sous son contrôle, dès lors qu'il constate le niveau adéquat de santé et de sécurité des produits.

Il est précisé que les équipements de protection individuelle et les dispositifs médicaux mis à disposition sur le marché dans les conditions définies aux points I et II sont destinés aux professionnels et ne doivent pas être commercialisés à destination des consommateurs.

Vous voudrez bien nous rendre compte de l'exécution de la présente instruction en adressant vos rapports sous le timbre de nos quatre ministères.

ANNEXE I

Equivalence des normes pour les équipements de protection individuelle (masques FFP)

Ces masques sont des équipements de protection individuelle qui doivent répondre au règlement (UE) 2016/425 du 9 mars 2016 relatif aux équipements de protection individuelle.
Le respect de la norme européenne EN 149+A1:2009 donne présomption de conformité aux exigences de ce règlement.
Ces masques sont notamment de types FFP1, FFP2 ou FFP3.

Type d'équipements de protection individuelle	Norme harmonisée européenne /classe de protection	Normes étrangères /classe de protection
Masque de protection	**NF EN 149 : 2001+A1:2009** « Appareils de protection respiratoire - Demi-masques filtrants contre les particules Exigences, essais, marquage »/FFP1	**Norme chinoise GB2626-2006** GB2626-2019/ KN 90 Norme chinoise GB/T 32610-2016/classe B
Masque de protection	**NF EN 149 : 2001+A1:2009** « Appareils de protection respiratoire - Demi-masques filtrants contre les particules Exigences, essais, marquage »/FFP1	**Norme australienne et néozélandaise AS/NZS** 1716:2012/ P1
Masque de protection	**NF EN 149 : 2001+A1:2009** « Appareils de protection respiratoire - Demi-masques filtrants contre les particules Exigences, essais, marquage »/FFP1	**Norme japonaise Japan JMHLW-** Notification 214, 2018/ DS1 ainsi que DL1
Masque de protection	**NF EN 149 : 2001+A1:2009** « Appareils de protection respiratoire - Demi-masques filtrants contre les particules Exigences, essais, marquage »/FFP1	**Norme brésilienne ABNT/NBR** 13698:2011/ PFF1

Table 1. Tableau d'équivalence entre les normes européennes et les principales normes étrangères applicables aux masques de type FFP1.

Type d'équipements de protection individuelle	Norme harmonisée européenne /classe de protection	Normes étrangères /classe de protection
Masque de protection	**NF EN 149 : 2001+A1:2009** « Appareils de protection respiratoire - Demi-masques filtrants contre les particules - Exigences, essais, marquage »/FFP2	**Norme américaine NIOSH 42** CFR 84/N95 ainsi que P95 et R95
Masque de protection	**NF EN 149 : 2001+A1:2009** « Appareils de protection respiratoire - Demi-masques filtrants contre les particules - Exigences, essais, marquage »/FFP2	**Norme chinoise GB2626-2006** GB2626-2019/KP95 ainsi que KN95 (particules non huileuses) (*) Norme chinoise GB/T 32610-2016 /classe A
Masque de protection	**NF EN 149 : 2001+A1:2009** « Appareils de protection respiratoire - Demi-masques filtrants contre les particules - Exigences, essais, marquage »/FFP2	**Norme australienne et néozélandaise AS/NZS** 1716:2012/P2
Masque de protection	**NF EN 149 : 2001+A1:2009** « Appareils de protection respiratoire - Demi-masques filtrants contre les particules - Exigences, essais, marquage »/FFP2	**Norme coréenne KMOEL - 2017-64**/1ère classe
Masque de protection	**NF EN 149 : 2001+A1:2009** « Appareils de protection respiratoire - Demi-masques filtrants contre les particules - Exigences, essais, marquage »/FFP2	**Norme japonaise Japan JMHLW-Notification 214,** 2018/DS2 ainsi que DL2
Masque de protection	**NF EN 149 : 2001+A1:2009** « Appareils de protection respiratoire - Demi-masques filtrants contre les particules - Exigences, essais, marquage »/FFP2	**Norme brésilienne ABNT/NBR** 13698:2011/PFF2
Masque de protection	**NF EN 149 : 2001+A1:2009** « Appareils de protection respiratoire - Demi-masques filtrants contre les particules - Exigences, essais, marquage »/FFP2	**Norme mexicaine NOM-116-200**9/N95 ainsi que P95, R95

Table 2. Tableau d'équivalence entre les normes européennes et les principales normes étrangères applicables aux masques de type FFP2

(*) Dans cette indication, l'utilisation d'un masque KN95 permet de garantir l'équivalence de protection à un masque FFP2. Toutefois, la couverture d'autres risques (comme certains agents chimiques) nécessitant une performance sur la filtration de particules huileuses nécessitera l'utilisation d'un masque KP95.

Type d'équipements de protection individuelle	Norme harmonisée européenne /classe de protection	Normes étrangères /classe de protection
Masque de protection	**NF EN 149 : 2001+A1:2009** « Appareils de protection respiratoire - Demi-masques filtrants contre les particules - Exigences, essais, marquage »/FFP3	**Norme américaine NIOSH 42** CFR 84/N99, ainsi que N100, P99, P100, R99, R100
Masque de protection	**NF EN 149 : 2001+A1:2009** « Appareils de protection respiratoire - Demi-masques filtrants contre les particules - Exigences, essais, marquage »/FFP3	**Norme chinoise GB2626-2006** GB2626-2019/KN100 ainsi que KP100
Masque de protection	**NF EN 149 : 2001+A1:2009** « Appareils de protection respiratoire - Demi-masques filtrants contre les particules - Exigences, essais, marquage »/FFP3	**Normes australienne et néozélandaise AS/NZS** 1716:2012/P3
Masque de protection	**NF EN 149 : 2001+A1:2009** « Appareils de protection respiratoire - Demi-masques filtrants contre les particules - Exigences, essais, marquage »/FFP3	**Norme japonaise Japan JMHLW-Notification 214,** 2018/DS3 ainsi que DL3
Masque de protection	**NF EN 149 : 2001+A1:2009** « Appareils de protection respiratoire - Demi-masques filtrants contre les particules - Exigences, essais, marquage »/FFP3	**Norme brésilienne ABNT/NBR 13698:2011**/PFF3
Masque de protection	**NF EN 149 : 2001+A1:2009** « Appareils de protection respiratoire - Demi-masques filtrants contre les particules - Exigences, essais, marquage »/FFP3	**Norme mexicaine NOM-116-2009**/ N99, ainsi que N100, P99, P100, R99, R100

Table 3. Tableau d'équivalence entre les normes européennes et les principales normes étrangères applicables aux masques de type FFP3.

ANNEXE 2

Equivalence des normes pour les dispositifs médicaux

Les masques dits « chirurgicaux » sont des dispositifs médicaux qui doivent répondre à la directive 93/42/CEE du 14 juin 1993 relative aux dispositifs médicaux.

Le respect de la norme européenne EN 14683:2019 donne présomption de conformité aux exigences de cette directive.

Ces masques sont de deux types : type I, II et IIR.

→ Les masques de type I sont définis dans la norme EN 14683:2019 comme des masques pouvant être utilisés « au minimum pour des patients afin de réduire le risque de propagation des infections, en particulier dans un contexte d'épidémie ou de pandémie ».

→ Les masques de type II ou IIR sont, d'après la norme, « principalement destinés à être utilisés par les professionnels de santé dans des blocs opératoires ou dans d'autres installations médicales aux exigences similaires ».

L'article 2 de la décision d'exécution (UE) 2020/437 de la Commission du 24 mars 2020 concernant les normes harmonisées relatives aux dispositifs médicaux élaborées à l'appui de la directive 93/42/CEE du Conseil, proroge la norme DM 14683 : 2005 (et versions suivantes) jusqu'au 30 septembre 2021.

Pour les masques répondant à la réglementation américaine

→ Un masque répondant aux exigences de la norme américaine ASTM F2100-19 level 1 respecte un niveau de santé et de sécurité » garantissant le respect de la législation européenne pour les masques à usage médical de type I selon la norme européenne EN 14683:2019 ;

→ Un masque répondant aux exigences de la norme américaine ASTM F2100-19 level 2 respecte un niveau de santé et de sécurité » garantissant le respect de la législation européenne pour les masques à usage médical de type IIR selon la norme européenne EN 14683:2019 ;

→ Un masque répondant aux exigences de la norme américaine ASTM F2100-19 level 3 respecte un niveau de santé et de sécurité » garantissant le respect de la législation européenne pour les masques à usage médical de type IIR selon la norme européenne EN 14683:2019.

Pour les masques répondant à la réglementation chinoise

→ Un masque répondant aux exigences de la norme chinoise YY/T 0969-2013 respecte un niveau de santé et de sécurité » garantissant le respect de la législation européenne pour les masques à usage médical de type I selon la norme européenne EN 14683:2019 ;

→ Un masque répondant aux exigences de la norme chinoise YY 0469-2011 respecte un niveau de santé et de sécurité » garantissant le respect de la législation européenne pour les masques à usage médical de type I selon la norme européenne EN 14683:2019.

ANNEXE 3

Equivalence des normes pour les équipements de protection individuelle (lunettes et visières de protection)

Ces lunettes et visières de protection sont des équipements de protection individuelle qui doivent répondre au règlement (UE) 2016/425 du 9 mars 2016 relatif aux équipements de protection individuelle. Le respect de la norme européenne EN 166:2001 donne présomption de conformité aux exigences de ce règlement.

De par leur conception/fabrication, et quelles que soient leurs variantes (écran facial, visière, lunettes...), ces produits ont pour objet de protéger les yeux, qui sont effectivement l'un des points d'entrée du virus. De tels produits peuvent prétendre à protéger le porteur contre la pénétration du virus par les yeux, sous réserve de respecter les contraintes réglementaires applicables aux EPI de catégorie III. Toutefois, ces produits ne peuvent pas prétendre bloquer la pénétration des aérosols par les voies aériennes supérieures (nez et bouche). Toute mention allant dans le sens d'une protection efficace des voies respiratoires par ce type de produit relèverait de la tromperie. Le port d'un masque FFP2 ou FFP3 sous la visière en question est ainsi indispensable pour une protection individuelle respiratoire car, en pratique, l'écran facial / la visière / les lunettes protège(nt) les yeux, tandis que le masque FFP2 ou FFP3 protège le nez et la bouche : ils sont complémentaires et il n'y a pas de rapport de substitution de l'un à l'autre.

Type d'équipements de protection individuelle	Norme harmonisée européenne /classe de protection	Normes étrangères /classe de protection
Lunettes de protection/ Visières de protection	**EN 166:2001** « Protection individuelle de l'œil — Spécifications »/ **7.2.4 Protection contre les gouttelettes et les projections liquides** marquage du symbole « 3 » (gouttelettes ou projections de liquide)	**Norme américaine ANSI / ISEA Z87.1** Marquage du symbole « D3 »
Lunettes de protection/ Visières de protection	**EN 166:2001** « Protection individuelle de l'œil — Spécifications »/ **7.2.4 Protection contre les gouttelettes et les projections liquides** marquage du symbole « 3 » (gouttelettes ou projections de liquide)	**Norme chinoise GB/T 14866**
Lunettes de protection/ Visières de protection	**EN 166:2001** « Protection individuelle de l'œil — Spécifications »/ **7.2.4 Protection contre les gouttelettes et les projections liquides** marquage du symbole « 3 » (gouttelettes ou projections de liquide)	**Norme australienne AS/NZS 1337**
Lunettes de protection/ Visières de protection	**EN 166:2001** « Protection individuelle de l'œil — Spécifications »/ **7.2.4 Protection contre les gouttelettes et lesprojections liquides** marquage du symbole « 3 » (gouttelettes ou projections de liquide)	**Norme canadienne CSA Z94.3** **Norme canadienne CSA Z94.5**
Lunettes de protection/ Visières de protection	**EN 166:2001** « Protection individuelle de l'œil — Spécifications »/ **7.2.4 Protection contre les gouttelettes et lesprojections liquides** marquage du symbole « 3 » (gouttelettes ou projections de liquide)	**Norme japonaise JIS T 8141** **Norme japonaise JIS T 8147**

12.4 ANSM answer to crisis 3D printing, April 10th 2020

ANSM - Fiche d'encadrement Impression 3D pour la fabrication de dispositifs médicaux dans le cadre de la crise du Covid-19

1. Introduction

Cette fiche d'encadrement a pour objectif de donner des lignes directrices pour accompagner la mise en œuvre de procédés de fabrication innovants tel que l'impression 3D dans un cadre de crise sanitaire pouvant conduire à des ruptures d'approvisionnement et ce, en dehors du cadre habituellement défini par la réglementation relative aux dispositifs médicaux (DM) en vue de leur mise sur le marché.

L'impression 3D est une technologie nouvelle qui, contrairement aux procédés classiques de fabrication, procède par dépôt de couches successives de matériaux jusqu'à obtenir des objets tridimensionnels. Ce procédé de fabrication, qui englobe également la conception numérique des objets à fabriquer, repose sur plusieurs familles de procédés de fabrication permettant des adaptations fines des objets fabriqués, aussi bien en termes de formes que de matériaux, fonctionnalités ou encore propriétés mécaniques.
La disponibilité de ces moyens de production, et la matière première disponible sont une ressource utile à la gestion de la crise, en permettant de compléter les sources d'approvisionnement classiques pour certains DM, la réalisation de consommables ou d'équipements de protection individuelle.

Dans le contexte exceptionnel COVID-19, il y lieu de s'appuyer sur le cadre réglementaire existant, comme un guide qui doit permettre d'assurer la sécurité des patients lors de l'utilisation de ces produits, tout en prenant en considération la rupture normative imposée par l'urgence sanitaire et l'esprit général de « bien faire » pour résoudre des problèmes où le pragmatisme l'emporte temporairement sur des théories d'évaluation validées. Il s'agit de considérer qu'une situation de crise peut conduire à une redéfinition temporaire du rapport bénéfice/ risque dans la mesure où l'absence de moyen usuel devient le comparateur (et non plus le produit princeps devenu innaccessible).

Le rôle des équipes soignantes et des établissements de santé est essentiel pour permettre un déploiement rationnel et une évaluation continue et diffuse, mais centralisable, de ces solutions de crise dès lors que la situation l'exige.

Ce qui est faisable dans un contexte de crise sanitaire

2.1. Considérations générales à prendre en compte par les porteurs de projets

Dans ce contexte nouveau de crise majeure il convient d'adopter certains principes et d'évaluer la possibilité de leur mise en place pour assurer une évaluation au fil de l'eau.

→ Les DM doivent être élaborés dans un objectif d'obtention d'une équivalence au produit « princeps» ;

→ Une évaluation clinique avant diffusion est souhaitable quand elle est envisageable extemporanément au début de la production. Dans ce sens, le fabricant est invité à rechercher un site et une équipe médicale de validation simplifiée en conditions cliniques d'utilisation.

→ Une coordination d'emblée pouvant être difficile à réaliser, il convient d'adopter au sein de chacun des sites et services utilisateurs une procédure de déploiement progressif du DM. La première utilisation chez un premier bénéficiaire doit faire l'objet d'un recueil initial de données tracées par un observateur identifiable (au mieux représenté par la personne contact du site pour le fabricant et en charge des déclarations d'évènements indésirables au fil de l'eau.

→ Un lien fiable doit être établi entre le fabricant et les utilisateurs pour le suivi de la dispensation et des données d'utilisation (indications, déroulement, adaptations, traçabilité datée et descriptive des évènements indésirables sans recherche immédiate d'imputabilité, ...) ;

→ Une analyse au fil de l'eau de ces informations devra être assurée par un acteur coordonnateur de façon à diffuser, au besoin, des informations utiles à l'adaptation des DM mis à disposition dans l'ensemble des sites utilisations.

→ L'ensemble des données recueillies (en respect des dispositions règlementaires de confidentialité) devra être centralisée pour une analyse continue permettant la diffusion d'alertes ou d'informations complémentaires éventuelle.

2.2. Dispositions applicables aux industriels.

Les industriels dont l'activité est la fabrication par impression 3D, quel que soit le mode de production, devront rechercher une dérogation de mise sur le marché au titre de l'article R 5211-19 auprès de l'ANSM à partir du plan de développement en annexe 1. Ces demandes ne seront recevables que pour des DM, dont le demandeur justifiera de la situation de rupture ou de tension d'approvisionement.

2.3. Dispositions applicables aux autres structures

Les autres structures, établissement de santé ou associatifs, appuieront leurs démarches sur les dispositions suivantes pour structurer et documenter leur projet.

→ Il semble évident que le niveau de technicité des pièces produites devra être adapté aux moyens et à la structure qui envisage de les produire.

→ Dans ce cadre, le niveau de documentation à rassembler devra également être proportionné au matériel fabriqué et en tenant compte des compétences, de l'expérience et la capacité « à faire » de la structure porteuse du projet.

→ Le recours à ces dispositifs fabriqués par impression 3D ne peut venir qu'en dernier recours et en l'absence de dispositifs conventionnels.

→ L'attention portée à la conception des objets 3D pour une utilisation clinique doit être maximale, en termes de performances essentielles.

→ Il est essentiel de s'associer à des professionnels de santé pour la conception de ces dispositifs. Ceci est particulièrement important pour les initiatives menées par des acteurs non professionnels du DM.

→ La phase de conception du projet 3D nécessite a minima la prise en compte des points suivants :

→ Être en capacité de documenter les choix de conception (matériau et design) permettant d'assurer la sécurité et la performance dans l'usage. Dans ce cadre, les exigences de sécurité et de performance requises dans le cadre de la réglementation relative aux DM et les normes applicables devraient être prises en références ;

→ Des essais fonctionnels simplifiés permettant de démontrer que la performance et la sécurité sont compatibles avec une utilisation dans un contexte clinique. Le dimensionnement des essais sera proportionné à l'usage du dispositif. Une documentation de réalisation d'essais fonctionnels permettant de vérifier performance et sécurité avant une utilisation clinique devra être établie ;

→ En supplément, pour les dispositifs en charge du maintien des fonctions vitales d'un patient, l'utilisation en condition clinique ne pourra se faire que sous la forme d'un protocole d'essais suivant les lignes directrices d'une évaluation clinique pour les DM. Dans la mesure du possible, une autorisation d'investigation clinique sera recherchée auprès de l'ANSM et du CPP. Pour les autres dispositifs, un protocole de suivi observationnel sera établi pour documenter les premières utilisations.

L'utilisation des solutions réalisées doit être mise en place en relation avec les personnels de santé
Le porteur du projet doit établir un lien permettant le recueil d'avis portant sur l'utilisation, notamment pour informer de difficultés ou d'incidents. Il assurera une traçabilité de la mise à disposition.

Le déploiement dans un service de soin ou un établissement doit être pro-

gressif et limité à quelques utilisations consécutives avec une observation précise du comportement du produit. Une attitude de prudence pratique, permettra d'ajuster l'utilisation et permettra de prendre en compte une courbe d'apprentissage.
Une traçabilité de l'utilisation de ces solutions sera réalisée par l'établissement de santé.

Toutes les demandes, qu'elles soient dérogatoires ou autres seront examinées par l'ANSM en urgence selon une procédure accélérée.

Annexe 1

Guide dans l'élaboration du projet

Il est rappelé quelques activités nécessaires à mettre en œuvre pour l'utilisation de ce type de procédé:
→ Valider les logiciels utilisés et inclus dans le procédé d'impression 3D
→ Valider le procédé de fabrication dans sa globalité
→ Assurer une maintenance du procédé pour permettre ses performances dans le temps
→ Contrôler les matériaux utilisés
→ Etablir les spécifications des produits fabriqués et des matériaux utilisés
→ Être en mesure de mettre en œuvre des procédés complémentaires (polissage, nettoyage, stérilisation) en fonction des dispositifs fabriqués
→ Contrôler les produits finis
D'un point de vue réglementaire pour le fabricant 3D
→ Description du dispositif
→ Tests mécaniques (référence aux normes lorsqu'elles existent ou référentiel interne si pas de norme)
→ Tests dimensionnels
→ Caractérisation des matériaux
→ Plan de test en condition simulé d'utilisation
→ Protocole d'utilisation clinique

La mise en œuvre de procédés 3D nécessitent des compétences professionnelles propres sur toutes les étapes de la chaine de production, depuis la conception numérique, l'impression 3D jusqu'à la stérilisation (si applicable) des DM fabriqués.

Annexe 2

Rappel réglementaire

D'un point de vue réglementaire, ce qu'il faut savoir:

→ Les DM fabriqués par impression 3D sont soumis aux mêmes obligations règlementaires que les DM fabriqués au moyen d'autres procédés de fabrication

→ Les DM fabriqués par impression 3D doivent être marqués CE avant leur mise sur le marché si la mise sur le marché est faite par un opérateur externe à l'établissement de soins, ou si il ne s'agit pas de DM sur mesure. Selon la classe de risque du DM, le marquage CE sera subordonné à l'intervention d'un organisme notifié.

→ Les établissements de santé peuvent fabriquer des DM par impression 3D pour les utiliser en leur sein, sous certaines conditions très limitatives et encadrées (et ce indépendamment du critère de fabrication en 3D)

→ Les établissements de santé ne pourront ainsi fabriquer et utiliser en leur sein des DM (sans transfert vers une autre entité juridique) que s'ils se sont assurés au préalable qu'aucun DM équivalent disponible sur le marché ne peut satisfaire aux besoins spécifiques du groupe cible de patients avec les niveaux de performance et de sécurité appropriés.

→ Les établissements de santé devront établir une documentation permettant de comprendre les installations de fabrication, les procédés de fabrication, la conception et les données sur les performances des DM qu'ils fabriquent. Ils devront également porter une attention particulière à la démonstration de la conformité aux exigences applicables, en particulier aux points suivants : propriétés chimiques, physiques et biologiques des matériaux, compatibilité des matériaux avec les tissus biologiques, incidence des procédés de fabrication sur les propriétés des matériaux (y compris les étapes de nettoyage, traitements de surface, stérilisation), maitrise des procédés de fabrication, propriétés mécaniques des dispositifs (résistance, usure, rupture, fatigue…) mais aussi aux performances précliniques et cliniques qui devront être démontrées.

→ Le règlement européen impose aux établissements de santé d'examiner l'expérience issue de l'utilisation clinique des DM et de prendre toutes les mesures correctives nécessaires. Ils devront donc mettre en place un plan d'amélioration continue afin de réduire les risques liés à l'utilisation des DM qu'ils fabriquent en 3D et agir le cas échéant sur les procédés de fabrication.

Toutefois, le règlement européen n'empêche pas les établissements de santé de fabriquer des DM par impression 3D à des fins de recherche en vue de la réalisation d'essais cliniques. Dans une telle hypothèse ils seront soumis à la réglementation applicable aux recherches impliquant la personne humaine.

12.5 Mission given to OMEDIT by AGEPS

ASSISTANCE PUBLIQUE HÔPITAUX DE PARIS

AGENCE GÉNÉRALE DES ÉQUIPEMENTS ET PRODUITS DE SANTÉ

AGEPS

75221 PARIS Cedex 05

92023 NANTERRE Cedex

Directeur de l'AGEPS

Ligne directe : 01.46.69.15.23
Secrétariat : 01.46.69.15.00/9228
Télécopie : 01.46.69.13.01

Paris, le 24/04/2020

Destinataires :

[redacted] pharmacien, praticien hospitalier, responsable de l'OMEDIT Île-de-France

[redacted] pharmacien, praticien hospitalier exerçant à l'OMEDIT

Réf : DIR/RC/HC/2020-0045
Objet : Lettre de mission

Je soussigné [redacted], directeur de l'AGEPS, conseiller technique du Directeur général de l'APHP en charge de la politique du médicament, après accord de Monsieur [redacted] chef du service EPBU, considérant la mission d'appui aux établissements de l'OMEDIT Île-de-France, missionne :

[redacted] pharmacien, praticien hospitalier, responsable de l'OMEDIT Île-de-France

[redacted], pharmacien, praticien hospitalier exerçant à l'OMEDIT

pour appuyer l'AGEPS dans le recours à l'utilisation de l'impression 3D pour la fabrication de dispositifs médicaux dans le contexte COVID-19.
Dans le cadre de cette mission elles me rendront compte directement.

1/ Nature de la mission :

- Proposer un scénario de recours à l'impression 3D pour la fabrication de dispositifs médicaux dans le contexte COVID-19 à l'AP-HP décliné sous forme de procédure
- Accompagner les parties prenantes dans l'application de ce scénario : prestataires, professionnels de santé, AGEPS

2/ Organisation de la mission :
Jusqu'à avis contraire, [redacted] et [redacted] travailleront 6 journées hebdomadaires (soit 1,2 ETP) à l'AGEPS, à Cochin ou en télétravail, à répartir entre elles et dans la semaine.

La mission ne donne lieu à aucune rémunération, les postes de [illegible] et [illegible] étant portés par l'AGEPS. Le Directeur de l'ARS Île-de-France est informé de cette mission.
La mission justifie que leur soient transmis tous les documents et informations utiles à la compréhension du dossier, au suivi et au reporting des différentes actions engagées en matière :

- D'analyse de besoin
- D'analyse de faisabilité
- D'activité de prototypage ou de production
- De tests et de contrôles
- De suivi observationnel et de signalement d'évènements indésirables

De leur côté [illegible] et [illegible] s'engagent à communiquer, informer la Direction de l'AGEPS et à organiser un reporting régulier de leur activité.

Les livrables attendus sont :
- la procédure de recours à l'utilisation de l'impression 3D pour la fabrication de dispositifs médicaux dans le contexte COVID-19 à l'AP-HP : 24 avril 2020
- la trame de dossier pour demande dérogatoire d'autorisation à l'ANSM de fabrication de dispositifs médicaux dans le contexte COVID-19 : 4 mai 2020
- l'organisation du système documentaire : 11 mai 2020

[illegible] CATELAND
Directeur de l'AGEPS

12.6 Protocol proposed by AGEPS to run 3D COVID

Procédure de recours a l'utilisation de l'impression 3d pour la fabrication de DM dans le contexte COVID-19

1. Objet et domaine d'application

La présente procédure a pour objet de décrire les modalités de couverture d'un besoin d'approvisionnement en DM, en complément des sources d'approvisionnement classiques, par l'utilisation de l'impression 3 D (procédé de fabrication innovant) comme solution d'ultime recours pour pallier à l'absence de disponibilité de dispositifs conventionnels, dans le contexte exceptionnel d'extrême urgence sanitaire, en application des lignes directrices définies par l'ANSM (Cf Annexe 1 : Fiche d'Encadrement de l'utilisation 3D pour la fabrication de DM dans le cadre de la crise du COVID-19 telle que publiée le 14 avril 2020).

Est exclue du champ d'application de cette procédure la production des EPI par impression 3D, non soumise à validation pharmaceutique.

2. RESPONSABILITE

Le régime de responsabilité applicable aux parties co-contractantes (AP-HP et BONE 3D) est régi par les dispositions contractuelles idoines du marché cité ci-dessous et du « Contrat de Licence Simple d'Exploitation - Production Impression 3D Etat d'Urgence Sanitaire COVID-19 » opposables aux parties.

BONE 3D

Prestataire, titulaire du marché 2020ACHC 203806 relatif à la fourniture de prestations de conception et fabrication de pièces sur imprimante 3D, opération d'impression 3D fournitures et prestations associées. AP-HP : Donneur d'ordre, responsable de la qualité et de la sécurité des pièces produites par son parc d'imprimantes 3D (dont elle a la propriété) mis à disposition du prestataire.

Définitions / Abréviations

AGEPS : Agence générale des équipements et des produits de santé (Pharmacie centrale AP-HP)

ANSM : Agence Nationale de Sécurité du Médicament et des produits de santé

CODIMS : Comité des Dispositifs Médicaux Stériles de l'AP-HP

EI : évènement indésirable

PUI : Pharmacie à Usage Intérieur

PAC : Plan d'amélioration continu
Le terme de « DM reproduit » utilisé ci-après désigne le DM produit par impression 3D, sur la base des éléments du DM princeps.

Description d'activité

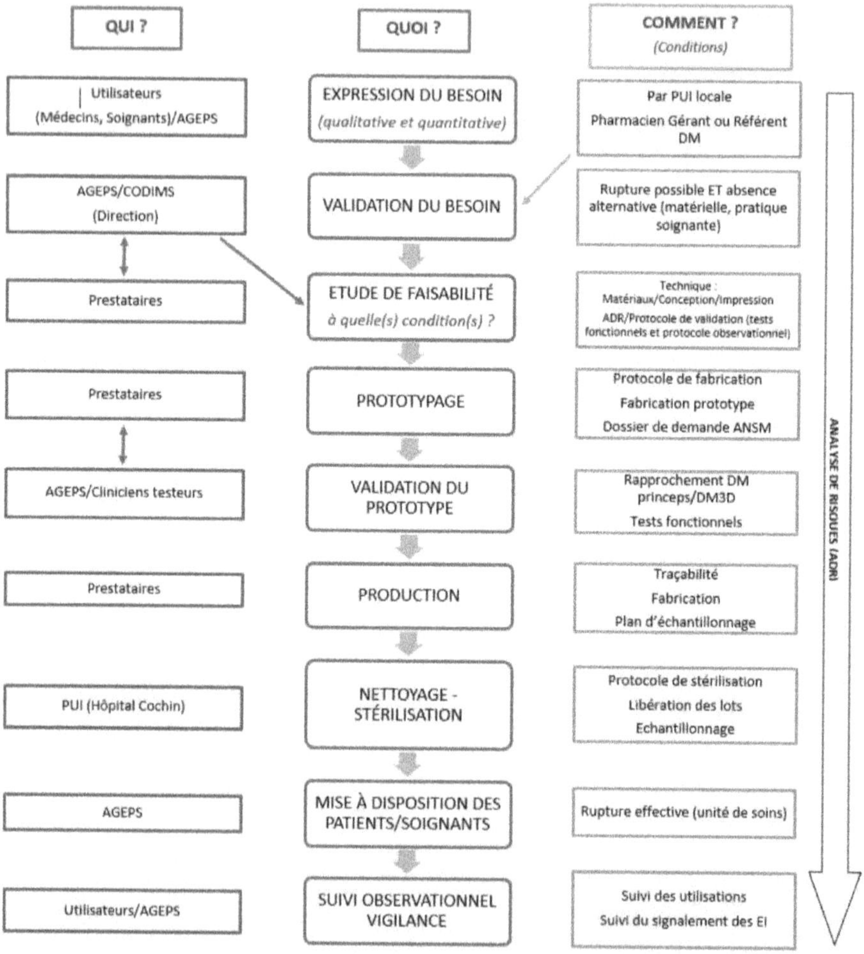

Logigramme 1. « Dispositif de gestion des besoins en approvisionnement DM COVID-19 Imp. 3D »

Description détaillée du circuit de validations et de production

Expression du besoin
Deux modalités d'expression du besoin

1. Besoin formulé par l'AGEPS

Nécessité absolue d'assurer la continuité d'approvisionnement d'un produit de santé (DM ou pièce) présentant un risque objectivé de rupture en l'absence de solution palliative à court terme (épuisement des stocks disponibles, absence d'alternative sur le marché (absence de produit de substitution chez le titulaire de marché, absence d'autres fournisseurs ou d'autres produits) et absence d'alternative thérapeutique soignante équivalente.

2. Besoin formulé par un ou des professionnels de santé (PM ou PNM) ET validé par le pharmacien gérant ou le pharmacien compétent en matière de DM de la PUI de rattachement

(critère : rupture d'approvisionnement objectivée dans les services de soins du GH concerné et communiquée préalablement à l'AGEPS)

Le besoin exprimé ne pourra être pris en compte qu'à la condition qu'« *aucun DM équivalent disponible sur le marché ne peut satisfaire aux besoins spécifiques du groupe cible de patients avec les niveaux de performance et de sécurité appropriés* ». L'expression du besoin décrit les qualités fonctionnelles du DM à reproduire (ex : transparence, souplesse, étanchéité...), la classe de risque du DM initial ainsi que les quantités estimées nécessaires pour satisfaire le besoin pour 1 mois.

Renouvellement de la demande

→ Toute nouvelle demande d'impression de quantités supplémentaires d'un DM auprès du prestataire suit le même circuit de validation.

→ Le prestataire ne déclenche aucune production sans validation du directeur de l'AGEPS.

Examen des conditions d'éligibilité

Sous couvert du directeur de l'AGEPS, le CODIMS, et ses experts le cas échéant, instruisent la demande, au regard des critères suivants :

« Rupture effective ou risque de rupture objectivé (épuisement des stocks disponibles, livraisons programmées reportées ou annulées, défaillance du ou des titulaires de marché imputable à des ruptures dans la chaîne de production ou d'approvisionnement)

« Absence d'alternative sur le marché (absence de produits disponibles sur le marché, absence de fournisseurs de substitution) et absence d'alternative thérapeutique soignante équivalente.

« Connaissance du procédé et du/des matériau(x) utilisé(s) pour l'impression du « DM reproduit »

La validation ne peut intervenir que par nécessité absolue d'assurer la continuité d'approvisionnement et donc des soins dans un contexte d'extrême urgence.
La demande validée de production d'un prototype est formalisée et transmise au prestataire. Le CODIMS et ses experts, sur la base d'une analyse de risques sommaire formalisent les paramètres qui devront obligatoirement être testés, les conditions de test, ainsi que les paramètres qui pourront faire l'objet d'un suivi en situation d'usage.

Etude de faisabilité

Après analyse du besoin exprimé, le prestataire réalise une étude de risques et en formalise le résultat. Cette étude de risques prend en compte la conformité aux exigences applicables (1) :

1. Propriétés chimiques, physiques et biologiques des matériaux,
2. Compatibilité des matériaux avec les tissus biologiques, prenant en compte la durée d'exposition
3. Incidence des procédés de fabrication sur les propriétés des matériaux (y compris les étapes de nettoyage, traitements de surface, stérilisation),
4. Maîtrise des procédés de fabrication,
5. Propriétés mécaniques des dispositifs (résistance, usure, rupture, fatigue…).
6. L'étude de faisabilité prend en compte l'examen des fonctionnalités attendues pour le prototype.

Prototypage

Selon le résultat de cette analyse de risques, le prestataire confirme la faisabilité et propose au directeur de l'AGEPS la réalisation d'un prototype.

Le Directeur de l'AGEPS valide la réalisation du prototype sur la base des résultats de l'analyse de risques et indique le nombre de prototypes à fournir. Les résultats de l'étude de risques, permettent de rédiger le protocole de tests fonctionnels.

Chaque fabrication de prototype donne lieu à l'élaboration d'une fiche navette intégrant son identification, son numéro de lot de production, une photo, les coordonnées du référent.

Validation du prototype

Le prestataire évalue la conformité du prototype aux spécifications attendues.

L'AGEPS procède ou fait procéder à l'évaluation de la conformité et de la sécurité du prototype:

Des échanges sont réalisés entre le prestataire et l'AGEPS en tant que de besoin.

Des tests d'usage (par exemple sur banc d'essai, sur mannequins, selon la nature du DM) sont réalisés conformément au protocole du CODIMS :

Ces tests donnent lieu à la production d'un rapport d'analyse comportant une des décisions suivantes : non validation, validation sous réserve de corrections ou validation.

Les modalités de nettoyage, stérilisation du dispositif reproduit doivent être analysées dès l'étape de prototypage.

Le rapport d'analyse est transmis au directeur de l'AGEPS. Selon les résultats des tests, le directeur de l'AGEPS valide ou non du lancement d'une production strictement proportionnée au besoin estimé pour l'ensemble des services de soins de l'AP-HP ayant confirmé un besoin et pour une durée strictement limitée à celle de la rupture d'approvisionnement.

La production est immédiatement suspendue en cas de déclaration(s) d'événement(s) indésirable(s) (dans le cadre du suivi observationnel mis en place dans les services cliniques testeurs ou dans les services utilisateurs après phase de tests) ou en cas de remise à disposition du DM princeps.

Examen du respect des exigences posées en termes d'hygiène et de stérilisation par la PUI du site d'implantation de la plateforme d'impression 3D

Examen des résultats du protocole de nettoyage, d'identification et de stérilisation :

→ Validation sous réserve de corrections ou validation par le pharmacien de la stérilisation du site d'implantation de la plateforme d'impression 3D.
→ Libération du lot
→ Gestion de l'échantillonnage à conserver en lien avec la PUI de Cochin.
→ Les résultats des contrôles sont transmis au directeur de l'AGEPS.

Organisation logistique

Les différentes étapes logistiques font l'objet d'une traçabilité qui doit permettre de connaître à tout moment la localisation des DM reproduits, et le cas échéant de retirer de la circulation ces DM lors d'un retour à un approvisionnement en DM de référence.

Mise en œuvre du suivi observationnel et matériovigilance

Un plan d'amélioration continue permettant de réduire les risques liés à l'utilisation des DM fabriqués en 3D et d'agir le cas échéant sur les procédés de fabrication est mis en place.

Organisation d'un suivi observationnel réalisé par les utilisateurs, sur la base d'un document-type et selon les orientations données par le CODIMS. Toute survenue d'un EI devra obligatoirement faire l'objet d'un signalement à l'échelon local de matériovigilance, l'échelon régional le cas échéant et, le cas échéant, d'une analyse des causes. Le directeur de l'AGEPS est destinataire de ce signalement. Ces EI doivent faire l'objet d'une traçabilité.

Système documentaire

Un système documentaire est construit, intégrant les résultats de l'analyse de risques des différents contrôles et résultats de suivi observationnel.

Le système documentaire comporte les éléments suivants :
→ installations de fabrication,
→ procédés de fabrication,
→ conception,
→ données sur les performances des DM fabriqués.

Documents établissant la conformité aux exigences applicables :
→ propriétés chimiques, physiques et biologiques des matériaux,
→ compatibilité des matériaux avec les tissus biologiques, selon la durée d'exposition
→incidence des procédés de fabrication sur les propriétés des matériaux (y compris les étapes de nettoyage, traitements de surface, stérilisation),
→ maitrise des procédés de fabrication,
→ propriétés mécaniques des dispositifs (résistance, usure, rupture, fatigue…).
→ notice d'utilisation proposée
→ examens du respect des exigences posées en termes de sécurité d'utilisation et de performances sur la base de tests réalisés sur prototype rapport des tests sur « banc d'essai » (sécurité et performance)
→ rapport des tests sur mannequin (sécurité et performance), le cas échéant
→ rapport des tests cliniques réalisés sur la base d'un protocole de suivi observationnel défini par le CODIMS

Cellule 3D

Le directeur de l'AGEPS constitue une cellule impression 3D positionnée à l'AGEPS pour déployer le scénario de recours à l'impression 3D pour la fabrication de dispositifs médicaux dans le contexte COVID-19 et accompagner les parties prenantes dans l'application de ce scénario : prestataires, professionnels de santé, AGEPS.

Rappel des lignes directrices de l'ANSM

Le workflow tel que décrit ci-dessus (acteurs métier, étapes clés de validation, supports documentaires) vise à satisfaire l'ensemble des conditions posées à la régularité du recours à cette solution palliative par l'ANSM, consistant en la mise en place d'un système d'assurance qualité proportionné aux objectifs poursuivis et bilan bénéfices/risques dans le contexte exceptionnel de la crise sanitaire COVID-19 (Cf annexe 1).

Règles de portée générale/ Principes fondamentaux

Dans le contexte exceptionnel COVID-19, il convient d'interpréter le cadre réglementaire existant avec pragmatisme (susceptible d'impliquer une redéfinition temporaire du rapport bénéfice / risque) afin d'assurer la sécurité des patients lors de l'utilisation des DM produits : Poursuivre un objectif d'équivalence au produit « princeps» ;

Aménager un dispositif d'évaluation clinique simplifiée en conditions cliniques d'utilisation avant diffusion ;

Etablir un plan de déploiement progressif du DM dont la déclinaison doit être adossée aux résultats d'analyse des données de suivi observationnel et de vigilance (DEI) ;

Formaliser et centraliser un dispositif d'amélioration continue permettant une réactivité d'adaptation des DM au regard des données d'utilisation enregistrées (indications, déroulement, adaptations, traçabilité datée et descriptive des évènements indésirables sans recherche immédiate d'imputabilité, ...) ;

Règles opposables au fabricant:

→ Niveau de documentation proportionné au matériel fabriqué
→ Impression DM 3D doit être une solution d'ultime recours
→ Conception ciblée utilisation clinique (performances essentielles)
→ Nécessaire co-conception en associant les professionnels de santé
→ Dispositions spécifiques à la phase de conception
→ Documentation des choix de conception
→ Essais fonctionnels simplifiés et proportionnés (performance-sécurité)
→ Protocole de suivi observationnel ou protocoles d'essais (DM en charge avec maintien des fonctions vitales)
→ Règlementation applicable (conditions limitatives-pré-requis) :
→ Absence de DM équivalent disponible sur le marché susceptible de satisfaire aux besoins spécifiques du groupe cible de patients avec les niveaux de performance et de sécurité appropriés
→ Documentation technique (enregistrements relatifs aux installations de fabrication, procédés de fabrication, à la conception et les données sur les performances des DM qu'ils fabriquent et de données attestant la conformité aux exigences applicables en matière de propriétés chimiques, physiques et biologiques des matériaux, compatibilité des matériaux avec les tissus biologiques, incidence des procédés de fabrication sur les propriétés des matériaux (y compris les étapes de nettoyage, traitements de surface, stérilisation), maitrise des procédés de fabrication, propriétés mécaniques des dispositifs (résistance, usure, rupture, fatigue...) mais aussi de performances précliniques et cliniques qui devront être démontrées.
→ Plan d'amélioration continue afin de réduire les risques liés à l'utilisation des DM fabriqués en 3D et adapter avec réactivité les procédés de fabrication.

12.7 Report of the first strategic meeting for the 2nd phase

COPIL 3D - 21/09/20

Présents
Membres

→ [illegible], DGA AP-HP
→ [illegible] Directeur de l'AGEPS
→ [illegible], Adjointe au Directeur de l'AGEPS
→ Dr Khonsari, référent médical du projet plateforme 3D
→ [illegible] DACSEL GHU Université Paris-Saclay, promoteur du projet fab-flab de BCT
→ [illegible] co-directeur plateforme iLumens
→ [illegible], réanimation

pédiatrique RPC, utilisateur de la 3D dans le cadre de projets
de recherche innovation
→ ~~Dr F. Simon~~, ORL Necker, utilisateur de la 3D pour la mise au point de modèles pédagogiques
→ ~~Christian Maus~~, représentant la structure ACHA
→ ~~Dr N. Martelli~~ pharmacien, encadrant d'une thèse relative à l'utilisation de la 3D pour
fabriquer des DM
→ ~~Pr E. Vibert~~, chirurgien hépatique, chaire d'innovation BOPA
→ ~~T. Duong~~, représentant l'OTTPI
→ ~~E. Salomon~~, directrice de projets DSI

Invités

→ ~~J. Adam~~, Bone 3D, prestataire conception-fabrication d'objets en 3D dans le cadre de la
plateforme 3D et transfert de compétence
→ ~~G. Fauchille~~, Humaniteam design, prestataire animation du fab-lab de BCT

Excusés

→ ~~Pr R. Salomon~~, président de la CME
→ ~~Pr Paubel~~, Chef du service évaluation pharmaceutique et bon usage, AGEPS

Déroulement de la séance

~~Mme Charmet Delcoutre~~ remercie les participants d'avoir accepté de siéger au sein de ce COPIL. Elle rappelle que la plate-forme 3D a été mise en place dans l'urgence dans un contexte de crise et sur un mode expérimental d'une durée de 4 mois, prolongée à 1 an. Elle indique que le rôle du COPIL sera de fixer les orientations de cette plateforme pour la poursuite de l'expérimentation, et à plus long terme, ainsi que ses modalités de fonctionnement. Mme le ~~Pr Paugam~~ rappelle les questions qui se posent au COPIL, car plusieurs initiatives cohabitent aujourd'hui à l'AP-HP, représentées par les membres présents. Elle souligne notamment l'enjeu du modèle organisationnel (concentration du parc ou déconcentration, concentration des acteurs ou déconcentration) et le modèle de production (objectifs, périmètre qualitatif et quantitatif).

M. le Dr Khonsari présente le bilan de la plateforme 3D, il indique qu'elle a été conçue pour être simple d'utilisation avec l'acquisition de machines faciles à utiliser et similaires, avec l'objectif de suppléer la fabrication d'EPI, ce qui a très bien fonctionné, et d'explorer la faisabilité des DM, ce qui s'est avéré plus complexe. Parallèlement à la production d'EPI, la plateforme a très vite été sollicitée par des services de son site d'accueil (Cochin), pour la production de pièces de maintenance dans le domaine du biomédical, d'outils sur mesure dans différents domaines, et notamment l'ergothérapie. Il constate que le bouche à oreilles fonctionne bien en interne du site, voire du GH, moins à l'échelle de l'AP-HP.

Il présente quelques productions marquantes : EPI d'ouverture des portes, porte-tubes, outil d'ouverture de bouteilles, modèle pédagogique.

De cette expérience en temps de crise et post-crise, il tire les conclusions suivantes :

→ La clé du bon fonctionnement de la production 3D est l'interaction directe soignant-ingénieur, au sein de la plateforme
→ La centralisation des machines permet de maximiser le potentiel de production, non pas tant pour une production de masse, mais pour pouvoir mener plusieurs productions en simultané.
→ La diversification des machines est nécessaire à une production plus diversifiée
→ Il est nécessaire de mieux faire connaître l'offre de service de la plateforme
→ Les 4 principaux axes de développement de la plateforme sont :
1. L'univers de la maintenance (pièces détachées)
2. Les objets à usage en contexte médical qui ne sont pas des DM
3. Les objets d'enseignement
4. Le DM mais c'est plus complexe et il reviendra sur ce sujet par la suite
→ Sur la base d'un bon projet, trouver des financements ne lui paraît pas impossible
→ De manière pragmatique, la plateforme a besoin d'une localisation physique

M. Adam complète avec une présentation de données de production : 20 000 pièces produites en 2 mois pendant la période de crise, et la diversité des services demandeurs sur Broussais, Cochin et Necker. Il insiste sur la nécessité d'un filtre pour sélectionner les projets à soutenir sur la plateforme, et sur l'opportunité à communiquer sur la constitution d'une banque de produits.

[illegible] et Mm[illegible] sentent une autre expérience, celle du Fab-Lab de Bicêtre. Celui-ci existe depuis 2 ans. L'ambition est différente et probablement complémentaire de celle de la plateforme, le projet est inspiré du lean-management et vise à donner accès aux agents à la conception de la solution à leurs problèmes, au plus proche du service. Celle-ci peut passer par la 3D, mais également d'autres techniques. L'accès aux équipement et l'analyse de la problématique sont accompagnés, mais l'objectif reste une appropriation des outils par les agents. La production ne vise pas à la sérialisation mais, soit à des réponses sur mesure à des problématiques, soit à la mise en place de prototype éventuellement reproductibles à plus large échelle, mais dans un autre cadre (partenariat industriel, ou pourquoi pas, plate-forme). Comme la plate-forme, les principales réalisations 3D portent sur des pièces de maintenance, des objets de facilitation du quotidien (adaptateurs de pied à perfusion sur brancard), et pendant la crise des EPI. Le Fab-lab souligne particulièrement l'intérêt de l'implication des agents dans l'évolution des solutions proposées, et leur adaptation au contexte local. La question des DM a été a priori écartée du fait des contraintes, mais de fait, le Fab-lab a été sollicité pour la recherche d'une solution de type DM sur laquelle le travail est en cours mais l'obstacle à lever sera la modalité de production du fait de l'impossibilité de remplir les conditions du DM.

Les points forts du Fab-lab sont
→ sa capacité à recueillir les besoins en proximité et à les analyser avec diverses gammes de réponses possible.
→ La logique de réapropriation de la conception voire de la réalisation par les acteurs de l'hôpital
Le point faible est sa petite taille qui limite la capacité d'absorption des sujets et qui a conduit à une communication très modérée.

Le ~~Dr Martelli~~ évoque ensuite la problématique spécifique des DM. Il souligne la difficulté à se positionner dans les critères de l'ANSM, en effet, les pénuries sont par nature imprévisibles à moyen terme et le temps de développement d'un DM répondant aux critères ANSM est très long, il est donc très difficile d'établir une banque de DM susceptibles de tomber en pénurie.

En revanche, il estime que la problématique est différente dans le domaine du DM sur mesure, fabriqué en tenant compte des spécificités individuelles d'un patient.

M. Adam et le Dr Khonsari abondent dans son sens, après quelques contacts à l'ANSM, ils sont arrivés à la même conclusion. En revanche, ils estiment réelles les perspectives en matière de production de DM sur mesure (osteosynthèse par exemple), qui sont souvent très coûteux, avec des marges importantes des fournisseurs. Ils relèvent que notamment les chirurgies ORL, Maxillo-faciale, dentaire, et orthopédique sont très concernées par ce sujet.

[illegible] précise que si on doit comparer le cout des produits achetés, il ne faut plus raisonner en coût marginal (consommables pour un produit) mais en coût complet (amortissement des machines, des locaux, ressources humaines, etc.)

Les membres du COPIL débattent de ces retours d'expérience qu'ils éclairent de leur propre expérience du sujet.

La conclusion de ces débats est la suivante

→ Sur la production hors DM : il est possible d'articuler plusieurs approches et plusieurs lieux d'émergence des problèmes à résoudre (par exemple expression du besoin et conception de la réponse au besoin au plus proche de l'utilisateur local, mutualisation de la solution trouvée, production plateformisée dès que nécessité d'une petite série, il serait utile de les fédérer pour que la prise en compte des sujets se fasse sur le lieu le plus adapté, et de construire un label « 3D AP ».

→ La mutualisation de l'accès aux équipements maximalise leur utilisation et concentre les expertises

→ Les projets portés en local (mais ceci est dépendant de porteurs d'initiative qui existent ou non) maximisent la capacité à repérer les sujets intéressants

→ Sur la production des DM, celle-ci doit se limiter au « sur-mesure », en priorisant ceux pour lesquels existe une valeur ajoutée qualitative ou économique du fait de l'investissement nécessaire (machines et assurance-qualité). Il est demandé de réaliser une analyse transversale des DM sur mesure à forte potentialité

→ AGEPS recherche les données de dépense (montants, nombre de commandes)

→ Plate-forme élabore projection de production et coût du projet

→ La plate-forme a quelques difficultés pratiques à résoudre : Qui valide les dépenses ? Sur quel budget ? Quel lieu pour l'avenir ? Quelles modalités de communication interne? Site intranet AP ? Tournée des sites.

12.8 Long-term 5-year plan for 3D printing within AP-HP

This document was produced by Khonsari the 28th of September, 2020 and sent to AGEPS for assessment. No answer was obtained until the end of December.

Politique d'impression 3D pour l'APHP

Feuille de route 2020-2025

1. Quel est le contexte actuel de l'impression 3D à l'APHP ?

→ L'APHP est le plus important groupe hospitalier d'Europe.

→ Il s'agit d'un groupe hospitalo-universitaire impliqué dans le soin et la formation.

→ Il n'y a pas actuellement de politique unifiée APHP d'engagement dans l'impression 3D.

→ L'impression 3D est aujourd'hui utilisée en routine pour les soins et l'enseignement.

→ Le retour d'expérience de la 'ferme' de Port-Royal (3DCOVID) va permettre de construire une offre unique au monde.

L'impression 3D est une technologie de prototypage devenue depuis quelques années un outil de production. Ses coûts d'utilisation se réduisent d'année en année, à mesure qu'augmente la facilité d'utilisation de cette technologie.

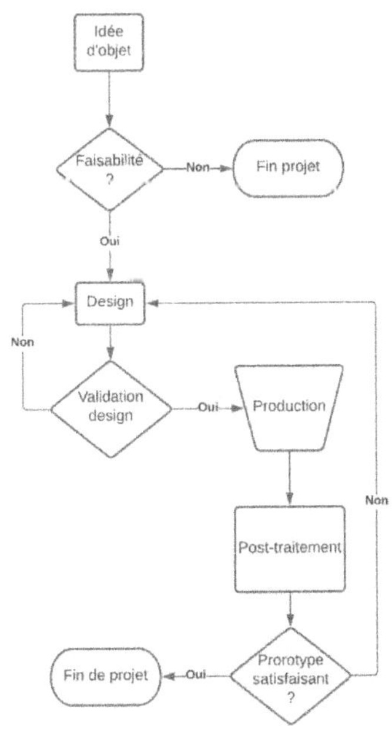

Logigramme 2. Le cycle de production d'un objet imprimé en 3D implique, de l'idée au produit.

Divers plastiques et métaux sont imprimables en 3D et certains de ces matériaux sont bio-compatibles.

L'impression 3D hospitalière permet de produire 5 catégories d'objets, qui correspondent à 5 missions de base d'une plateforme de santé:
→ des objets médicaux innovants à la demande des soignants,
→ des dispositifs médicaux sur mesure,
→ des dispositifs médicaux en petites séries,
→ des objets de maintenance pour la vie de tous les jours des services techniques des hôpitaux,
→ et des objets d'enseignement pour les patients et le soignants.

Ces objets peuvent améliorer les performances professionnelles et les conditions de travail de très nombreuses catégories d'employés d'une structure comme l'APHP: médecins,infirmiers, pharmaciens, chirurgiens, odontologistes, kinésithérapeutes et bien d'autres.

Grâce à un financement de mécénat COVID (groupe Kering), l'APHP dispose depuis avril 2020 d'une structure d'impression 3D industrielle composée de 60 imprimantes dépôt de fil (Stratasys série F123), ainsi que d'une expérience unique au monde de l'impression 3D médicale forgée au cours de la crise du COVID19. Nous devons aujourd'hui pérenniser l'intégration de cette technologie au sein de notre structure, construire la gouvernance de la plateforme d'impression et définir ses missions à long terme.

2. Quels sont les principes de gouvernance de l'impression 3D à l'APHP ?

Principe #1 - Unité de lieu

Une plateforme centrale doit fédérer des sites d'impression satellites. Cette unité de lieu permettra de valider les exigences règlementaires pour la production de dispositifs médicaux (selon RE 2017/745) et concentrera les besoins. Elle permettra également de valoriser les initiatives d'impression 3D déjà en place au sein de l'APHP en créant un réseau. L'unité de lieu permettra enfin de stimuler l'innovation en réunissant soignants, ingénieurs et techniciens sur un même site.

Principe #2 - Binôme soignant / ingénieur

Ce binôme est au cœur de la démarche d'innovation des soignants. Il est secondé de trois partenaires cruciaux:
→ spécialiste de la règlementation (pharmacien ou master en affaires règlementaires)
→ spécialiste de la propriété intellectuelle (OTT&PI)
→ et spécialiste de la logistique (cadre).

Principe #3 - Partenariat public / privé

L'expertise en impression 3D médicale est en grande partie industrielle. Le partenariat public / privé implique des entreprises spécialistes de l'impression 3D pour les prestations ingénieur, la maintenance et la gestion du parc machines.

Principe #4 - Cinq missions de base

L'unité de lieu et des moyens de production permet de concentrer sur un site unique cinq missions complémentaires (voir aussi paragraphe 1) :
→ production de matériel médical,
→ production de dispositifs médicaux sur mesure,
→ production de dispositifs médicaux en petites séries,
→ contribution à la maintenance des hôpitaux,
→ et production de matériel d'enseignement.

Principe #5 - Implications universitaires et sociales

La mission de formation de la plateforme de l'APHP inclut :

→ la formation à l'échelle nationale et internationale de soignants et d'ingénieurs aux principes du dessin 3D et de l'impression,
→ la création d'outils d'enseignement pour les patients et les soignants.
Cette mission peut s'intégrer dans le cadre de la création d'un service ou d'une unité fonctionnelle pouvant accueillir des internes et des médecins / pharmaciens en post-internat.
Le caractère unique au monde de l'initiative mise en place pendant la crise du COVID a par ailleurs stimulé le lancement de deux types de projets entrant dans le cadre des missions universitaires et sociales de la plateforme :
→ développement international – reproduction du principe de la 'ferme' de Port-Royal,
→ développement artistique – utilisation de la plateforme pour des projets créatifs participant à la vie hospitalière.

Principe #6 - Valorisation

La plateforme est un vecteur d'innovation :

→ le principe de la plateforme elle-même fera l'objet de valorisation dans le déploiement international de 'fermes',
→ les projets valorisables ayant vu le jour au sein de la plateforme feront l'objet de licences exploitées par le couple public/privé,
→ des offres d'enseignement seront développées (sur le modèle du DU existant 'Planification chirurgicale et médecine personnalisée'), pour les médecins, odontologistes, pharmaciens, kinésithérapeutes et autres catégories de soignants, selon deux modalités
1. Enseignement des technologies 3D elles-mêmes (modélisation, impression, règlementation),
2. Enseignements utilisant des outils produits par la plateforme (modèles anatomiques, simulateurs chirurgicaux).

3. Questions liées à l'unité de lieu et au fonctionnement de la plateforme

Les machines acquises dans le cadre de la crise du COVID sont actuellement à l'Abbaye de Port-Royal et devront être déplacée fin 2020.

Le site d'installation final de la plateforme devra respecter les principes suivants
→ lieu attractif central dans Paris, au sein d'une structure hospitalière et/ou

universitaire,
→ en partie de plein-pied, permettant l'installation de toute ou partie du parc de Port-Royal
→ permettant la diversification des structures de production: stéréolithographie, frittage de poudre, impression métal avec respect des contraintes techniques,
→ possible mise en conformité pour la production de dispositifs médicaux.

Le coût d'aménagement de ce lieu unique selon les normes de production de dispositifs médicaux est estimé à 200k€.

Pour la diversification du parc machines, deux options seront à considérer :

→ Option 1 – rachat de toute ou partie du parc actuel d'imprimantes FDM (60 machines) par un prestataire privé et mise à disposition de technologies diversifiées (SLA, SLM, SLS) par ce même prestataire, de manière partiellement décentralisée,

→ Option 2 – achat de machines par l'APHP pour compléter le parc existant, qui sera maintenu (SLA : 15k€; SLS : 150k€ ; SLM : 350k€).

Pour la gestion de la plateforme, une prestation du partenaire privé devra inclure :
→ 4 personnes à plein temps pour le dessin, l'impression et les déplacements sur les différents site de l'APHP et de l'Université, assurant les principes 2 à 6 définis ci-dessus,
→ 2 personnes à mi-temps pour la gestion des problèmes plus complexes de maintenance et d'ingéniérie,
→ La gestion des matières premières avec facturation à l'euro l'euro des achats. Cette prestation est évaluée à 100k€ mensuels, ce qui représente un forfait de moins de 3,000€ mensuels par hôpital de l'APHP.

4. Questions liées à la production de dispositifs médicaux

Deux types de dispositifs médicaux pourront être produits par la plateforme :
→ dispositifs médicaux sur mesure
→ dispositifs médicaux en petites séries.

La production de dispositifs médicaux sur mesure nécessite une mise en conformité de la chaîne de production qui sera assurée par un prestataire externe. Trois types de dispositifs médicaux sur mesure vont être produits comme preuve de concept :`
→ matériel d'ostéosynthèse sur mesure pour la chirurgie orthognathique,
→ plaques de cranioplastie sur mesure en PEEK
→ attelles et masques de compression sur mesure.

La prévision de coût de la mise en conformité de toutes les chaînes de production est de 200k€ pour la chaine de production, avec 50k€ à prévoir pour l'ajout d'une nouvelle technologie d'impression.

Chaque nouvelle catégorie de dispositif médical dont la production sera décidée nécessitera un investissement spécifique de 150k€ pour la constitution des dossiers règlementaires.

La production dé dispositifs médicaux en petites séries fait suite à l'action de la plateforme de crise. Dans le cadre d'une crise sanitaire, certaines contraintes règlementaires sont levées pour permettre de répondre à des pénuries de matériel. La mission de la plateforme est de préparer 3 dossiers pour des dispositifs médicaux en série, qui pourront être soumis à l'ANSM en cas de crise sanitaire et qui serviront de preuve de concept. Ces trois dispositifs sont :

→ joints de réanimation (série de 15 modèles de diamètres différents),
→ porte-fil de chirurgie cardiaque,
→ valve de Boussignac.

La prévision de coût de constitution des dossiers pour ces 3 dispositifs médicaux en série est de 30k€ par objet.

5. Missions académiques et sociétales

→ Les missions d'enseignement de la plateforme reprendront la structure du diplôme d'université déjà mis en place à l'Université de Paris (Planification Chirurgicale et Médecine Personnalisée) pour offrir une structure de formation aux soignants de l'APHP et aux cadres des plateformes mises en place à l'international.

→ Dans le cadre de partenariats public/ privé, divers objets d'enseignement pour les patients et les soignants seront développés et valorisés.

→ Une structure d'Unité Fonctionnelle permettra d'accueillir des médecins, pharmaciens et odontologistes en formation à divers niveaux (internes, chefs de clinique - assistants en chirurgie, en pharmacie, en radiologie, etc), qui participeront à la production des dispositifs médicaux ainsi qu'à l'innovation avec les soignants.

→ Des projets artistiques avec résidence sur site d'artistes prendront la continuité des deux projets actuels (Olga Kisseleva et Laurent Saksik / Alain Blondel), avec un budget dédié.

Une prévision de coût annuel pour la résidence artistique est de 50k€.

6. Bilan financier du projet (en k€)

Prévision de coût des travaux d'aménagement du site	200
Prévision de coût de diversification du parc machines	0 / 500
Prévision du coût du contrat de prestation / an	1200
Prévision de coût de la mise en conformité des chaînes de production	200
Prévision de coût de constitution des dossiers de 3 DM sur mesure	450
Prévision de coût de constitution des dossiers de 3 DM en série	90
Prévision de coût de la résidence artistique et sociales	50
TOTAL	2190 / 2690

12.9 Scientific publications of the 3D COVID team

→ **Thierry B, Célérier C, Simon F, Lacroix C, Khonsari RH**
How and why use the EasyBreath surface snorkeling mask as a personal protective equipment during the COVID-19 pandemic?
Eur Ann Otorhinolaryngol Head Neck Dis 2020;137:329-331

→ **François PM, Bonnet X, Kosior J, Adam J, Khonsari RH.**
3D-printed contact-free devices designed and dispatched against the COVID-19 pandemic: The 3D COVID initiative.
J Stomatol Oral Maxillofac Surg 2020;26:S2468-7855(20)30157-9.

→ **Delbarre M, François PM, Adam J, Caruhel JB, Froussart-Maille F, Khonsari RH**
3D-printed shields for slit lamps produced during the COVID-19 pandemic
Ann 3D Printed Med 2021;1:100004

→ **Laliève L, Adam J, Nataf P, Khonsari RH**
3D-printed suture guide for thoracic and cardiovascular surgery produced during the COVID19 pandemic
Ann 3D Printed Med 2021;1:100005

→ **Khonsari RH**
L'impression 3D de crise : preuve de concept de l'initiative de Port-Royal durant la pandémie de COVID-19
Réalités en Chirurgie Plastique 2020;39:11-15

→ **Bertrand J, Khonsari RH**
L'impression 3D sanitaire d'urgence. Les travaux de la 'ferme' de Port-Royal. Gestions Hospitalières 2021;605 :232-236

→ **Khonsari RH, Adam J, Benassarou M, Bertin H, Billotet B, Bouaoud J, Bouletreau P, Garmi R, Gellée T, Haen P, Ketoff S, Lescaille G, Louvrier A, Lutz JC, Makaremi M, Nicot R, Pham-Dang N, Praud M, Saint-Pierre F, Schouman T, Sicard L, Simon F, Wojcik T, Meyer C; French Society of Stomatology, Maxillo-Facial Surgery and Oral Surgery (SFSCMFCO).**
In-house 3D printing: Why, when, and how? Overview of the national French good practice guidelines for in-house 3D-printing in maxillo-facial surgery, stomatology, and oral surgery.
J Stomatol Oral Maxillofac Surg 2021 2021;122:458-461

→ **Khonsari RH, Oranger M, François PM, Mendoza-Ruiz A, Leroux K, Boussaid G, Prieur D, Hodge JP, Belle A, Midler V, Morelot-Panzini C, Patout M, Gonzalez-Bermejo J.**
Quality versus emergency: how good were ventilation fittings produced by additive manufacturing to address shortages during the COVID19 pandemic? PLoS ONE 2022;17:e0263808.

→ **Khonsari RH**
Digital fabrication in craniofacial surgery In Mallakpour S, Hussain CM (eds). Medical additive manufacturing: Concepts and fundamentals. Elsevier: Amsterdam. 2023 (in the press)

12.10 Online supplementary materials

Most of the designs presented in chapters 7 and 8 will be available for download on the online platform of the 'Phase 2' AP-HP 3D printing facility. All 3D files will be in STL format. Printing specifications are provided in chapters 7 and 8, with the printer type, raw materials and settings. Please share them freely and mention 'AP-HP 3D COVID project; Khonsari RH (2023) Emergency medical 3D printing.

Composed in Minion Pro and in Basic Sans.

Design and Layout
Emma Blanc-Tailleur

February 2023

Plateforme 3D COVID, Abbaye de Port-Royal, Hôpital Cochin, Paris, 21.I.2021. Encre de Chine sur papier, 50 x 65 cm. Collection particulière. © Christelle Téa

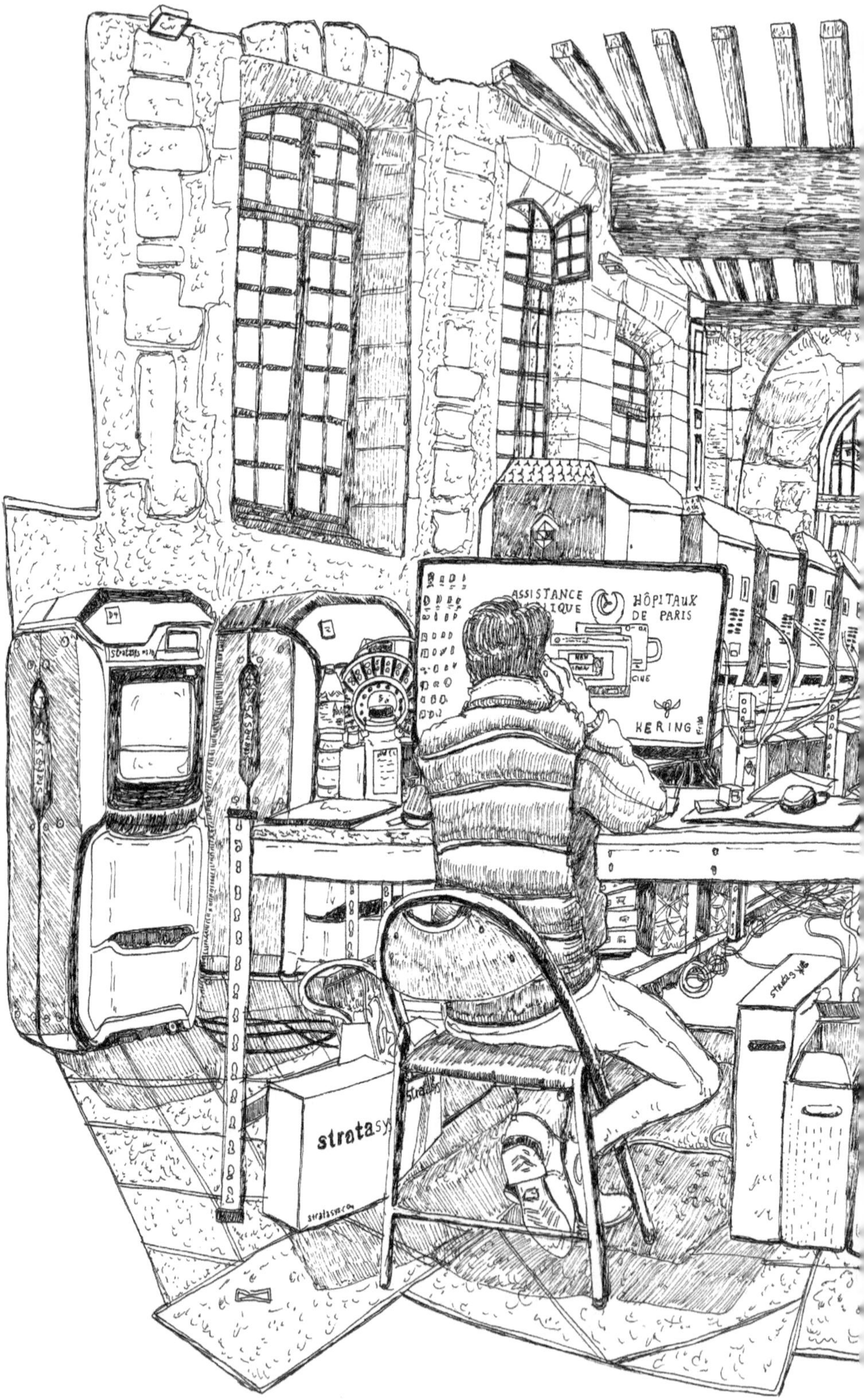

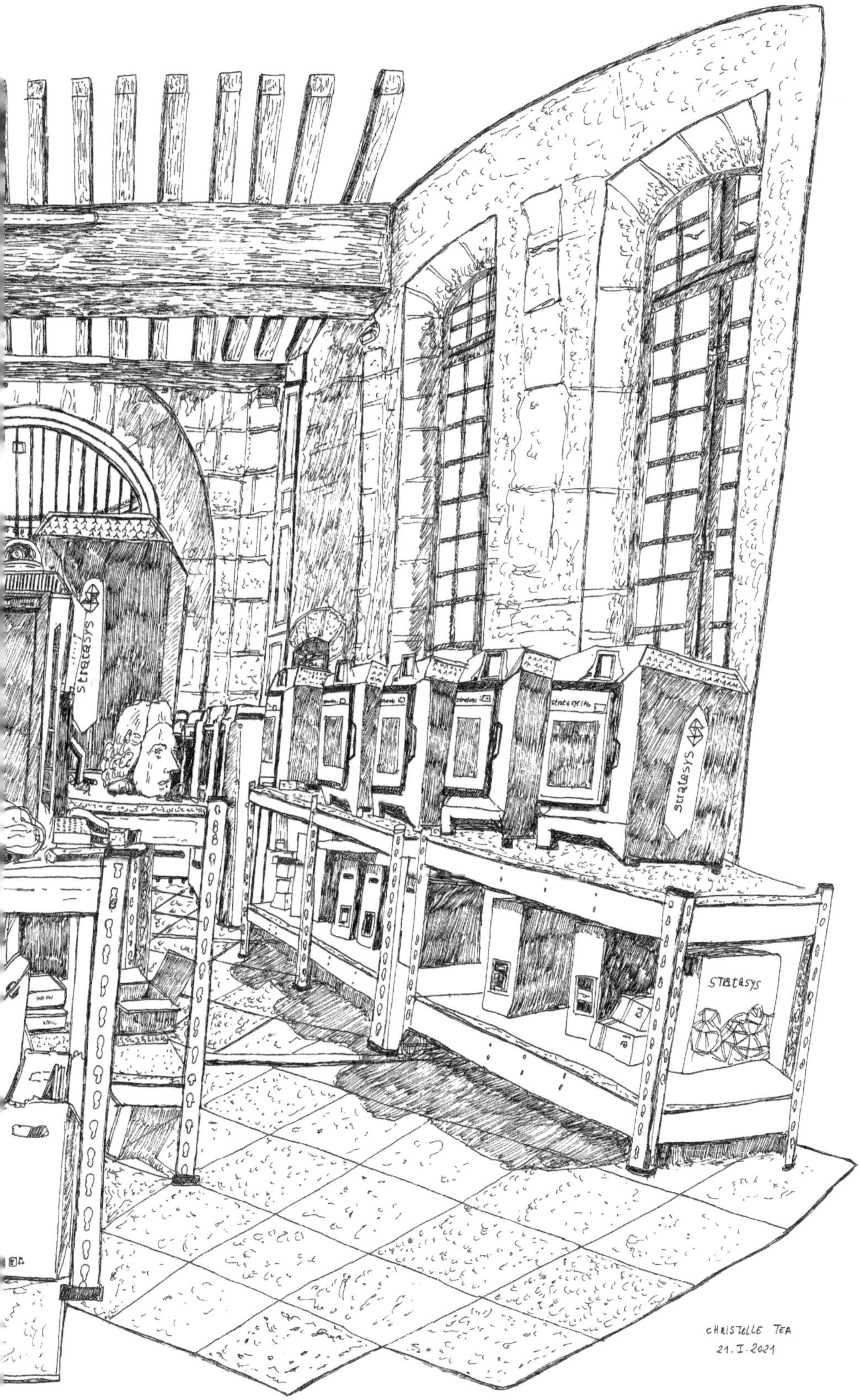
stratasys
stratasys
Stratasys
CHRISTELLE TEA
21. I. 2021

Structures éditoriales du groupe L'Harmattan

L'Harmattan Italie
Via degli Artisti, 15
10124 Torino
harmattan.italia@gmail.com

L'Harmattan Hongrie
Kossuth l. u. 14-16.
1053 Budapest
harmattan@harmattan.hu

L'Harmattan Sénégal
10 VDN en face Mermoz
BP 45034 Dakar-Fann
senharmattan@gmail.com

L'Harmattan Cameroun
TSINGA/FECAFOOT
BP 11486 Yaoundé
inkoukam@gmail.com

L'Harmattan Burkina Faso
Achille Somé – tengnule@hotmail.fr

L'Harmattan Guinée
Almamya, rue KA 028 OKB Agency
BP 3470 Conakry
harmattanguinee@yahoo.fr

L'Harmattan RDC
185, avenue Nyangwe
Commune de Lingwala – Kinshasa
matangilamusadila@yahoo.fr

L'Harmattan Congo
219, avenue Nelson Mandela
BP 2874 Brazzaville
harmattan.congo@yahoo.fr

L'Harmattan Mali
ACI 2000 - Immeuble Mgr Jean Marie Cisse
Bureau 10
BP 145 Bamako-Mali
mali@harmattan.fr

L'Harmattan Togo
Djidjole – Lomé
Maison Amela
face EPP BATOME
ddamela@aol.com

L'Harmattan Côte d'Ivoire
Résidence Karl – Cité des Arts
Abidjan-Cocody
03 BP 1588 Abidjan
espace_harmattan.ci@hotmail.fr

Nos librairies en France

Librairie internationale
16, rue des Écoles
75005 Paris
librairie.internationale@harmattan.fr
01 40 46 79 11
www.librairieharmattan.com

Librairie des savoirs
21, rue des Écoles
75005 Paris
librairie.sh@harmattan.fr
01 46 34 13 71
www.librairieharmattansh.com

Librairie Le Lucernaire
53, rue Notre-Dame-des-Champs
75006 Paris
librairie@lucernaire.fr
01 42 22 67 13

www.ingramcontent.com/pod-product-compliance
Lightning Source LLC
Chambersburg PA
CBHW071430230926
51846CB00001B/168
* 9 7 8 2 1 4 0 3 4 7 7 5 7 *